Fractals' Physical Origin and Properties

ETTORE MAJORANA INTERNATIONAL SCIENCE SERIES

Series Editor:
Antonino Zichichi
European Physical Society
Geneva, Switzerland

(PHYSICAL SCIENCES)

Recent volumes in the series:

Volume 36 NEW TECHNIQUES FOR FUTURE ACCELERATORS II: RF and Microwave Systems
Edited by M. Puglisi, S. Stipcich, and G. Torelli

Volume 37 SPECTROSCOPY OF LIGHT AND HEAVY QUARKS
Edited by Ugo Gastaldi, Robert Klapisch, and Frank Close

Volume 38 MONTE CARLO TRANSPORT OF ELECTRONS AND PHOTONS
Edited by Theodore M. Jenkins, Walter R. Nelson, and Alessandro Rindi

Volume 39 NEW ASPECTS OF HIGH-ENERGY PROTON–PROTON COLLISIONS
Edited by A. Ali

Volume 40 DATA ANALYSIS IN ASTRONOMY III
Edited by V. Di Gesù, L. Scarsi, P. Crane, J. H. Friedman, S. Levialdi, and M. C. Maccarone

Volume 41 PROGRESS IN MICROEMULSIONS
Edited by S. Martellucci and A. N. Chester

Volume 42 DIGITAL SEISMOLOGY AND FINE MODELING OF THE LITHOSPHERE
Edited by R. Cassinis, G. Nolet, and G. F. Panza

Volume 43 NONSMOOTH OPTIMIZATION AND RELATED TOPICS
Edited by F. H. Clarke, V. F. Dem'yanov, and F. Giannessi

Volume 44 HEAVY FLAVOURS AND HIGH-ENERGY COLLISIONS IN THE 1–100 TeV RANGE
Edited by A. Ali and L. Cifarelli

Volume 45 FRACTALS' PHYSICAL ORIGIN AND PROPERTIES
Edited by Luciano Pietronero

Volume 46 DISORDERED SOLIDS: Structures and Processes
Edited by Baldassare Di Bartolo

Fractals' Physical Origin and Properties

Edited by

Luciano Pietronero
University of Rome "La Sapienza"
Rome, Italy

Springer Science+Business Media, LLC

Library of Congress Cataloging in Publication Data

Special Seminar on Fractals (1988: Erice, Italy)
Fractals' physical origin and properties / edited by Luciano Pietronero.
p. cm—(Ettore Majorana international science series. Physical sciences; v. 45)
"Proceedings of the Special Seminar on Fractals, held October 9–15, 1988, in Erice, Sicily, Italy."—T.p. verso.
Includes bibliographical references.
ISBN 978-1-4899-3501-4
1. Fractals—Congresses. I. Pietronero, L. (Luciano) II. Title. III. Series.
QA614.86.S64 1988 89-49259
514'.74—dc20 CIP

ISBN 978-1-4899-3501-4 ISBN 978-1-4899-3499-4 (eBook)
DOI 10.1007/978-1-4899-3499-4

Proceedings of a Special Seminar on Fractals,
held October 9–15, 1988, in Erice, Sicily, Italy

PREFACE

This volume contains the Proceedings of the Special Seminar on: FRACTALS held from October 9-15, 1988 at the Ettore Majorana Centre for Scientific Culture, Erice (Trapani), Italy.

The concepts of self-similarity and scale invariance have arisen independently in several areas. One is the study of critical properites of phase transitions; another is fractal geometry, which involves the concept of (non-integer) fractal dimension. These two areas have now come together, and their methods have extended to various fields of physics. The purpose of this Seminar was to provide an overview of the recent developments in the field. Most of the contributions are theoretical, but some experimental work is also included.

During the past few years two tendencies have emerged in this field: one is to realize that many phenomena can be naturally modelled by fractal structures. So one can use this concept to define simple models and study their physical properties. The second point of view is more microscopic and tries to answer the question: why nature gives rise to fractal structures. This implies the formulation of fractal growth models based on physical concepts and their theoretical understanding in the same sense as the Renormalization Group method has allowed to understand the critical properties of phase transitions.

By comparing this volume to the one of the Trieste Symposium of 1985 ("Fractals in Physics", edited by L. Pietronero and E. Tosatti, North--Holland, Amsterdam, New York, 1986), it is clear that there has been substantial progress. Some problems have been clarified and many of the open ones are now much better posed. Nevertheless, some crucial questions have still to be answered. This makes the field healthy and the subject a pleasant one to work on.

It is a pleasure to thank Prof. Antonino Zichichi, Director of the E. Majorana Centre for having made this meeting possible and Dr. Alberto Gabriele and Dr. Pinola Savalli for the warm and efficient organization. Finally our thanks go to the following institutions that have generously sponsored the Seminar: Deutsche Forschungsgemeinschaft; Italian Ministry of Education; Italian Ministry of Scientific and Technological Research, and the Sicilian Regional Government.

Luciano Pietronero
Editor

CONTENTS

Part 4. Application of Fractal Growth Models to Physical Phenomena

Part 5. Diffusion and Vibrations on Fractals

Part 6. Diffusion Fronts and Invasion Percolation

Part 7. Random Surfaces

Part 8. Large Scale Distribution of Matter in the Universe

Part 1

Multifractals and Turbulence

A CLASS OF MULTINOMIAL MULTIFRACTAL MEASURES WITH NEGATIVE (LATENT) VALUES FOR THE "DIMENSION" $f(\alpha)$

Benoit B. Mandelbrot

Physics Department, IBM T.J. Watson Research Center,
Yorktown Heights NY 10598
Mathematics Department, Yale University, New Haven CT 06520

ABSTRACT

As is well known, fractals are *sets* of points that possess is the property of being invariant by dilation. When a fractal set is exactly self-similar, or is self-similar in a statistical sense, a central role is played by a positive quantity called *fractal dimension*, which need not be an integer, and which generalizes the "ordinary" dimension.

In this paper, a further generalization of dimension is introduced and motivated. When its value is positive, it effectively falls back on known definitions of fractal dimension. But its motivating virtue is that *its value can be negative*, in which case it quantifies and measures usefully the loose idea of "degree of emptiness" of an empty set.

Self-similar multifractals are also geometric objects invariant by dilation, but they *are not sets*. They are *measures*, a notion well illustrated by the concrete distributions of probability, of mass or of turbulent dissipation. They are described by a function $f(\alpha)$.

This paper shows that negative dimensions are needed to investigate the statistical properties of certain random self-similar multifractals, namely those for which $f(\alpha) < 0$ for some α's, called *latent* (= present, but hidden). The positive $f(\alpha)$'s define a "typical" distribution for the measure, while the negative $f(\alpha)$'s rule the variability between different samples from the same ensemble or population. Moments whose order lies beyond certain thresholds q^*_{max} and q^*_{min} are called *latent*. Their sample values are extremely sample dependent. Negative dimensions are best investigated using "supersamples."

In addition to negative f's, the multifractals investigated here involve a critical exponent $q_{bottom} < 0$, such that population moments of exponent q less than q_{bottom} are infinite. The corresponding sample moments are extremely "ill-behaved."

The "ordinary" multifractals, whose simplest example is the binomial, are called "manifest" by the author. Compared to them, the multifractals studied in this paper exhibit two "anomalies" that play a central role in the approach to multifractals the author has been developing since 1968. Their study requires nothing but elementary manipulations, making them the simplest examples of the anomalies in question.

Currently, the most active applications of negative dimensions are to the distribution of the dissipation of turbulence and to the distribution of the hitting probability along the boundary of a DLA cluster, which is an example of harmonic measure.

Fractals' Physical Origin and Properties
Edited by L. Pietronero
Plenum Press, New York

1. NEGATIVE DIMENSION AND INTRODUCTION TO MULTIFRACTALS

1.1. A generalized "latent" fractal dimension that can be negative. Examples

First, we restate the familiar "intersection rule" for fractal dimensions, and its equally familiar exception. Then we restate a suggestion made in Mandelbrot 1984 Section 2.1, and buttress it by new arguments and concrete illustrations.

1.1.1. *Generic intersection rule.* Take two sets S_1 and S_2 (either Euclidean or fractal) in a Euclidean space of ordinary (embedding) dimension E. Denote their codimensions by $E - \dim(S_1)$ and $E - \dim(S_2)$. "Generically," the intersection S of S_1 and S_2 satisfies

$$E - \dim(S) = E - \dim(S_1) + E - \dim(S_2).$$

Major exception to the rule. When $E - \dim(S_1) + E - \dim(S_2) > E$, the value of this expression does not matter: the intersection S is generically empty.

1.1.2. *A way to redefine dimension, which avoids this exception, hence simplifies but also enriches the intersection rule. The example of points, lines, planes and the like.* Compare the intersection of two lines and the intersection of a line by a plane. Both sets are "generically" of dimension 0, in agreement with the intersection rule and its exception. Yet, one would like to discriminate more finely between these various ways of being of dimension 0, by expressing numerically the idea that the intersection of two lines is "emptier" than the intersection of a line by a plane. If one could get rid of the exception to the intersection rule, one may perhaps be allowed to say that these two sets have the respective dimensions -1 and 0.

This loose idea can indeed be given precise and down-to-earth meanings. The root of the explanation is that one cannot observe an unbounded space, containing strict points, lines or planes. One can only observe a bounded "window" of space, containing small blobs, thin sticks and thin shells.

A generalized box dimension that is -1. A set of (Euclidean or fractal) dimension D_B requires $N(b) \sim b^{D_B}$ boxes of side $r = b^{-1}$ to be covered. The familiar box dimension D_B simply measures *the rate of increase* of $N(b)$ with b. One should be able to generalize D_B as describing the rate of either increase or *decrease* of "something that is like $N(b)$." This something could not be an integer, hence could not be a number of boxes. But let us show that it could be an ensemble or population expectation $\langle N\rangle$, which need not be an integer. To simplify the algebra, focus on a square window in the plane, whose side is L, and which includes a random point-like blob of side $1/b$ and a random line-like strip of width $1/b$. When the strip intersects the blob, $N = 1$; otherwise, $N = 0$. Intersection occurs when the distance between the point and the line is $< b$, which happens with probability $\sim b/L$. Thus, $\langle N\rangle = L/b$, and for large L/b we obtain the value

$$D_B = \log(1/b)/\log b = -1.$$

A generalized sausage codimension that is 3 in the plane. The familiar sausage of S is the set of points which lie within a distance ε of a point in S. Hence, the sausage of the union of S_1 and S_2 is the union of the sausages of S_1 and S_2. But what about the intersection? When S_1 and S_2 intersect, the intersection of the sausage and the sausage of the intersection scale in the same way as $\varepsilon \to 0$. When the sets S_1 and S_2 fail to intersect, only the intersection of the sausages continues to be defined. In the present example of a point and a line in the plane, its area is $\sim \varepsilon^2$ with a probability $\sim \varepsilon/L$, and 0 otherwise. Hence the expected area of the intersection is $\sim \varepsilon^3/L$. The exponent can be used to define a *generalized sausage codimension*. Its value is 3, hence $D_{MB} = -1$.

1.1.3. *The preceding reasoning extends to fractal sets. The example of the birth-and-death cascades on the interval* [0, 1]. The k-th cascade stage begins with dyadic cells of length 2^{-k}. Each cell is subdivided into 2 dyadic halves, and each dyadic half either "lives," with the probability $p < 1$, or "dies," with the probability $1 - p$. One defines a "birth and death process" [5, Chapter 23] by thinking of mother cells as dying and giving birth to N daughter cells. Here $N=0$ with the probability $(1-p)^2$, $N=1$ with the probability $2p(1-p)$, and $N=2$ with the probability p^2. Thus, $\langle N \rangle = 2p$.

When $\langle N \rangle > 1$, so that $D = \log_2 \langle N \rangle > 0$. It is known that this process has a positive probability of generating a non empty set, which one can call a *birth and death fractal dust*. For this set, D is the value of all useful forms of fractal dimension. But it is also known that a "bloodline" can die out, the probability being one when $D < 0$, and between 0 and 1 when $D > 0$.

We now propose to say that $D = \log_2 \langle N \rangle$ *in all cases*, even if $D < 0$.

Imbedding a "dead" birth and death fractal set as a one dimensional cut through a proper "living" birth and death set. Start with the E-dimensional cube $[0, 1]^E$, and apply the same birth and death process to each its 2^E sub cubes. Now, $\langle N_E \rangle = 2^E p$, and one can choose E to be large enough to insure $2^E p > 1$, hence $D_E = \log_2 \langle N_E \rangle > 0$. That is one can interpret every birth and death set on the line as a cut.

1.1.4. *The essential role of randomness. The term, "latent."* It must be underlined that the above expressions for D_B and D_S refer to a random ensemble or population of constructions. A negative generalized D says nothing about any individual set. Mandelbrot 1984 proposes for negative dimensions of the term *latent*, which in Latin means *present but hidden*, and implies that some operation is needed to *express* or *reveal* them. What *hides* them is the fact that, as the blob size or the sausage radius $\varepsilon \to 0$, there is an increasingly overwhelming probability that the sets to which negative dimensions often become empty. But they can be *revealed*, by taking a sufficient number of samples, namely, a number that increases with $1/\varepsilon$ and $|D|$. Since they can be revealed, they were *present* all along.

1.1.5. *Limitations of the Hausdorff-Besicovitch dimension D_{HB}.* The proposed generalizations add to the notion of fractal dimension. Overall complication increases, because one tries to tame yet another facet of reality, using geometric information that is available but otherwise discarded. To extend D_{HB} to negative values would be impossible. Furthermore, randomness is totally foreign to D_{HB}: In the case of random sets, D_{HB} applies to samples and not to populations. The example of D_{HB} had led us in the past to resist attempts to define a fractal dimension for a population. More important, they fulfilled no need, but we shall see that a need has now been created by the multifractals.

As the intuitive contents of fractal dimension expands, it continues to become increasingly clear that physics requires more than D_{HB}. Hausdorff and Besicovitch have provided us with a nearly ready-made notion that could be made into a useful tool of physics. But this tool proved to lack versatility and to be hard to use, and it keeps being thoroughly modified and diversified.

1.2. Continuity and singularity for measures. Scaling requirements that define a self-similar multifractal. A possible definition of self-similarity that allows $f(\alpha) < 0$

For the reader having even a moderate acquaintance with multifractals, the novelty of this paper is that it deals with random multifractal constructions in which two important features can be investigated without hand-waving and without extraneous complication. The first is that $f(\alpha) < 0$ for some α's, and the second is that population moments diverge when q is below a threshold q_{bottom}. Within the alternative approach to multifractals of Frisch and Parisi 1985, Halsey et al. 1986, these features are "anomalous," but in fact they are essential to the understanding of randomness in multifractal measures.

1.2.1. *Singular measures.* The set that supports a multifractal measure *can* be itself a fractal, but it *need not* be one. In this paper, extraneous complications will be eliminated by assuming that the support is the "time interval" $[0, 1]$, though we eventually need to move up to a higher dimensional Euclidean space. Also, the multifractals we consider are singular measures, that is, they correspond to distributions of mass that are continuous but fail to have a density. A measure carried by subsets of $[0, 1]$ is called *continuous* when the measures $\mu(dt)$ contained in the intervals $[t, t+dt]$ decrease to 0 with dt. Such a measure fails to have a density if $\mu(dt)$ fails to be "of the order of dt.".

1.2.2. ***A measure is a self-similar multifractal, when it satisfies certain geometric scaling relations. Statements of a widely held form of these scaling requirements.***

A) There exists an exponent α, function of t, such that one can say that

$$\mu(dt) \text{ is of the order of } (dt)^{\alpha}.$$

B) The set of values of t where α takes a certain value is a fractal. That is, the number of intervals characterized by α takes the form

$$N(dt) = (dt)^{-f(\alpha)}.$$

This means that $-\log N(dt)/\log(dt)$, which is ≥ 0 and is formally a fractal dimension, should not depend upon dt and should be a function $f(\alpha)$ of α.

This version of requirement B) turns around an argument Frisch & Parisi 1983 had based on an analysis of the multifractals presented in Mandelbrot 1974. Based on this version of B), and on yet another version (to be discussed in Section 1.5), the belief has spread that a multifractal is always and necessarily characterized by a function $f(\alpha) \geq 0$ of a variable $\alpha > 0$. Within a wider framework, however, this belief is unwarranted if the multifractal is random, and the goal of this paper is • A) To give examples to demonstrate that it is necessary to allow $f(\alpha) < 0$. • B) To explain the role of $f(\alpha) < 0$ in these examples.

1.2.3. *Generalized form of the scaling requirements that allow a random measure to be called a self-similar multifractal.* To prepare for a necessary generalization of the idea of self-similar measure, form the ratio

$$\frac{N(dt)}{(1/dt)} = dtN(dt) = (dt)^{-f(\alpha)+1} = (dt)^{-\rho(\alpha)}, \text{ with } \rho(\alpha) = f(\alpha) - 1.$$

Clearly, this ratio is the relative frequency, among $1/dt$ intervals of length dt, of the intervals in which a certain value of α occurs. Thus, the above second requirement for a measure to be self-similar, as written in Section 1.2.2, simply expresses that

$$\frac{\log(\text{probability of } \alpha)}{\log dt} \text{ is a function } \rho(\alpha).$$

The goal of this paper is to show that this last expression implies a generalized definition of $f(\alpha)$. As further preparation, observe that this expression can be said to be based upon a plot of the probability distribution of the random measure $\mu(dt)$ in doubly logarithmic coordinates. The plotting proceeds in two steps, each followed by renormalization. *First*, we work on $\mu(dt)$, replacing it by $\log \mu(dt)$ and renormalizing by dividing by $\log dt$, to obtain an abscissa that is a random variable A (read as capital α). *Second*, we work on the probability density of A, call it $p(\alpha)$. We replace it by $\log p(\alpha)$ and again renormalize by dividing by $\log dt$.

A definition of self-similar multifractals: We shall say that a measure $\mu(dt)$ on $[0, 1]$ is a self-similar multifractal if, as $dt \to 0$, the transformed and renormalized density $\log p(\alpha)/\log dt$ converges to a limit $\rho(\alpha)$.

The function $f(\alpha)$ is then defined starting from $\rho(\alpha)$, as $f(\alpha) = \rho(\alpha) + 1$.

1.3. Summary of the paper, and applications where one expects $f < 0$

1.3.1. *Summary*. A definition is only as good and useful as the variety of examples it allows. In this light, the introductory Section 2.3 will confirm that the definition given at the end of Section 1.2.3 is indeed satisfied by the "tamest" of all multifractals, which are the binomial measures; in that case, find $f(\alpha) \geq 0$ for all α.

Then Section 3 will show that this definition also allows for random self-similar measures for which $\alpha_{min} = 0$, $\alpha_{max} = \infty$ and $f(\alpha) < 0$ for some α's. A negative $f(\alpha)$ fails to be an "ordinary" fractal dimension, but is a "latent" dimension in the sense of Section 1.1. The examples in Section 3 have been chosen so that their definitions are natural, while the calculations are absolutely elementary throughout.

After that, Section 4 interprets the meaning of both positive and the negative values of this generalized $f(\alpha)$. The results being the newest in this paper, they deserve being summarized here. They concern the sample variability of the measures $\mu(dt)$, with particular accent on $\mathbf{A}_{max}$ and $\mathbf{A}_{min}$. It is found that a "typical" sample is described by the positive $f(\alpha)$'s. On the other hand, the sample variability is primarily ruled by the latent $f(\alpha)$'s. Section 4.5 shows ways to estimate latent $f(\alpha)$'s from the variability within "supersamples" obtained by pooling many samples together. In order to come increasingly close to $\alpha_{min} = 0$ or to $\alpha_{max} = \infty$, it is naturally necessary to pool data from increasingly long supersamples.

Section 5 generalizes Section 3, and Section 6 describes briefly a second class of interesting multifractals with latent α's.

1.3.2. *On the goals of fractal geometry.* One reason to estimate fractal dimensions and $f(\alpha)$'s is to do physics. Another reason is to compare messy data with theories. because $f(\alpha)$ is a window on a generating mechanism. It is important, therefore, to know that the positive values of $f(\alpha)$ fail to exhaust all that one should attempt to extract from the data. The negative $f(\alpha)$ need not remain latent = hidden. Revealing them tells us about the generating process, i.e., about what to expect from other random samples of the same process. In particular, they give us firmer grounds for the comparison between distinct sets of data, or for the proper fitting of a model to the data.

1.3.3. *The best understood occurrence of $f(\alpha) < 0$ concerns turbulence.* The early papers on multifractals, namely those we wrote from 1968 to 1976, have been primarily (but not exclusively) motivated by the study of the spatial distribution of dissipation in turbulence. This topic has again become extremely active in recent years, and negative $f(\alpha)$'s have proven to be of the most direct importance. Thus, Meneveau and Screenivasan 1987 had investigated the $f(\alpha)$ of dissipation along one dimensional cuts through 3d turbulence, and had concluded that the simplest binomial (Section 2) provides a good fit. Under our prodding, however, a more careful study was carried out (e.g., Prasad et al 1988). It has shown that the binomial fit was based on a method of estimating $f(\alpha)$ that automatically cancels the negative values.

1.3.4. *Interesting open issues concerning the sign of $f(\alpha)$ occur in the study of harmonic measure on DLA.* The study of diffusion limited aggregation and other fractal aggregates has drawn the physicists' attention to the harmonic measure observed when the Laplace equation is solved in a domain whose boundary is a fractal curve. Early work has assumed (without even saying) that $f(\alpha) \geq 0$ and that moments of all orders are finite. However, many authors have carried out formal calculations that suggest it is necessary to allow for $f(\alpha) < 0$. Now, Blumenfeld and Aharony 1989 give evidence that the population moments fail to converge for q below a threshold q_{bottom} about -1. They conclude that the harmonic measure *cannot* be multifractal. In our opinion, this conclusion may only express that the definition of multifractality via moments is unnecessarily narrow and should be avoided. We shall not discuss data, but we shall exhibit simple random examples for which sample moments for $q < q_{bottom}$ (where $q_{bottom} < 0$) "misbehave" because the corresponding population moments fail to exist.

1.3.5. Other uses of multifractals in physics have become very broad, but this is not the proper place, either to survey them, or to test whether they would benefit from the understanding of the notion of latency. Several authors have approached the issue of $f(\alpha) < 0$ from angles different from ours, have shown that restricting multifractals to $f(\alpha) \geq 0$ leads to self-contradiction (Cates and Deutsch 1987), or is otherwise not acceptable (Fourcade et al. 1987, Fourcade and Tremblay 1987). But we have already said that this paper has its sources in different applications.

1.4. The classification of multifractals in a wider perspective

1.4.1. *A wider perspective.* To summarize Section 1.2.3 in one phrase, the generalization from fractals to multifractals involves the passage from geometric objects that fractal geometry characterizes primarily by one number, namely, a fractal dimension, to geometric objects that must be characterized primarily by some function. To achieve broadest generality, while staying closest to familiar mathematical notions, the easiest is to use a "probability" distribution that has been plotted on doubly logarithmic coordinates and then renormalized suitably to yield a function denoted by $\rho(\alpha)$.

In this general framework, α is the renormalized logarithm of a measure which can range from $-\infty$ to $+\infty$, and $\rho(\alpha)$ is the renormalized logarithm of a probability density, which can range from $-\infty$ to 0. However, the range of variation may be narrower for both α and $\rho(\alpha)$. Hence, as shown in Mandelbrot 1988, 1989a, one can distinguish several levels of complication. Sections 1.4.4 and 1.5 tackle the same issue in terms of moments.

1.4.2. *The purely manifest random or non random multifractals.* At the lowest level of generality and complication, $\alpha > 0$, and $\rho(\alpha) \geq -1$ for every possible α. These multifractals' properties largely "manifest" themselves in every sample. In a purely manifest multifractal, the variable α is the Hölder exponent; it is a proper measure of singularity strength. For each α, the function $-\rho(\alpha)$ is a fractal codimension, hence the function $f(\alpha) = \rho(\alpha) + 1$ is a fractal dimension. Thus, the generalization from fractal sets to the manifest multifractal measures involves the passage *from one or a finite number of fractal dimensions to an infinite number of fractal dimensions,*

The main features of the manifest multifractals are present in the non random binomial measures (to be sketched in Section 2 for the sake of completeness), or in the multinomial measures (Mandelbrot 1988, 1989a). Purely manifest multifractals bring us one step beyond fractals along the path that leads away from the integer-valued dimensions of Euclid. Now we discuss a second and third steps beyond the first.

1.4.3. *The two levels of "anomalous" random multifractals involve latent f's and virtual α's.* Within the framework of Frisch and Parisi 1985 or Halsey et al. 1986, to be non-manifest is an "anomaly." However, Mandelbrot 1974, 1988, 1989a,b show that anomalies can and do occur and are important, both in theory and in practice.

The *"anomaly" of the latent f*'s. There exist random multifractal measures such that $\alpha > 0$, but $\rho(\alpha) < -1$ for some values of α, which we have proposed to call "latent," meaning *present* but hidden. As to $f(\alpha) = \rho(\alpha) + 1$, it is an ordinary fractal dimension when it is positive, but when it is negative it is a fractal dimension in the generalized sense described in Section 1.1.

The *"anomaly" of the virtual α*'s. This is the topic Mandelbrot 1989b investigates in detail, again using the simplest examples. There exist random multifractal measures such that $\rho(\alpha)$ is not only defined for $\alpha > 0$, but also for all $\alpha < 0$, which Mandelbrot 1988, 1989a have proposed to call "virtual" α's. Of course, α cannot be a Hölder exponent when it is negative (because a Hölder exponent is positive by definition).

A matter of terminology. In our mind, "latent" refers to the function f when $f(\alpha) < 0$, and "virtual" refers to the variable α when $\alpha < 0$. This would subdivide the category of "latent f" into "latent f, but Hölder α" and "virtual α." But in cases where there is no ambiguity we shall shorten "latent, but" to "latent."

1.4.4. *The two levels of anomalous multifractals involve the possibility for moments to be either latent, or divergent.* After $f(\alpha)$, which reflects the *distribution* of the measure of $\mu(dt)$, we examine *moments* of this measure. Under wide conditions, self-similar multifractals have the following property:

the ensemble or population q-th moment $\langle \mu^q(dt) \rangle$ scales like $(dt)^{\tau(q)+1}$,

$\tau(q)$ is a function that is related to $f(\alpha)$ by Legendre and inverse Legendre transforms. One condition under which this "power law" behavior holds without question is when the multifractal is manifest. Define the sample value of $\langle \mu^q(dt) \rangle$ as the sum $dt \sum \mu^q(dt)$ over $1/dt$ intervals of length dt. When α is manifest, the sample sum converges to $\langle \mu^q(dt) \rangle$. But $\langle \mu^q(dt) \rangle$ can misbehave in either of two ways.

The manifest moments. Suppose that $\alpha < \alpha^*_{min}$ and/or for $\alpha > \alpha^*_{max}$. The Legendre relations associate to α^*_{min} and α^*_{max} the exponents q^*_{max} and q^*_{min}. We propose that the moments such that $q^*_{min} < q < q^*_{max}$ be called *manifest*. The reason is that we shall show that they manifest themselves in "typical" samples.

The "anomaly" of latent moments. For $q < q^*_{min}$ and/or $q > q^*_{max}$, we propose that the moment of order q be called latent. Its population value may be finite or infinite. When α is latent, the sample sum $\sum \mu^q(dt)$ behaves very erratically, and the typical sample fails to suffice to estimate the population $\langle \mu^q(dt) \rangle$.

The "anomaly" of divergent moments. An additional features of latent multifractals, such as the examples in Sections 3 and 5, is that one has

$$\langle \mu^q(dt) \rangle < \infty \text{ if (and only if) } q > q_{\text{bottom}}, \text{ where } q_{\text{bottom}} < 0.$$

In addition, the virtual multifractals, such as of the limit lognormal multifractal of Mandelbrot 1989b, are such that $\langle \mu^q(dt) \rangle = \infty$ if (and only if) $q < q_{crit}$, where $q_{crit} > 0$.

Those various anomalies involve subtle and new concepts and arguments, without which the topic is full of paradoxes. Therefore, this paper focuses on examples for which exact calculations are totally elementary.

1.5. An alternative tentative definition of self-similar multifractals using the expression deduced from sample moments. Practical pitfalls

Logically, the topic of this Section is part of Section 1.4., but it has been separated for emphasis. Sections 1.2.2 and 1.2.3 examine the notion of self-similarity for a measure, and describe two versions of requirement B). As many readers know, this condition has also been written down in a different third way, by requiring that

(*) the q-th moment of $\mu(dt)$ within a sample scales like some power of dt;
$\sum \mu^q(dt)$ scales like dt to the power $\tau_{\text{sample}}(q)$.

As a matter of fact, the notations used here, q for the power and $\tau(q)$ for the function in Section 3.4, had been contributed by Hentschel and Procaccia 1983 for an expression that they call $\tau(q)$, but we must call $\tau_{\text{sample}}(q)$. In the manifest multifractals, relation (*) is a consequence of the definition proposed in Section 1.2.3. Hence, relation (*) can indeed serve to define a multifractal, but at heavy cost: by narrowing the scope of this notion to the manifest multifractals. In this special case, the direct definition of $f(\alpha)$ given in Section 1.2.3 can be replaced by an indirect definition that starts with $\tau(q)$ and uses Legendre and inverse Legendre transforms.

However, by excluding latent f and virtual α, which the definition in Section 1.1.3. allows, condition (*) fails to be an acceptable definition of multifractality. The basic symptom of the inadequacy of (*) is often noted but rarely diagnosed as serious. The symptom is that in many cases (*) is verified accurately when q is positive and small, but (*) becomes increasingly rough as q increases, or is negative and not close to 0. Many computer programs have been written to extract information from sample moments, to evaluate the corresponding $\tau_{\text{sample}}(q)$, and then to proceed to $f(\alpha)$ by Legendre. When the moments are unstable and messy, these computer programs blindly "stabilize" them. But messy sample moments may be trying to tell us that the population moments are latent or divergent. We return to this issue in Section 4.7.

2. PRELIMINARIES: BINOMIAL MEASURES ON THE INTERVAL [0, 1]

For the sake of completeness, Sections 2.1 and 2.2 repeat standard material concerning the binomial measures. This prepares for important points made in sections 2.3 and 2.4. The binomial measure rewards careful study. Let us therefore draw attention to the extensive additional material found in Mandelbrot 1989a, Section 5.

2.1. Construction of the binomial measures on [0, 1]

These multifractals form a family that depend upon a single parameter m_0, variously called a *multiplier* or a *mass*. One assumes that m_0 satisfies $0 < m_0 < 1$ and $m_0 \neq 1/2$, and one defines $m_1 = 1 - m_0$.

The "initiator" of the construction is the interval [0, 1] containing a mass taken as unity. The basic "generating step" is to spread mass over the halves of every dyadic interval, with the relative proportions m_0 and m_1 placed to the left and to the right. Thus, the first stage yields the mass m_0 in [0, ½] and the mass m_1 in [½, 1]. Each later stage consists in taking the mass yielded by the preceding stage, and multiplying it by either m_0 or m_1. Therefore, we deal with a *multiplicative process*. After k stages, suppose that $t = 0.\beta_1\beta_2 \ldots \beta_k$ is the development of t in the counting base $b = 2$, and let φ_0 and φ_1 denote the relative frequencies of 0's and 1's in the binary development of t. Then the binomial measure is defined as the measure such that the dyadic interval $[dt] = [t, t + 2^{-k}]$ of length $dt = 2^{-k}$ receives the mass

$$\mu(dt) = m_0^{k\varphi_0} m_1^{k\varphi_1}.$$

By construction, $\mu(dt)$ satisfies the property of self-similarity, as generalized from sets to measures.

2.2. Derivation of the function $f(\alpha)$

The Hölder exponent $\alpha = \log \mu(dt)/\log(dt)$. In the present case, it is obvious that

$$\alpha = \alpha(\varphi_0, \varphi_1) = -\varphi_0 \log_2 m_0 - \varphi_1 \log_2 m_1,$$

and $0 < \alpha_{\min} = -\log_2 m_0 \leq \alpha \leq \alpha_{\max} = -\log_2 m_1 < \infty$.

The box dimension. The number of intervals leading to φ_0 and φ_1 is $N(k, \varphi_0, \varphi_1) = k!/(k\varphi_0)!(k\varphi_1)!$. One can use N to form the expression

$$\delta(k, \varphi_0, \varphi_1) = -\frac{\log N(k, \varphi_0, \varphi_1)}{\log(dt)} = -\frac{\log[k!/(k\varphi_0)!(k\varphi_1)!]}{\log(dt)}.$$

This δ takes the form $-\log N/\log r$ that characterizes the box dimension of a set. Hence one can call δ a *box fractal dimension.* More precisely, since the boxes are cells in a dyadic grid, it is a *grid fractal dimension.* For large k, the replacement of the factorial by the leading term in the Stirling approximation shows that

$$\lim_{k\to\infty} \delta(k, \varphi_0, \varphi_1) = \delta(\varphi_0, \varphi_1), \text{ with } \delta(\varphi_0, \varphi_1) = -\varphi_0 \log_2 \varphi_0 - \varphi_1 \log_2 \varphi_1.$$

Derivation of a function $f(\alpha)$. Eliminating φ_0 and φ_1 between α and δ, we obtain a function written in parametric form. It will be denoted as $f(\alpha)$, a notation contributed by Halsey et al. 1985.

2.3. Restatement of Section 2.2 in terms of a limit theorem on the rescaled doubly logarithmic plots of probability densities. Derivation of the function $\rho(\alpha)$

The binomial measures are, of course, *not* random. Yet it is important, and also easy to reinterpreted the combinatorics in Section 2.2 in probabilistic terms. The interplay between non randomness and randomness is a general fact in fractal geometry, where for example a non random Cantor set becomes a random set when examined from a randomly selected origin.

2.3.1. *Mass in a dyadic cell of length 2^{-k} that has been picked at random among the 2^k such cells.* The probability of hitting a cell that corresponds to a prescribed α, or to the equivalent φ_0 and φ_1, will be denoted by $\Pr\{A=\alpha\}$. As said earlier, A is to be read as "capital alpha": we follow the probabilists' custom of denoting a random variable by a capital letter, and a sample value of this variable by the corresponding small letter.

Of course, $\Pr\{A=\alpha\}=2^{-k}N(k, \varphi_0, \varphi_1)$. The first result concerning $\Pr\{A=\alpha\}$ is a *law of large numbers.* Write $\langle\alpha\rangle=(1/2)(-\log_b m_0-\log_b m_1)$. Then, we have, for, $k\to\infty$.

$$\Pr\{A=\alpha\}=1 \text{ for } \alpha=\langle\alpha\rangle \text{ and } \Pr\{A=\alpha\}\to 0 \text{ for all } \alpha\neq\langle\alpha\rangle.$$

The next usual step in probability theory is to "renormalize" A in such a way that its distribution has a nontrivial limit for $k\to\infty$, that is, a limit that is neither 0 nor 1. But we are not free to take this step here, and (besides) it does not yield much of interest.

2.3.2. *Probabilistic restatement of the manipulations in Section 2.2.* These manipulations consist in renormalizing $\Pr\{A=\alpha\}$. Indeed, it suffices to define

$$\rho(k, \varphi_0, \varphi_1)=-\frac{\log \Pr\{A=\alpha\}}{\log dt}=-\frac{\log 2^{-k}N(k, \varphi_0, \varphi_1)}{\log dt}.$$

Obviously, $\rho(k, \varphi_0, \varphi_1)=\delta(k, \varphi_0, \varphi_1)-1$, with δ as in Section 2.2. Hence,

$$\lim_{k\to\infty}\rho(k, \varphi_0, \varphi_1)=\rho(\alpha)=f(\alpha)-1.$$

2.3.3. *Importance of the probabilistic reinterpretation of $f(\alpha)$.* First, the fractal codimension $-\rho(\alpha)$ comes up as a new form of already familiar probabilities, and only requires the further development of old intuitions. Far more important, as Sections 3 and 5 will show, the argument that yields $\rho(\alpha)$ has far broader domain for application than the argument that yields the "ordinary," positive, fractal dimension.

2.4. Tail dimensions and tail probabilities, and a prefactor

The following observation will be needed in Section 4. When $\alpha>\langle A\rangle$, the value dimension is $f(\alpha)$ is not only the fractal dimension of the set where $A=\alpha$, but also the fractal dimension of the set where $A>\alpha$. The limit $\rho(\alpha)=\lim_{k\to\infty}-\log\Pr\{A=\alpha\}/\log dt$ is also equal to $\lim_{k\to\infty}-\log\Pr\{A>\alpha\}/\log dt$.

Therefore, $\Pr\{A=\alpha\}=F\Pr\{A>\alpha\}$, where F is a prefactor that "varies slowly" with k, in the sense that $\log F/\log dt\to 0$ with dt. Very roughly, $\Pr\{A=\alpha\}\sim\Pr\{A>\alpha\}$.

The preceding paragraphs remain true when all the inequalities are inverted.

2.5. On the distinction between the asymptotic and the preasymptotic roles of $f(\alpha)$, from the viewpoint of the asymptotic and pre-asymptotic properties of the distribution of $\mu(dt)$. Significance of $f(\alpha)$ in the manifest case

Many readers of this paper know *how* to evaluate $f(\alpha)$, but, before we continue, it is good to add a word about *what* $f(\alpha)$ means and *why* it should be evaluated. The function $f(\alpha)$ plays two roles. The first role, that of a "spectrum of singularities," is an asymptotic property meaningful only for $dt\to 0$. The second role of $f(\alpha)$ is less widely appreciated but essential. It concerns its relevance to the histograms of the measure $\mu(dt)$ for various $dt>0$. These roles are hard to tell apart in the binomial case, or whenever $f(\alpha)$ for all $\alpha>0$, but that they separate sharply when some $f(\alpha)<0$.

3. A RANDOM MULTIFRACTAL MEASURE WITH UNIFORMLY DISTRIBUTED MULTIPLIERS

This Section and Section 5 replace the non-random multiplier m_0 of a binomial measure by a random number M_0 in $[0, 1]$. We assume that mass is conserved in the measure-generating cascade, therefore the multiplier m_1 is always replaced by $M_1 = 1 - M_0$. The random variables M_0 and M_1 are not independent. This Section picks the simplest form of M_0, and shows that $\rho(\alpha)$ is fully determined by the distribution of M_0.

However, Section 4.6 will show that a knowledge of the distribution of M_0 and of the resulting $\rho(\alpha)$ is not enough. It does not suffice to determine the measure itself, and either the "typical" histogram, or the extent of sample variability.

3.1. The simplest example: a random base 2 multifractal measure with multipliers uniformly distributed on $[0, 1]$

A sample is illustrated by Figures 1 and 2. When M_0 is uniformly distributed on $[0, 1]$, the same is true of M_1, and the ratio $R = M_1/M_0 = 1/M_0 - 1$ satisfies

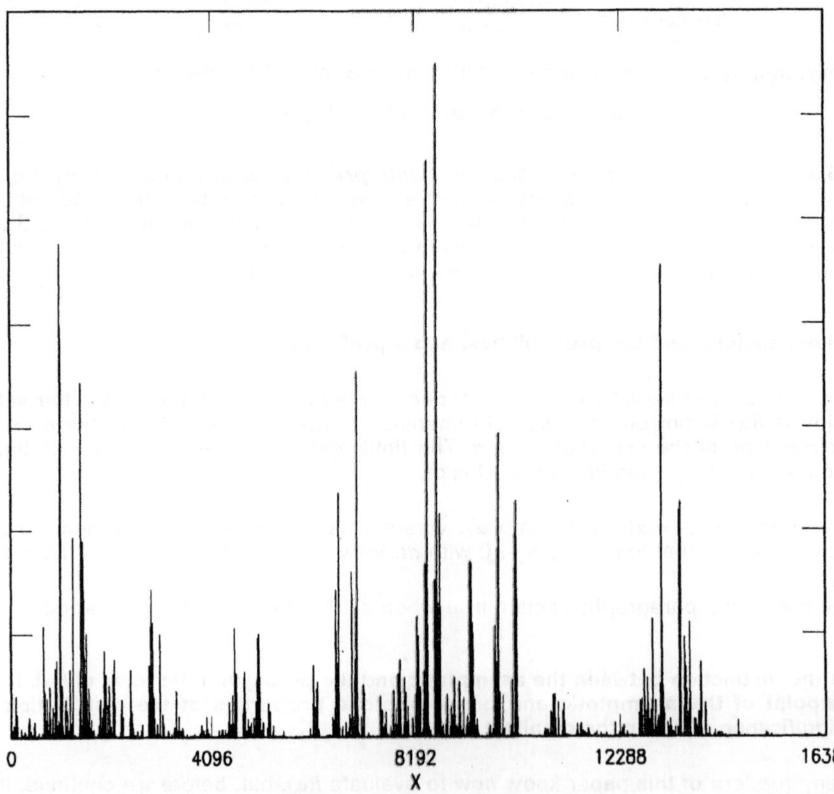

Figure 1. Sample of the random binomial multifractal $\mu(dt)$ introduced in Section 3.1. Here, $k = 14$, so there are 16384 data. The scales are linear. The most striking feature is that, even by the standard of the binomial multifractals, the present random $\mu(dt)$ seems far from being stationary. In particular, large μ's are very "ragged," in a very sample-dependent fashion.

$\Pr\{R > r\} = (1 + r)^{-1}$, hence R has an infinite expectation and infinite moments of order $q \geq 1$. The same is true of $1/R$. This fact expresses that one may find a great inequality between $\mu([0, 1/2])$ and $\mu([1/2, 1])$.

By a repetition of this scheme, the dyadic cell of length $dt = 2^{-k}$, starting at $t = 0.\eta_1\eta_2 \ldots \eta_k$ is given the mass

$$\mu(dt) = M(\eta_1)M(\eta_1, \eta_2) \ldots M(\eta_1, \ldots \eta_k).$$

Here, the successive random multipliers M for given t are identically distributed and independent uniform random variables. Furthermore,

$$\mathbf{A} == \log \mu(dt)/ \log dt = -(1/k)[\log_2 M(\eta_1) + \log_2 M(\eta_1, \eta_2) \ldots].$$

Thus, $\mathbf{A}$ is the average of k independent random variables. Let us show that its limit distribution for $k \to \infty$ can be obtained explicitly, and is far from being "intuitive."

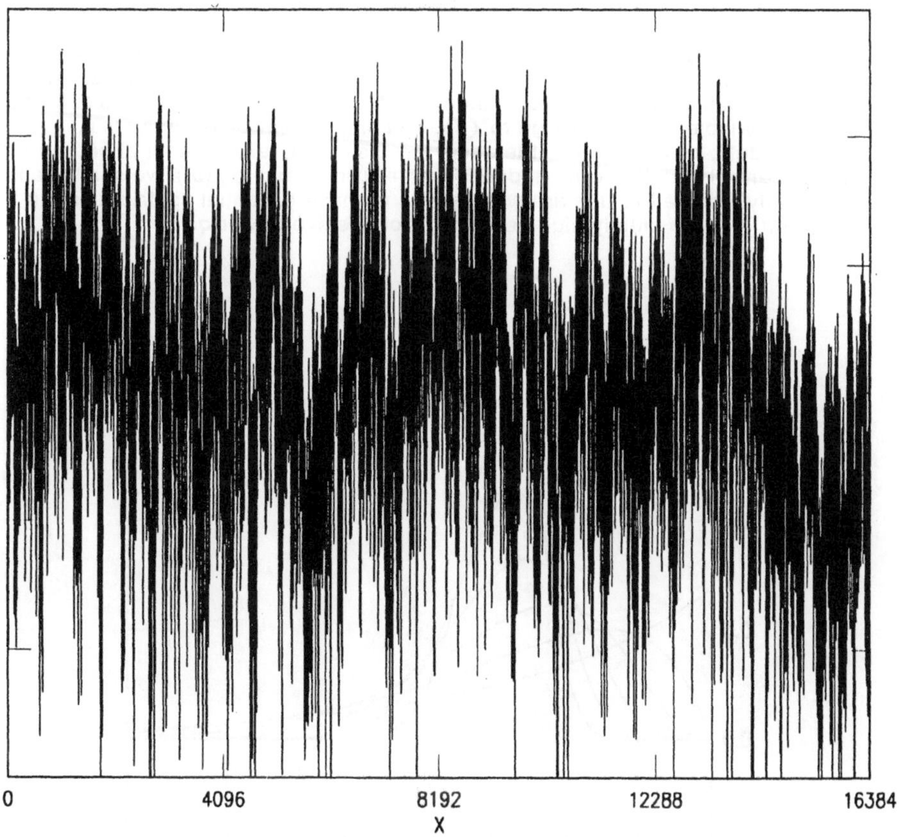

Figure 2. The apparent non stationarity of Figure 1 is further emphasized here, by using a logarithmic ordinate. For example, there is a probability of 1/100 of finding that the two halves of the overall sample (or the dyadic subintervals of any other dyadic interval) carry masses that are, *overall*, in the ratio of more than 100 to 1. This expresses the fact that, as shown in Section 3.1, the random variables M_0/M_1 and M_1/M_0 have infinite expectations.

3.2. The probability densities $p_k(y')$ and $p^*_k(\alpha)$

The variable M being uniformly distributed on $[0, 1]$, one has $\Pr\{M < m\} = m$. Therefore, the tail probability $\Pr\{X > x\}$ of $X = -\log_2 M$ and its probability density $p(x)$ are both exponential: Denoting $\log_e 2 \sim .6931$ by δ,

$$\Pr\{X > x\} = 2^{-x} = \exp(-\delta x) \text{ and } p(x) = \delta \exp(-\delta x).$$

The sum Y of k such exponential variables is a "Gamma variable" with the density

$$p_k(y) = \delta(\delta y)^{k-1} e^{-\delta y} / \Gamma(k).$$

Hence, $\mathrm{A} = Y/k$ has the probability density (shown on Figures 3 and 4)

$$p^*_k(\alpha) = \delta k(\delta k \alpha)^{k-1} e^{-\delta k \alpha} / \Gamma(k).$$

Figure 3 shows that, as k increases the graph of $p^*_k(\alpha)$ becomes increasingly close to the familiar shape called "Gaussian ogive," centered on $\langle X \rangle = 1/\delta \sim 1.4426$. This is to be expected, since $\langle X \rangle < \infty$ and $\langle X^2 \rangle < \infty$, hence $Y/\sqrt{k}$ obeys the classical central limit theorem and converges to a Gaussian. As a matter of fact, Y/k obeys the law of large numbers, and converges almost surely to the non random limit $\langle \mathrm{A} \rangle = \langle X \rangle$, making the density of Y/k converge to a delta function by a sequence of narrowing ogives. As a result, the most probable value, the expectation, and the other usual parameters of location of the random variable A all converge to $\langle X \rangle$. This limit behavior is "universal," that is, it holds very widely; hence, it tells little about A. Instead, it tells us a lot about the limitations of the central limit theorem. Indeed, if we return from α to $\mu(dt)$, we shall see that those "negligibly" few tail values are so huge, as to make essential contributions to the moments $\langle \mu^q(dt) \rangle$ of sufficiently high negative or of positive power q.

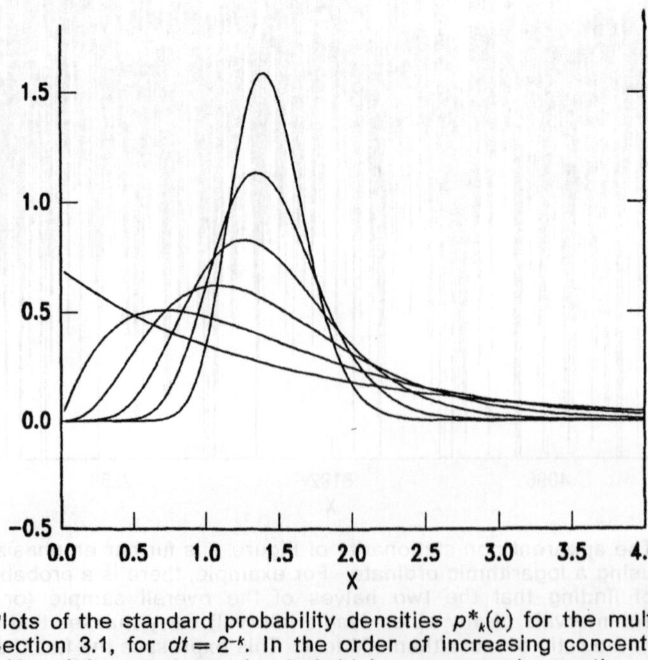

Figure 3. Plots of the standard probability densities $p^*_k(\alpha)$ for the multifractals in Section 3.1, for $dt = 2^{-k}$. In the order of increasing concentration near $\langle \mathrm{A} \rangle = \langle X \rangle$, we have $k = 1$ (which corresponds to the exponential distribution of X), then $k = 2$, 4, 8, 16 and 32.

In other words, while all the distributions that converge to the Gaussian to become close to each other in *some* ways, they *fail* to become close to each other from the way that interests us in the study of multifractals. We must make fine distinctions between distributions that the central limit theorem describes as indistinguishable.

3.3. The function $\rho(\alpha)$

To make these distinctions, let us again try the quantity that has served well in the non random binomial case, namely (Figure 5)

$$\rho_k(\alpha) = \frac{\log_2 p^*_k(\alpha)}{k}.$$

The truncated Stirling formula $\log \Gamma(k) \sim (k - 1/2) \log k - k + (\log 2\pi)/2$ yields the large k approximations

$$\rho_k(\alpha) = \log_2(\alpha\delta) - \alpha + 1/\delta - \frac{\log_2(2\pi k \alpha^{-2})}{2k}.$$

Now the peculiar expression $\rho_k(\alpha)$ is motivated by the following obvious fact:

$$\text{as } k \to \infty, \quad \rho_k(\alpha) \to \rho(\alpha) = \log_2(\alpha\delta) - \alpha + 1/\delta.$$

Since $\rho'(\alpha) = -1 + 1/\alpha\delta$, we verify that $\rho'(\alpha) = 0$ for $\alpha = \langle \mathrm{A} \rangle = 1/\delta$, at this point, $\rho(\alpha)$ attains its maximum $\rho(\langle\alpha\rangle) = 0$. We also see that $\rho'(\alpha) = 1$ for $\alpha = 1/2\delta = \langle \mathrm{A} \rangle/2 \sim .7213$. More generally, $\rho'(\alpha) = q$ for $\alpha = 1/(q+1)\delta$, which requires $q > -1$.

3.4. The ensemble moments $\langle M^q \rangle$ and the function $\tau(q) = -\log_2\langle M^q \rangle - 1$

Since the moments of our measure are $\langle M^q \rangle = \int_0^1 x^q dx$, we have

$$\text{for } q > -1, \quad \langle M^q \rangle = 1/(q+1); \quad \text{for } q \leq -1, \quad \langle M^q \rangle = \infty.$$

We shall say that $q_{\text{bottom}} = -1$ is the *lower critical* q for this multiplier.

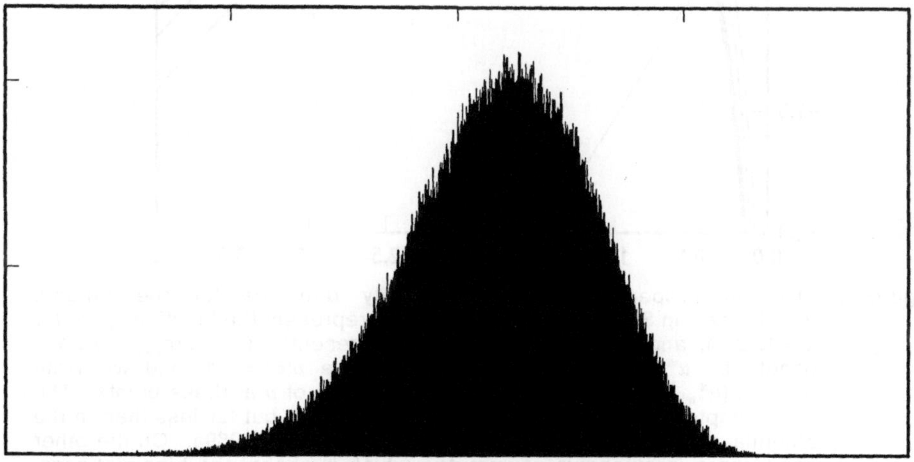

Figure 4. Sample histogram of 2^{14} values of $\mu(dt)$ (Figure 1.) The "fat tails" are non universal, and contain all the interesting information.

(This notion of criticality for M differs from the notion of criticality for Ω, which is discussed in Section 8 of Mandelbrot 1989. In particular, a critical q_{crit} can be encountered even when $\langle M^q \rangle < \infty$ for all q.)

Next, define the function $\tau(q)$ by writing the moments of the measure $\mu(dt)$ in the form

$$\langle \mu^q(dt) \rangle = \left[\langle M^q \rangle \right]^k = (dt)^{1+\tau(q)}.$$

The far reaching importance of $\tau(q)$ in the study of multifractals has first been noted in Mandelbrot 1974, where $-\tau(q)$ is denoted by $\varphi(h)$. In the present case

$$\tau(q) = -\log_2 \langle M^q \rangle - 1 = \log_2(q+1) - 1.$$

The Legendre and inverse Legendre transforms. One can verify that $\tau(q)$ and $\rho(\alpha)+1$ are related by these transforms. This is a special case of a theorem of H. Cramèr (originally published in 1936; see Deutschel and Stroock 1989; Mandelbrot 1989a contains further references). Compared to Frisch & Parisi 1983 and Halsey et al. 1986, the present context shows two new features. A) The Legendre relations are being applied in a more general setting that allows $f(\alpha) < 0$ for some α's. B) They concern $\tau(q)$ as defined on the basis of a population expectation, while the usual heuristic derivation via steepest descents concerns $\tau_{sample}(q)$, as defined on the basis of actual samples (Sections 1.5 and 4.7).

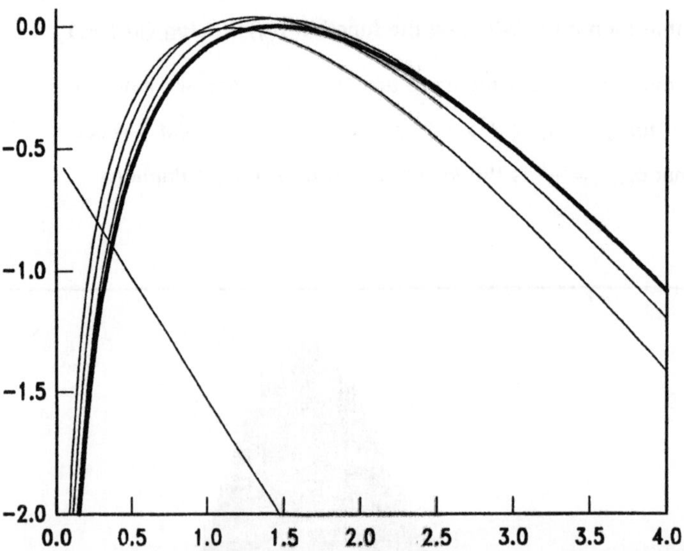

Figure 5. Plots of properly rescaled probability densities for the random multifractals in Section 3.1. The thin lines represent the functions $\rho_k(\alpha)$ for $k = 1$, 2, 4, and 16. The thicker line represents $\rho(\alpha) = \lim_{k\to\infty} \rho_k(\alpha)$. We denote by α^*_{min} and α^*_{max} the points where $\rho(\alpha) = -1$, and we write $q^*_{max} = f'(\alpha^*_{min})$ and $q^*_{min} = f'(\alpha^*_{max})$ for the slope of ρ at these points. The pre-asymptotic $\rho_k(\alpha)$ overshoots $\rho = 0$ for large k, but far less than in the binomial case illustrated by Figure 3 of Mandelbrot 1989a. On the other hand, there is extensive asymmetry, which is absent the binomial case. For example, the value that maximizes $\rho_k(\alpha)$ increases with k. This is a possible source of bias.

3.5. Negative values of $f(\alpha)$, and the distinction between *manifest* and *latent* α's and q's.

Negative values of $f(\alpha)$. The random multifractals of Section 3 satisfy $\alpha_{min} = 0$ and $\alpha_{max} = \infty$, with $f(\alpha_{min}) = -\infty$ and/or $f(\alpha_{max}) = -\infty$. In the Frisch & Parisi formalism, this possibility is not available, hence its occurrence introduces a very important theme.

A new and important distinction. In Section 1.4.2., α's such that $f(\alpha) \geq 0$ are called *manifest*, and α's such that $f(\alpha) < 0$ are called *latent*. The functions $\tau(q)$, D_q, and $f(q)$ that have been computed on the basis of manifest values of α will be called "manifest $\tau(\alpha)$ and $f(\alpha)$ and D_q" and denoted by $\tau^*(q)$, D^*_q, and $f^*(\alpha)$, the latter being simply $f(\alpha)$ with a narrower range of definition.

Crossover values from the manifest to the latent α's and q's.

$$\alpha^*_{min}, \text{ defined by } f(\alpha^*_{min}) = 0, \text{ is } \alpha^*_{min} = 0.3346.$$
$$\alpha^*_{max}, \text{ defined by } f(\alpha^*_{max}) = 0, \text{ is } \alpha^*_{max} = 3.3864.$$
$$f'(\alpha^*_{min}) = q^*_{max} = 3.310674 < \infty.$$
$$f'(\alpha^*_{max}) = q^*_{min} = -.626635 > -\infty.$$

Latent moments. The latent α's contribution to the population moments and to the functions $\tau(q)$, $\tau^*(q)$, D_q and D^*_q. When q satisfies $q^*_{min} < q < q^*_{max}$, latent α's contribute nothing to $\tau(q)$, so that $\tau^*(q) = \tau(q)$ and $D^*_q = D_q$. By the Legendre transform, the derivatives of $\tau(q)$ are the two ends of the manifest range are α^*_{max} and α^*_{min}.

However, for $q \to \infty$, $\tau^*(q) \sim q\alpha^*_{min}$, and $q \to -\infty$, $\tau^*(q) \sim q\alpha^*_{min}$. Because of the convexity properties of $\tau(q)$, this means that $\tau^*(q)$ shoots off from $\tau(q)$ along its tangents at q^*_{min} and q^*_{max} (Figure 6).

The overall shape of the graph of $\tau(q)$ is very unexpected, while the shape of the graph of $\tau^*(q)$ looks familiar to anyone acquainted, for example, with the multinomial measures. The same holds for D_q: the elimination of the latent α's replaces an extremely unexpected shape by one familiar from multinomial measures. Therefore, the estimates of $\tau(q)$ or D_q are equal to the corresponding $\tau^*(q)$ and D^*_q are truncated and biased.

4. TYPICAL HISTOGRAMS. THE SAMPLE VARIABILITY OF THE HISTOGRAMS. SUPER-SAMPLING

If $f(\alpha) = \rho(\alpha) + 1$ were necessarily an "ordinary" fractal dimension, as many authors believe, the very idea that $f(\alpha) < 0$ would be self-contradictory. This being granted, this Section shows how negative $f(\alpha)$'s express themselves. These are the first results in this area. The basic "rule" is that the role of $f(\alpha)$ is fully determined by its sign.

However (disappointingly), this rule suffers exceptions. These exceptions depend on detailed characteristics of the generating process that did not have to be pinned down up to this point, because they do not affect $\rho(\alpha)$. Thus, our findings are not final but should motivate a more detailed study of negative $f(\alpha)$'s.

4.1. Summary of Section 4. Introduction to three forms of randomness

In different calculations, we shall let randomization take either of two forms, to be called "complete." and "stratified," with an additional wrinkle.

4.1.1. *Complete randomness* (Sections 4.3 and 4.5). One can assume each dyadic splitting of an each individual cell to carry its own random M_0. (If so, each of the $M(\eta_1 \ldots \eta_k)$ of Section 3.1 depends upon all the $\eta_1 \ldots \eta_k$.)

Given $\rho(\alpha)$, the property of the resulting measure are simple in form and attractive in substance. The manifest $f(\alpha)$'s are shown to be fractal dimensions that describe a *typical* level of sampling variability of $\mu(dt)$ within a *single* sample. They can be said to define a "typical" histogram that is achieved asymptotically as $k \to \infty$. The latent $f(\alpha)$'s are shown to describe sampling variability around this typical level.

Thus, in order to obtain increasingly reliable information concerning increasingly negative $f(\alpha)$'s, the only generally valid method is to pool data from increasingly many statistically independent samples. This task makes it necessary to move up from ordinary samples to what we shall call "supersamples." They make it possible to expand the exploration of the latent portion of $f(\alpha)$ as far as desired. The interesting fact is that these diverse aspects of the sample distribution of the $\mu(dt)$ are mutually interrelated by their very fact that they are ruled by different portions of the same function $\rho(\alpha)$. Altogether, the whole range of $\rho(\alpha)$ is the proper way of characterizing a multiplicative measure.

4.1.2. *A non stratified canonical cascade* (Section 4.4). The arguments we shall present for the completely random cascade will be approximate, but we shall immediately proceed to describe relevant facts concerning a slightly different problem, whose solution suggests that the results referred to in Section 4.1.1 are exact.

4.1.3. *Stratified randomness* (Section 4.6). Unfortunately, those who expect the world to be simple, hence manageable by simple mathematics, will be disappointed. A sharp separation of the role of $f > 0$ and $f < 0$ *fails to be a universal property* because it ceases to hold when randomization is "stratified." Stratification means that M_0 is the same for all cells at the same level of the cascade, and $M(\eta_1 \ldots \eta_k)$ only depends upon the η_k corresponding to the cascade stage k. This assumption may seem artificial, but has the virtue of allowing useful exact calculations, and yields very different results for the typical histogram and sample variability.

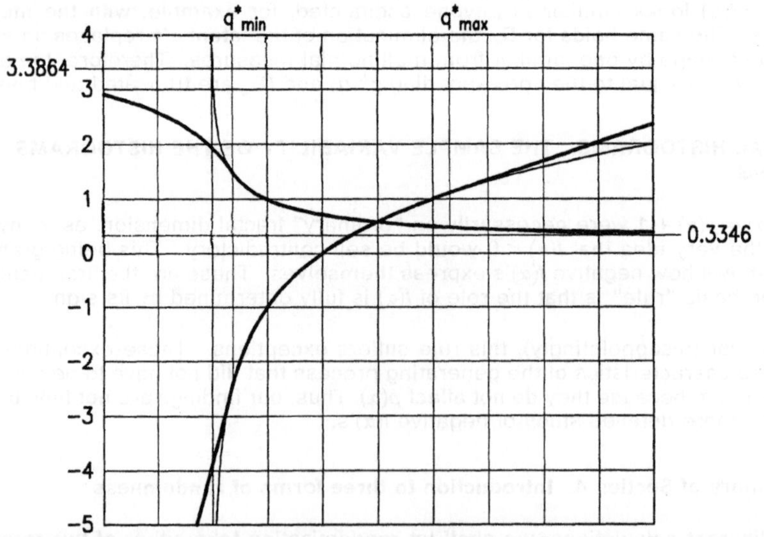

Figure 6. Full and truncated versions of $\tau(q)$ and of D_q for the random multifractal in Section 3.1. For q between q^*_{min} and q^*_{max}, the monotone increasing bold curve represents the "full" $\tau(q) = \log_2(q+1) - 1$, and the decreasing bold curve represents the "full" $D_q = \tau(q)/(q-1)$. For $q > q^*_{max}$ and for $q < q^*_{min}$, these full functions are represented by thin lines. The thick lines represent the "manifest" functions $\tau^*(q)$ and D^*_q obtained by considering the manifest α's exclusively. The manifest $\tau^*(q)$ are straight lines of the forms $\alpha^*_{max}q$ and $\alpha^*_{max}q$, tangent to the full curve $\tau(q)$.

Section 4.7 recalls that brutal estimation of $f(\alpha)$ from a sample, using the Legendre path, would yield $f(\alpha) > 0$ in all cases, therefore would hide the rich structure we now proceed to describe in detail.

While the example of Section 3 is worth keeping in mind, much of this section holds for far more general multifractals. Therefore, the arguments will be stated in terms of a general base b instead of the base $b = 2$, and of an unspecified function $\rho(\alpha)$.

4.2. The range of sampling variability of $\mu(dt)$ in purely manifest multifractals

The plainest multifractals. Let us begin with background observations that concern multifractals, such that $\alpha_{min} > 0$ and $\alpha_{max} < \infty$, and such that the construction proceeds by successive splitting of $[0, 1]$ (or any other support) into b equal parts. The characteristic examples are the binomial (Section 2.1) and the multinomial (Mandelbrot 1989a). After k stages of a construction of base b, one can observe b^k values of $\mu(dt)$, with $dt = b^{-k}$. Section 2.3 argues that it is useful to handle them as if they formed a random sample; in particular, one can draw a histogram using the rescaled doubly logarithmic coordinates α and $\rho(\alpha)$. This histogram exhausts the "sample." Therefore, the values $\alpha_{min} > 0$ and $\alpha_{max} < \infty$ are actually attained in every case, even if k is small. When dt is not of the form b^{-k}, A_{min} and A_{max} differ slightly from these absolute extrema.

Purely manifest random multifractals. Let us continue to assume that $\alpha_{min} > 0$, $\alpha_{max} < \infty$, and $f(\alpha) \geq 0$. Obviously, the sample random interval $[\mathrm{A}_{min}, \mathrm{A}_{max}]$ lies entirely within the population interval $[\mathrm{A}_{min}, \mathrm{A}_{max}]$. A full proof is not available, but there is no doubt that, for large k, the sample interval becomes effectively identical to this population interval, that is, it ceases to be subject to sample variability.

4.3. Typical behavior and variability of $\mu(dt)$ within a single sample. Even when there are latent α's, one has a "typical" first approximation determined by the positive $f(\alpha)$'s, and $\mathrm{A}_{min} = \alpha^*_{min}$ and $\mathrm{A}_{max} = \alpha^*_{max}$. But the distributions of A_{min} and A_{max} are mostly ruled by the latent portions of $f(\alpha)$

4.3.1. *The "typical" range $[\mathrm{A}_{min}, \mathrm{A}_{max}]$ when some α's are latent. Very rough evaluation, under the approximating assumption that the b^k data are statistically independent.* A single sample, if examined for $dt = b^{-k}$, yields b^k values of $\mu(dt)$. We know that they are *not* statistically independent, but it is useful to first suppose that they are.

An heuristic argument then suggests that one can estimate the probability $\Pr\{\mathrm{A} = \alpha\}$ if, and only if, the number of occurrences of this value α has the expectation at least equal to 1. This yields the condition $\Pr\{\mathrm{A} = \alpha\} b^k \geq 1$. For extremely large k, this condition reads $b^{k\rho(\alpha)+k} \geq 1$, yielding $\rho(\alpha) \geq -1$ or $f(\alpha) \geq 0$. In the notation of Section 3.5, the final result is marvelously simple: $\mathrm{A}_{min} \sim \alpha^*_{min}$ and $\mathrm{A}_{max} \sim \alpha^*_{max}$.

For moderately large k, modifications are needed: $\rho(\alpha)$ should be replaced by $\rho_k(\alpha)$ in the terminology of Section 3.3. This decreases A_{min}, making it less extreme, i.e., closer than α^*_{max} to $\langle \mathrm{A} \rangle$. But this also decreases A_{max}, making it farther than A^*_{min} from $\langle \mathrm{A} \rangle$. The discrepancy is visible on the graph.

If this were the last word, negative $f(\alpha)$'s would fail to affect observed $\mu(dt)$, and the empirical estimation of negative $f(\alpha)$'s would be impossible on the basis of the $\mu(dt)$. Very naively, it seems one could expand the sample size by simply increasing k. But of course this would not affect the range of α's, because the definition of α involves a division by $\log(dt)$. The only way out is to face negative dimensions.

4.3.2. *The typical position and the distribution of the range $[\mathrm{A}_{min}, \mathrm{A}_{max}]$ when some α's are latent. Exact derivation, under the approximating assumption that the b^k data are statistically independent.* Under this assumption, the distribution of A_{max} is classical in the theory of "extreme values" of probability theory. The inequality $\{A_{max} < \alpha\}$ holds if, and only if, b^k independent inequalities of the form $\{\mathrm{A} < \alpha\}$ hold simultaneously. Hence,

$$\Pr\{A_{max} < \alpha\} = [\Pr\{A < \alpha\}]^{b^k}.$$

The case of very large k. Now take account of a fact noted in Section 2.4 concerning the tail probability $\Pr\{\alpha > \langle A \rangle\}$. One can without harm neglect the slowly varying prefactor so that $\Pr\{A > \alpha\} \sim$ probability density $\sim b^{k\rho(\alpha)}$. One can also assimilate $\rho_k(\alpha)$ to $\rho(\alpha)$. It follows that

$$\Pr\{A_{max} > \alpha\} \sim 1 - [1 - b^{k\rho(\alpha)}]^{b^k} \sim 1 - \exp\{-b^{k[\rho(\alpha)+1]}\}.$$

Since k is large

$$\Pr\{A_{max} > \alpha\} = \begin{cases} \sim 1 & \text{when } \rho(\alpha) < -1, \text{ i.e., } \alpha < \alpha^*_{max} \\ \sim b^{k[\rho(\alpha)+1]} & \text{when } \rho(\alpha) > -1, \text{ i.e., } \alpha > \alpha^*_{max}. \end{cases}$$

A first conclusion from these relations is that, for every ε, the probability $\Pr\{|A_{max} - \alpha^*_{max}| > \varepsilon\}$ converges to 0 as $k \to \infty$. Probabilists say that $A_{max} \to \alpha^*_{max}$ "in distribution." This is a confirmation and slight sharpening of the very rough "typical range" of Section 4.4.1. But in addition, by adding that $\Pr\{A_{max} > \alpha\} \sim$ probability density $p(\alpha_{max})$, we reach the more refined conclusion that

$$\log p(\alpha_{max}) / \log dt \to \rho(\alpha) + 1.$$

That is, $\rho(\alpha) + 1$ is the $\rho(\alpha)$ function of A_{max}, to be denoted by $\rho_{max}(\alpha)$. Precisely the same argument applies to A_{min}. Overall, the graphical expression of this result is that one obtains the $\rho(\alpha)$ functions of A_{max} and A_{min} as follows: Translate the $\rho(\alpha)$ function of A *up* by unity, discard the middle portion, denote the portion to the right as $\rho_{max}(\alpha)$ and assign it to A_{max}, denote the position to the left as $\rho_{min}(\alpha)$ and assign it to A_{min} (The $\tau(q)$ functions of corresponding to the limits of $\Pr\{A_{min} > \alpha\}$ and $\Pr\{A_{max} < \alpha\}$ are not continuous).

Corrections for moderately large k. One should not neglect the slowly varying prefactor of Section 2.4., and one should not hasten to assimilate $\rho_k(\alpha)$ to $\rho(\alpha)$.

4.4. A canonical completely random cascade, and reasons to expect the results of Section 4.3 to be exact. Branching Brownian motions and Kolmogorov-Fisher waves

A rigorous treatment of the distribution of A_{max} is not available for the multifractals of Section 3.1. But it happens that a closely related problem has been fully investigated in the literature, and yields precisely the same result. This related problem involves a variant multifractal generating cascade that is interesting on its own rights.

The most sensitive novel feature is that the multipliers M_0 and M_1 within each cell cease to be constrained to add to 1, and are made independent. Therefore the addends $-\log M_0$ and $-\log M_1$ become independent. The original cascade of Section 3.1 is called *conservative* in Mandelbrot 1988, 1989a (*microcanonical* in the terminology of Mandelbrot 1974). The variant cascade is called *canonical.*

It is easy to see that replacing conservative randomness by canonical randomness changes $\mu(dt)$, but leaves $\rho(\alpha)$ unchanged. This is one of many ways in which $\rho(\alpha)$ determines $\mu(dt)$ incompletely. (A more interesting example will be examined in Section 4.6). On the other hand we believe that the change from conservative to canonical leaves the distribution of A_{max} and A_{min} is the same.

A second novelty involves the instants when a cell splits and its mass is distributed between two subcells. Section 3.1 assumes that the time spans between successive splittings are equal to 1 on the scale of k's. But one can also assume these spans to be exponentially distributed. This change brings a touch of realism, together with some complication, and the resulting model deserves study. But our calculations suggest very strongly that the distribution of A_{max} and A_{min} is unaffected.

A third innovation is that one assumes that the variables $-\log M_0$ and $-\log M_1$ are Gaussian. The resulting problem was posed in McKean 1975, where it is shown that the solution reduces to that of a traveling wave equation that A.N. Kolmogorov and R.A. Fisher has encountered in genetics in 1937. Bramson 1978, 1983 reexamines the issue, and finds that the very large k heuristic (Sections 4.3.1 and 4.3.2) is correct to first order in α. Additional logarithmic terms are present, but they only affect the correction one needs for large but finite k.

Between our problem and the Kolmogorov-Fisher waves, the most critical difference concerns the replacement of conservation by canonicity. We have already mentioned our belief that this does not affect A_{max}, *at least* to the first order. If this belief is disproved, the relative importance of the canonical model will increase.

Query to mathematicians. The equation underlying our cascade differs from the Kolmogorov-Fisher equation, and deserves attention.

4.5. The notion of "supersample" made of an increasing number $N = b^{k(N-1)}$ of independent samples of a random measure $\mu(dt)$. As the supersample size N grows, the variability of the range $[\mathrm{A}_{min}(E), \mathrm{A}_{max}(E)]$ is controlled by increasingly latent portions of $f(\alpha)$

Section 4.3 was concerned with squeezing information about $f(\alpha)$ from a single sample of our multifractal measure. Now we shall examine what is gained if we can pool data from many statistically independent samples, so as to increase the sample size from b^k to a larger value and create a "supersample."

4.5.1. *A good reason for writing the number of independent samples as $N = b^{(E-1)k}$, hence the supersample size as b^{Ek}.* The notation is meant to suggest that one thinks of E as an embedding dimension. After the fact, this notation will be justified after we show that the effectiveness of supersampling turns out to be measured by the value of $E = 1 + (1/k)\log_b N$. We shall indeed show that, in order to achieve a given desired "supersampling effect" E, any increase in the number of pieces b^k within each sample should be accompanied by an increase in the number $N = b^{(E-1)k}$ of distinct samples.

In terms of original motivation, our notation E is due to awareness of the fact that negative $f(\alpha)$'s can also have another, logically distinct cause. Indeed, as shown in Mandelbrot 1989b and in Section 8 of Mandelbrot 1989a, random multifractals with latent α's may also appear in random low-dimensional cuts through a higher-dimensional measure that need not be random and can be completely conventional. "Generically," one should expect the overall original measure to include cells of higher or lower measure, "hotter" or "colder", than the hottest or coldest cells along the 1-dimensional cut. Therefore, a natural way of extending the range of observable α's is to consider the original measure in its original imbedding space, or at least through higher-dimensional cuts. In the present paper, we do not deal with a random cut, nevertheless supersampling amounts to investigating our measure "as if" it were not expressed along $[0, 1]$, but across a cube in a space of dimension E.

We proceed with the same approximations and exact arguments as in Section 4.2.

4.5.2. *An estimate of the range of variability of $[\mathrm{A}_{min}(E), \mathrm{A}_{max}(E)]$ within a supersample. Very rough evaluation under the assumption that the b^{KE} data are statistically independent.* Define $\mathrm{A}_{max}(E)$ as the largest value of in a sample of size $N = b^{E-1}$. The very rough argument already used in Section 4.2 now suggests that it may be possible to estimate $\Pr\{\mathrm{A}_{max}(E) = \alpha\}$ if, and only if, $\Pr\{\mathrm{A} = \alpha\} b^{Ek} \geq 1$, that is, $b^{k\rho(\alpha)+kE} \geq 1$. Hence $\rho(\alpha)$ can be estimated on the condition that $\rho(\alpha) \geq -E$. This condition, much weaker than $\rho(\alpha) \geq -1$, is satisfied in an interval to be denoted by $[\alpha^*_{min}(E), \alpha^*_{max}(E)]$. Thus, an increase in the sample size allows, in addition to the α's such that $f(\alpha) \geq 0$, to estimate all $f(\alpha)$'s such that $-E + 1 \leq f(\alpha) < 0$.

4.5.3. *Distribution of the range $[\mathrm{A}_{min}(E), \mathrm{A}_{max}(E)]$ under the assumption that the b^{Ek} values in our sample are statistically independent.* By the argument in Section 4.2,

$$\Pr\{A_{max}(E) > \alpha\} \sim 1 - [1 - b^{k\rho(\alpha)}]^{Nb^k} \sim 1 - \exp\{-b^{k[\rho(\alpha)+E]}\}.$$

As $k \to \infty$, we obtain the result that

$$\Pr\{A_{max}(E) > \alpha\} = \begin{cases} \sim 1 & \text{when } \rho(\alpha) > -E, \text{ i.e., } \alpha < \alpha^*_{max}(E) \\ \sim b^{k[\rho(\alpha)+E]} & \text{when } \rho(\alpha) < -E, \text{ i.e., } \alpha > \alpha^*_{max}(E) \end{cases}$$

The same rule applies to $A_{min}(E)$.

4.6. The ranges $[A_{min}, A_{max}]$ and $[A_{min}(E), A_{max}(E)]$ when randomness is stratified

Before we get carried away by the simplicity of the conclusion of Sections 4.3 and 4.4, let us show that this domain of validity fails to include the multifractals characterized by the same function $\rho(\alpha)$, but stratified randomness.

4.6.1. *A step by step procedure to identify exactly the interval dt that yields α_{min} (resp., α_{max}).* It suffices at each dyadic subdivision to follow the half that is assigned the larger mass, namely the half for which $M > 1/2$, so that $-\log M < 1$ (resp., the smaller mass, for which $-\log_2 M > 1$). It follows that the random variable $\max\{-\log_2 M_0, -\log_2 M_1\}$ is simply identical in distribution to $1 + \log_2 M_0$, and is exponentially distributed. Hence, the random variable A_{max} has precisely the same distribution as $1 + A$. To obtain the curve of $\rho_{max}(\alpha)$, it suffices to translate the $\rho(\alpha)$ curve of Section 3.4 to the right by 1. The translated $\rho_{max}(\alpha)$ lies entirely to the right of $\alpha = 1$.

As to the random variable $\min\{-\log_2 M_0, -\log_2 M_1\}$, it is an exponential truncated to $[0, 1]$. The A_{min} being the average of k such variables, one has $0 \leq \alpha_{min} \leq 1$, so that the graph of $f_{min}(\alpha)$ lies entirely between $\alpha = 0$ and $\alpha = 1$. It is conveniently separated from the graph of $f_{max}(\alpha)$. Its exact form hardly matters, but it could easily be obtained using algebra that will become familiar in Section 5.

4.6.2. *Typical values and fluctuations.* One conclusion is that, as $k \to \infty$, both α_{max} and α_{min} converge almost surely to their expectations. $A_{max} \to \langle A \rangle + 1 = 2.4426$, which is smaller than the estimate under the assumption of independence, namely $\alpha^*_{max} = 3.3864$. Similarly, $A_{min} \to -1 + 1/\log_e 2 = .4426$, which is larger than the estimate under the assumption of independence, namely $\alpha^*_{min} = .3346$. Of course, we know that, in the multifractal context, neither behavior denies the extreme variability of A^*_{max} and A_{min} that is characterized by $f_{max}(\alpha)$ and $f_{min}(\alpha)$.

4.6.3. *When randomization is stratified, there is a strong negative interdependence between A_{min} and A_{max}.* Suppose a big sampling fluctuation occurs at *any stage of the cascade.* This occurrence will multiply half of the sample by a small factor, the other half being multiplied by a factor close to 1. This means that an extreme value of M_0 at any one cascade stage will suffice to create extreme values of both A_{min} and A_{max}.

Let a sample be called "typical" if no small M_0 is encountered at any stage. If so, replacing any M_0 by a very small value would have as effect to split the typical histogram into two halves, one of which is translated a little towards smaller α's and the second is translated substantially towards larger α's. Therefore, a single extreme value is sufficient to broaden the histogram of α's along the α scale. This variability and this negative interdependence occur because of very small M_0's, hence occur because of the presence of latent tails.

4.6.4. *Exact distribution of the range $[A_{min}(E), A_{max}(E)]$ when randomization is stratified.* We deal with the largest of $b^{(E-1)k}$ statistically independent quantities $A_{max}(1)$, each of which we know to be of the form $A + 1$. The already twice-used extreme values argument yields

$$\Pr\{A_{max}(E) > \alpha\} = 1 - [1 - b^{k\rho(\alpha-1)}]^N \sim 1 - \exp[-Nb^{k\rho(\alpha-1)}]$$
$$= 1 - \exp\{-b^{k[\rho(\alpha)+E-1]}\}.$$

$$\langle M^q \rangle = \frac{(1-\varepsilon)^{q+1} - \varepsilon^{q+1}}{(1-2\varepsilon)(q+1)}; \tau(q) = -1 + \log_2(1-2\varepsilon) + \log_2|q+1| - \log_2|(1-\varepsilon)^{q+1} - \varepsilon^{q+1}|.$$

The two non constant logarithmic terms of $\tau(q)$ are singular at $q=-1$, but their difference is a smooth monotone function. So is the graph of D_q. Furthermore,

$$\max D_q = -\log_2(1-\varepsilon) = \alpha_{\max}, \text{ and } \min D_q = -\log_2\varepsilon = \alpha_{\min}.$$

These last two features of D_q are formally the same as in the standard binomial case, except that m_0 has been replaced by ε.

As to the graph of $f(\alpha)$, its parametric representation in terms of q is

$$\alpha(q) = \frac{1}{q+1} - \frac{(1-\varepsilon)^{q+1}\log(1-\varepsilon) - \varepsilon^{q+1}\log\varepsilon}{(1-\varepsilon)^{q+1} - \varepsilon^{q+1}}$$

$$f(q) = q\alpha(q) + 1 - \log_2(1-2\varepsilon) - \log_2|q+1| + \log_2|(1-\varepsilon)^{q+1} - \varepsilon^{q+1}|.$$

The resulting $f(\alpha)$ has the conventional feature of being contained between the vertical lines with the abscissas $\alpha_{\min} > 0$ and $\alpha_{\max} < \infty$. Furthermore, the manifest "bell" is fairly conventional also, the more so as ε is increased, especially if one does not pay attention to the slopes at $\alpha^*_{\min}$ and $\alpha^*_{\max}$. For $\varepsilon = .1$ or $\varepsilon = .2$, the bell is clearly asymmetric, and certainly could not be $f(\alpha)$ of a binomial. But for $\varepsilon \geq .3$, the bell is effectively symmetric. For $\varepsilon = .45$, it should prove hard to tell such a measure from the $f(\alpha)$ of a binomial measure. But the latent tails, present in our measure, are absent from the binomial.

The difference between the case of small ε and $\varepsilon = 0$ (Section 3) draws special comment. The manifest $f(\alpha)$'s are indistinguishable. But sample variability i.e., to the extent of apparent non stationarity, is greater for $\varepsilon = 0$ than for ε small. This difference is determined by the latent portions of $f(\alpha)$.

5.2. Base 2 with a non uniform distribution of the multiplier

Our first step is to change the probability density of m_0 from being uniform to be equal to

$$\frac{\Gamma(2\eta+2)}{[\Gamma(\eta+1)]^2} m^\eta (1-m)^\eta,$$

where the exponent η satisfies $\eta \neq 0$. This η need not be an integer, and the only restriction is $\eta > -1$. In comparison with the preceding section, the values of m_0 and m_1 tend to be even more unequal when $\eta < 0$, and to be less unequal when $\eta > 0$.

$$\langle M^q \rangle = \frac{\Gamma(2\eta+2)}{[\Gamma(\eta+1)]^2} \int_0^1 m^{\eta+q}(1-m)^\eta dm = \frac{\Gamma(2\eta+2)}{\Gamma(\eta+1)} \frac{\Gamma(\eta+q+1)}{\Gamma(2\eta+q+2)}$$

As usual, $\tau(q) = -1 - \log_2\langle M^q \rangle$. Hence, $q_{\text{bottom}} = -1 - \eta$. This q_{bottom} is still negative, but can be as close to 0 as desired. We obtain $f(\alpha)$ through Cramèr's Legendre path, as $f(\alpha) = \min_q[q\alpha - \tau(q)]$. The minimum occurs when $\alpha = \alpha(q)$, with

$$\alpha(q)\delta = (\Gamma'/\Gamma)(\eta+q+1) - (\Gamma'/\Gamma)(2\eta+q+2),$$

where (Γ'/Γ) denotes the derivative of $\log\Gamma(x)$.

The next step is to take q a parameter, and to write $\alpha(q) = \tau'(q)$ and $f(\alpha) = q\alpha(q) - \tau(q)$, so that both α and f are functions of the parameter q. This procedure is nicely expressed in the important thermodynamic interpretation of the Legendre formalism, in which $1/q \sim$ temperature, $\alpha \sim$ energy, and for entropy. Indeed, we obtain entropy as function of energy by using temperature as parameter. (The simplest of many ways of introducing the thermodynamical interpretation is given in Mandelbrot 1989a.)

When $\eta = 1$, one can write $\tau(q)$ and $f(\alpha)$ in elementary closed form. The lower critical q is -2, and the ratio M_1/M_0 has infinite moments of order $q \leq -2$.

5.3. Limit cases of Section 5.2 for $\eta \to -1$ and $\eta \to \infty$

A virtue of the generalization in Section 5.1 is that it provides a one-parameter interpolation between two interesting limits. For $\eta \to \infty$, one has the non random uniform measure on $[0, 1]$. For η very close to -1, M can be either 0 or 1. Since we work in the base $b = 2$, this means that the limit measure concentrate in one randomly chosen point of $[0, 1]$.

A scaling property valid for $\eta \to -1$. Write $\varepsilon = 1 + \eta$. When ε is very small, $D_1 = \alpha(1)$ is also very small. Indeed, one can apply near 0 the standard Gamma function approximations $\Gamma(z) \sim 1/x$ and $(\Gamma'/\Gamma)(x) \sim 1/\alpha$, obtaining $\alpha(1)\delta = \varepsilon$. All values $q > 1$ occur in a portion of $f(\alpha)$ that rises very sharply from the point of coordinates 0 and $-\infty$ to the point of coordinates $\alpha(1)$ and $\alpha(1)$, very close to the origin. Similarly, $f(\alpha)$ is positive but very small from $\alpha \sim \varepsilon$ until α approaches the value where $f(\alpha) = 1$, which is $\alpha(0) = \langle\alpha\rangle = 1/2\varepsilon\delta$. Except near $\alpha = 0$, $|q| < \varepsilon$ except for $\alpha < 2\alpha^*_{\min}$. Replotting $f(\alpha)$ in terms of $\alpha^* = \alpha/\varepsilon$ and $q^* = q/\varepsilon$ yields

$$\alpha^*(q^*)\delta = \frac{1}{1+q^*} - \frac{1}{2+q^*}; \quad f^*(\alpha^*) = q^*\alpha^*(q^*) + \log_2(2+q^*) - \log_2(1+q^*)$$

Extrapolating the limit distribution to $q^* \to \infty$, yields

$$\alpha^* \sim 1/\delta q^{*2} \text{ and } f^* \sim 1/\delta q^*, \text{ hence } f^*(\alpha^*) \sim \sqrt{\delta\alpha^*}.$$

For $\eta \to \infty$, *the convergence of our measure to Lebesgue measure is extremely slow.* For example, write $m = 1/2 + \varepsilon$ and consider the quantity $[4m(1-m)]^\eta = [(1-4\varepsilon^2)]^\eta$. Its graph is bell-shaped, and the width of its bell can be defined as the value of ε where it reduces to e^{-1}. This happens when $\exp(-4\varepsilon^2\eta) = e^{-1}$, that is, for $\varepsilon = 1/2\sqrt{\eta}$. This width decreases slowly as $\eta \to \infty$. The slowness of this convergence means that a variable m_0 may be modelled by a random M_0 with a suitable η.

5.4. Base $b = 2$ with a different non uniform distribution for the multiplier

To obtain a family of measures that ranges up to the non degenerate binomial, it suffices to start with a multiplier M^*_0 having the density M_0

$$\frac{\Gamma(\eta+\theta+2)}{\Gamma(\eta+1)\Gamma(\theta+1)} m^\eta(1-m)^\theta.$$

The maximum of μ^*_0 occurs for $\eta/m = \theta/(1-m)$. Then we introduce a multiplier M_0 that is equal to either M^*_0, or $1 - M^*_0$, with equal probabilities. Everything is derived from

$$\langle M^q\rangle = \frac{\Gamma(\eta+\theta+2)}{2}\left[\frac{\Gamma(\eta+q+1)}{\Gamma(\eta+1)} + \frac{\Gamma(\theta+q+1)}{\Gamma(\theta+1)}\right]\frac{1}{\Gamma(\eta+\theta+q+2)}.$$

5.5. Base $b > 2$

To construct a multinomial measure of base $b > 2$, we require b masses m_β $(0 \leq \beta \leq b-1)$. Denote by Φ the point whose coordinates are the frequencies φ_β of the digits β in the base-b development $0.\eta_1\eta_2 \ldots \eta_k$. Every b-adic interval characterized by Φ contains the measure $\prod m_\beta^{k\varphi_\beta}$.

The "1974 multifractals" introduced in Mandelbrot 1974 allow a multiplier M that is not limited to the finite collection of prescribed m_β's, but may be a more general random variable > 0. The multiplier relative to the cell indexed by β $(0 \leq \beta \leq b-1)$ will be denoted by M_β.

The simpler of two kinds of 1974 multifractals assume that mass is conserved while it is spread around within a cell. This leads to the strong "conservation" rule that at every cascade stage, our b random multipliers M_β must satisfy $\sum M_\beta = 1$. To create a useful geometric intuition of these rules, consider the b-dimensional representative point $\mathcal{M}$ whose coordinates are M_β. This random point $\mathcal{M}$ is restricted to lie in an "admissible domain" that is the portion of b-dimensional space defined by $M_\beta \geq 0$ and $\sum M_\beta = 1$.

This section assumes that our point is uniformly distributed on this admissible domain. This distribution is symmetric, which implies that coordinates M_β have the same distribution for every β. Clearly, $0 \leq M \leq 1$ and $\Pr\{M > m\} = (1-m)^{b-1}$. Hence,

$$\langle M^q \rangle = (b-1)\int_0^1 x^q(1-x)^{b-2}dx = \frac{\Gamma(q+1)\Gamma(b)}{\Gamma(q+b)} = \frac{(b-1)!}{(q+1)(q+2)\ldots(q+b-1)}.$$

The dependence of $\langle M^q \rangle$ upon q is very much like in Section 5.2, but simpler, because here b is an integer. Again, $q_{\text{bottom}} - 1$. In particular, $\langle M \rangle = 1/b$.

5.6. A combined generalization

In the case $b > 2$, the representative point $\mathcal{M}$, instead of being uniformly distributed in its admissible domain, can be given a density proportional to $m_0^\gamma m_1^\gamma m_2 \ldots m_{b-1}^\gamma$.

6. A MULTIPLICATIVE CASCADE, AND A SIMPLE "TRIO" MULTIFRACTAL

This very brief section is added for its intrinsic interest, and also to insure that Mandelbrot 1989c can be considered a summary of this paper. Figure 7 is not quite the same as Figure 1 of that summary.

Construction. Let a cascade begin with mass equal to 1, uniformly spread over $[0, 1]$, and let the k-th cascade stage share the mass in a cell of length b^{-k} between two halves of length b^{-k-1} in either of 3 ways: half and half; in the ratios m_0 and $m_1 = 1 - m_0$ with $m_0 \geq 1/2$, or in the ratios m_1 and m_0. This multiplies the mass in either half by a random variable M that is m_0, $1/2$, or $m_1 = 1 - m_0$, with the respective probabilities

$$\Pr\{M = m_0\} = 1/8, \quad \Pr\{M = 1/2\} = 6/8, \quad \text{and } \Pr\{M = m_1\} = 1/8.$$

By a repetition of this scheme, the dyadic cell $[dt]$ of length $dt = 2^{-k}$ that starts at $t = 0.\eta_1\eta_2\ldots\eta_k$ determines k identically distributed and independent random multiplier variables M, and one has

$$\mu_1(dt) = M(\eta_1)M(\eta_1, \eta_2)\ldots M(\eta_1, \ldots \eta_k)$$
$$\mathrm{A}_k = \log \mu_1(dt)/\log dt = -(1/k)[\log_2 M(\eta_1) + \log_2 M(\eta_1, \eta_2)\ldots].$$

To know $\mu_1(dt)$ is to know for all k the probability density $p_k(\alpha)$ of A_k.

The main finding, again, is that

$$\rho_k(\alpha) = (1/k)\log_2 p_k(\alpha) \text{ converges for large } k \text{ to}$$
$$\rho(\alpha) = -1 + \text{ the Legendre transform of } \tau(q) = -\log_2\langle M^q \rangle - 1.$$

The proof uses Cramèr's theorem. Again, $f_1(\alpha) < 0$ is traced to our having defined $\tau(q)$ through the expectation $\langle M^q \rangle$, instead of the usual "partition function" $\sum \mu_1^q(dt)$.

The resulting $\rho(\alpha)$ is drawn on Figure 7. First remark: α ranges from $\alpha_{\min} = -\log_2 m_0$ to $\alpha_{\max} = -\log_2 m_1$, which is a familiar feature in binomial measures. Second feature: $f_1(\alpha)$ ranges from -2 to 1, which brings in the striking novelty that $f_1(\alpha)$ is negative for $\alpha^*_{\max} < \alpha \leq \alpha_{\max}$ and $\alpha_{\min} \leq \alpha < \alpha^*_{\min}$.

Imbedding the trio measure as a one dimensional cut through a "conventional" multinomial measure in 3d space. Now consider the following cascade on a cube subdivided into $2^3 = 8$ cubes. Each cascade stage begins with the mass m; the share of a randomly picked "hot" cube is $mm_0/8$, and the share of a randomly picked "cold" cube is $mm_1/8$ and the share of each of the 6 remaining cubes is $m/8$. This construction leads to a multinomial spatial multifractal $\mu_3(d\mathbf{x})$. The Legendre formalism enters (in the familiar Frisch-Parisi interpretation to yield $f_3(\alpha) = \rho(\alpha) - 3 = f_1(\alpha) + 2$.

Embedding the trio measure in 4d space. Since $2^4 = 16$, our cascade divides a mass of m between 16 cubes: two hot ones receive $mm_0/16$, and two cold cubes receive $mm_1/16$, while the 12 remaining cubes receive $m/16$. The Legendre formalism yields $f_4(\alpha) = \rho(\alpha) - 4 = f_1(\alpha) + 3$.

Conclusion. The function $\rho(\alpha) = f_E(\alpha) - E$ is the same for $E = 1$ and $E = 3$, and ranges from -3 to 0. Furthermore, α itself depends on E, but $\alpha - E$ does not.

The conventional interpretation of $f_1(\alpha)$. It is known that $f_3(\alpha)$ is the fractal dimension of the 3d set where the Hölder exponent of $\mu_3(d\mathbf{x})$ is α. Applying the intersection rule with its exception (Section 2) to multifractals, the positive values of $f_3(\alpha) - 2$ are the dimensions of the sets where the Hölder α of $\mu_1(dt)$ is α. The negative $f_3(\alpha) - 2$ are simply brought to 0. We claim that this is a waste of valuable information.

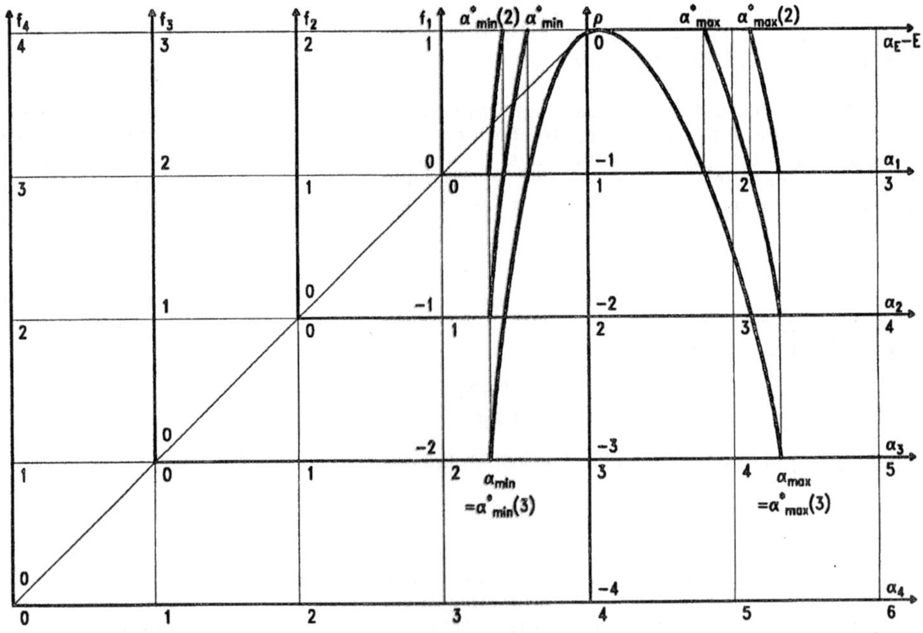

Figure 7. Illustration of the trio measures defined in Section 6, with $m_0 = .2$. To make it possible for a single "ogive" (bold curve) to represent simultaneously the four functions $\rho(\alpha)$, $f_1(\alpha)$, $f_2(\alpha)$, $f_3(\alpha)$ and $f_4(\alpha)$, four distinct sets of coordinate axes have been drawn (bold lines). The additional bold curves to the right (resp., to the left) of the ogive relate to the distributions of $A_{max}(2)$, $A_{max}(3)$, and $A_{max}(4)$ (resp., of $A_{min}(2)$, $A_{min}(3)$, and $A_{min}(4)$), as defined in the text. The value of α^*_{max} is a gross underestimate of α_{max}.

References

Blumenfeld, R. and Aharony, A. 1989. Breakdown of multifractal behavior in diffusion limited aggregates. *Phys. Rev. Lett.* **62**, 2977-2980.

Bramson, M. D. 1978. Maximal displacement of branching Brownian motions. *Communication of Pure and Applied Mathematics* **31**, 531-581.

Bramson, M. D. 1983. Convergence of solutions of the Kolmogorov equation to travelling waves. *Memoirs of the American Mathematical Society* **44**, No. 285.

Cates M.E. and Deutsch, J.M. 1987. Spatial correlations in multifractals. *Phys. Rev. A* **35**, 4907.

Chhabra, A., and Jensen, R.V. 1989. Direct determination of the $f(\alpha)$ singularity spectrum. *Phys. Rev. Lett.* **62**, 1327.

Deutschel, J.D. and Stroock D.W. 1989. *Large Deviations*. New York: Academic Press.

Fourcade, B., Breton, P. and Tremblay, A.-M.S. 1987. Multifractals and critical phenomena in percolating networks: Fixed point, gap scaling and universality. *Phys. Rev. B* **36**, 8925.

Fourcade, B. and Tremblay, A.-M.S. 1987. Anomalies in the multifractal analysis of self-similar resistor networks. *Phys. Rev. A* **36**, 2352.

Frisch, U. and Parisi, G. 1985. Fully developed turbulence and intermittency in *Turbulence and Predictability in Geophysical Fluid Dynamics and Climate Dynamics*, International School of Physics "Enrico Fermi," Course 88, edited by M. Ghil. North-Holland, Amsterdam, p 84.

Halsey, T.C., Jensen, M.H., Kadanoff, L.P., Procaccia, I. and Shraiman, B.I. 1986. Fractal measure and their singularities: The characterization of strange sets. *Phys. Rev. A* **33**, 1141.

Hentschel, H.G.E. and Procaccia, I. 1983. The infinite number of generalized dimensions of fractals and strang attractors. *Physica (Utrecht)* **8D**, 435.

Mandelbrot, B.B. 1974. Intermittent turbulence in self-similar cascades; divergence of high moments and dimension of the carrier. *J. Fluid Mech.* **62**, 331; also *Comptes Rendus* **278A**, 289, 355.

Mandelbrot, B.B. 1982. *The Fractal Geometry of Nature*. New York: W.H. Freeman.

Mandelbrot, B.B. 1984. Fractals in physics: squig clusters, diffusions, fractal measures and the unicity of fractal dimension. *J. Stat. Phys.* **34**, 895.

Mandelbrot, B.B. 1988 An introduction to multifractal distribution functions, in *Fluctuations and Pattern Formation* (Cargèse, 1988). H.E. Stanley and N. Ostrowsky, Dordrecht-Boston: Kluwer, 1988, 345-360.
NOTE: This paper is entirely superseded by Mandelbrot 1989b. In particular, the treatment of Section 3.5 is impossibly hasty and contains an error; most of its material is presented better and more accurately in Mandelbrot 1989b and the present text.

Mandelbrot, B.B. 1989a. Multifractal measures, especially for the geophysicist. *Pure and Applied Geophysics* **131**, nos. 1/2.
NOTE: The treatment of α_H in Section 8 of this paper is in error, and Figure 5 is incomplete. Updated presentations are given in Mandelbrot 1989b, which the reader is advised to study before Section 8 of Mandelbrot 1989a.

Mandelbrot, B.B. 1989b. Limit lognormal multifractal measures, in: *Frontiers of Physics: Landau Memorial conference* (Tel Aviv, 1988). Edited by Errol Gotsman, New York: Pergamon.

Mandelbrot, B.B. 1989c. Negative fractal dimensions and multifractals, in: *Proceedings of Stat Phys 17*. Edited by Constantino Tsallis. *Physica A*.

Mandelbrot, B.B. (forthcoming). *Fractals and Multifractals: Noise, Turbulence and Galaxies* (Selecta, Vol. 1). New York: Springer.

McKean, H. P. 1975. Application of Brownian motion to the equation of Kolmogorov-Petrovskii-Piskunov. *Communication of Pure and Applied Mathematics*, **28**, 323

Meneveau, C. and Sreenivasan, K.R. 1987. Simple multifractal cascade model for fully developed turbulence. *Phys. Rev. Lett.* **59**, 1424.

Meneveau, C. and Sreenivasan, K.R. 1989. Measurement of $f(\alpha)$ from scaling of histograms, and applications to dynamic systems and fully developed turbulence. *Physics Letters A* **137**, 103-112.

Prasad R.R., Meneveau, C. and Sreenivasan, K.R. 1988. Multifractal nature of the dissipation field of passive scalars in fully turbulent flaws. *Phys. Rev. Lett.* **61**, 74.

SOME ASPECTS OF THE FRACTAL APPROACH TO THE FULLY DEVELOPED TURBULENCE

Angelo Vulpiani

INFN Sezione di Roma and GNSM-CISM Unità di Roma
also Dipartimento di Fisica, Università de L'Aquila
Piazza dell'Annunziata 1, 67100 L'Aquila

TO THE MEMORY OF MY FATHER

1. BASIC CONCEPTS

It is well known that at low Reynolds numbers (R_e) an incompressible fluid behaves in a laminar way (i.e. roughly speaking the evolution is regular and stable). On the contrary, at very large Reynolds numbers there is a highly chaotic and irregular behaviour. The regime $R_e \gg R_{crit}$ is called fully developed turbulence, where R_{crit} is the value of R_e at which the onset of turbulence appears i.e. there is a transition from laminar to chaotic flow. We underline that for R_e slighly larger than R_{crit} there are often only temporal chaos and highly spatial coherent structures. In the limit $R_e \gg R_{crit}$ the chaotic behaviour involves

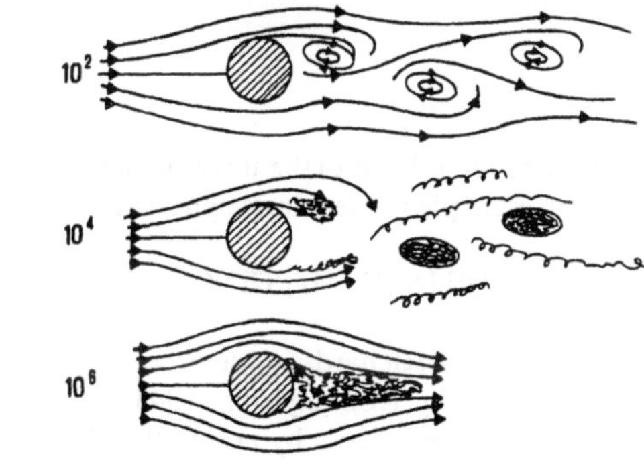

Fig. 1. Schematic pictures of the behaviour of a fluid around a cylinder at different Reynolds numbers.

Fractals' Physical Origin and Properties
Edited by L. Pietronero
Plenum Press, New York

fluctuations on a so small scale of space and time that it seems possible only a description in terms of the statistical properties of the flow. An idea of the increasing chaos with R_e is given by Fig.1.

In this paper we treat just the eulerian aspect of the turbulence (i.e. the chaotic behaviour of the eulerian velocity field) and we do not discuss the lagrangian turbulence (i.e. the chaotic motion of particles in the fluid). Let us recall that one can have chaotic motion of particles also without the eulerian turbulence (see Henon 1966 and Falcioni et al. 1988).

In principle one could build up the statistical mechanics of turbulence on the basis of the Navier-Stokes (N-S) equations:

$$\begin{cases} \partial_t \underline{u} + (\underline{u} \cdot \underline{\nabla})\underline{u} = - 1/\rho \, \underline{\nabla}\, p + \nu \, \Delta \, \underline{u} + \underline{f} \\ \underline{\nabla} \cdot \underline{u} = 0 \quad + \text{ initial and boundaries conditions} \end{cases} \tag{1.1}$$

where $\underline{u}$ is the velocity field, ρ the density, p the pressure, ν the kinetic viscosity and $\underline{f}$ an external force. Unfortunately, each analytical theory of turbulence, i.e. an approach which makes use of eq. (1.1), unavoidably encounters closure problems.

These difficulties are typical of all nonlinear equations. An analogous situation is present in the gas kinetic theory with the B-B-G-K-Y hierarchy (see Huang 1987). We do not consider here these approachs (for a general reference see Leslie 1973). However, an approximate understanding of a large number of statistical properties (at least on small scales) does not require a direct use of the N-S equations since the identification of the fundamental physical mechanism is sufficient.

Richardson (1922 and 1926) was the first who put forward some penetrating ideas on the physical mechanism acting at large R_e. In his assumption the fully developed turbulence consists essentially in a hierarchy of "eddies" (i.e. turbulent structures or disturbances) on different scales. Eddies of a certain scale are the result of the unstability of eddies at a larger scale, and in their own turn, they generate smalle eddies by their unstability. One has, in this scenario, a <u>cascade process</u> of eddy breaking-down in which there is a transmission of energy of the overall flow to motions of smaller and smaller eddies up to the smallest scale η where the fragmentation process is stopped by dissipation.

This physical picture is nicely expressed in the following rhyme (page 66 of Richardson 1922):

Big whorls have little whorls;
Which feed on their velocity:
And little whorls have lesser whorls:
And so on to viscosity
(In the molecular sense).

Let us recall that these considerations are related to the three dimensional case since in the bidimensional situations a quite different phenomenology appears as discussed in section 5.

2. KOLMOGOROV THEORY AND THE INTERMITTENCY PROBLEM

The qualitative and general ideas of Richardson have been further developed and formulated in a more precise language by Kolmogorov (1941). Kolmogorov made an addition to the assumptions on the cascade process by noting that, because of the chaotic nature of the enery transfer among the eddies, the orienting effect of the mean flow must be weakened with each breaking down. Consequently it is natural to expect that at spatial scales much smaller than the external length (i.e. the typical length of the mean flow) and time scales much smaller than the typical time of the mean flow, the velocity fluctuations are homogeneous, isotropic and quasi-steady. At sufficiently small-scale the turbulence is thus characterized by the mean flux of energy $\bar{\varepsilon}$ (from the overall flow to the smallest eddies) and by the dissipation. Moreover, if the scale length is not too small it is natural to assume that the viscosity play no role, because the dissipation term in the N-S equations is negligible.

In a more quantitative way Kolmogorov formulated the two following hypotheses:

1) The statistical properties of the velocity difference $\Delta\underline{V}(\underline{r}) = \underline{u}(\underline{x}+\underline{r}) - \underline{u}(\underline{x})$ are universal isotropic function only of r, ν and $\bar{\varepsilon}$, in the case $r \ll L$.
2) If $L \gg r \gg \eta$ (the so-called inertial range) these statistical properties are independent of ν.

The two hypotheses lead immediately, by dimensional analysis, to an explicit form for the moments of $|\Delta\underline{V}(\underline{r})|$ for r in the inertial range:

$$< |\Delta\underline{V}(\underline{r})|^p > \sim (\bar{\varepsilon} r)^{p/3} \tag{2.1}$$

where $< \cdot >$ now denotes a spatial average. Moreover the dissipation length (i.e. the scale at which the dissipation is able to compete with the nonlinear transfer) is

$$\eta = (\nu^3/\varepsilon)^{1/4} \sim R_e^{-3/4} L \tag{2.2}$$

Let us stress that the basic assumption in the K41 theory is that $\bar{\varepsilon}$ should be the only relevant parameter in the cascade process. This hypothesis is reasonable only if the energy transfer

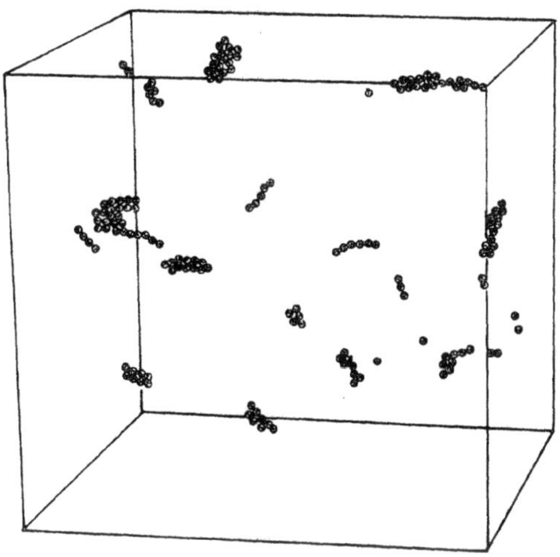

Fig.2. Numerical simulation (Siggia 1981) shows the structure of the zones containing the energy dissipation. The 95% of the energy dissipation is concentrated in the dark regions.

(or the energy dissipation density) $\varepsilon(\underline{x})$ does not strongly fluctuate with varying $\underline{x}$ and over a scale r which one is looking at. The assumption on the smooth behaviour of $\varepsilon(\underline{x})$ seems to be not satisfied since experiments (Batchelor and Townsend 1949) evidenciate strong intermittent bursts, both in space and time. For details on experimental studies see for ex. Kuo and Corrsin (1971 and 1972). Fig. 2 obtained by a direct simulation of the N-S equations (Siggia 1981) shows that $\varepsilon(x)$ is concetrated in a tiny region of the space. Experiments at large Reynolds number (Anselemet et al 1984) show scaling laws in the inertial range:

$$< | \Delta \underline{V}(\underline{r})|^p > \sim r^{\zeta(p)} \tag{2.3}$$

but with $\zeta(p) \neq p/3$. The disagreement between the experimental values of $\zeta(p)$ and the K41 predictions is small for not too large $p(\leq 4 \div 5)$ and increases with p. In the following we shall compare the experimental data with the estimates obtained by fractal and multifractal models.

These considerations on small-scale intermittency led Kolmogorov and Obukhov (Kolmogorov 1962, Obukhov 1962 and Yaglom 1966) to modify the K41. In their approach (called log-normal model) the fluctuations of energy dissipation are distributed according to a log-normal distribution. We do not discuss it here since it is not directly relevant to our purpose and because of the peculiarity of the log-normal distribution (see Mandelbrot 1972)

3. FRACTAL AND MULTIFRACTAL MODELS FOR INTERMITTENCY

The K41 theory assumes that each point $\underline{x}$ of the fluid has the same "singularity" structure:

$$\Delta V_{\underline{x}}(r) \sim r^h \qquad h = 1/3 \tag{3.1}$$

It is easy to see that (3.1) is equivalent to assume that $\varepsilon(\underline{x})$ is smoothly distributed in a region of R^3. Let us define the eddy turnover time and the kinetic energy per unit mass at scale r:

$$t(r) \sim r/(\Delta V(r)) \tag{3.2}$$

$$E(r) \sim \Delta V(r)^2 \tag{3.3}$$

The transfer rate of energy per unit mass from the eddy at scale r to smaller eddies is then given by

$$\tilde{\varepsilon}(r) = \frac{E(r)}{t(r)} \sim \frac{\Delta V(t)^3}{r} \tag{3.4}$$

Since $\tilde{\varepsilon}_{\underline{x}}(r) = \frac{1}{r^3} \int_{\Lambda_{\underline{x}}(r)} \varepsilon(\underline{y})\, d^3\underline{y}$ ($\Lambda_{\underline{x}}(r)$ is a cube of edge r around $\underline{x}$),

one has by (3.4) and (3.1)

$$\int_{\Lambda_{\underline{x}}(r)} \varepsilon(\underline{y})\, d^3\underline{y} \sim r^3 \qquad (3.5a)$$

A simple way to modify the K41 consists in assuming that the active turbulent structures cover a homogeneous fractall S (with fractal dimension D<3) on which $\varepsilon(x)$ is uniformly distributed.

Let us remark that in turbulence we do not use the word fractal in the exact mathematical sense. Indeed in the "true" limit $r \to 0$, because of the dissipation, one probably finds no singular structures. $r \to 0$ means r in the inertial range and the regions containing the large part of ε ($\underline{x}$) are a "physical" approximation of a fractal structure. In this approach (called absolute curdling (Mandelbrot 1974, Frisch et al 1978) one replaces (3.5a) with

$$\int_{\Lambda_{\underline{x}}(r)} \varepsilon(\underline{y})\, d^3\underline{y} \sim \begin{cases} r^D & \text{if } \underline{x} \in S \\ 0 & \text{otherwise} \end{cases} \qquad (3.5b)$$

or in an equivalent way:

$$\Delta V_{\underline{x}}(r) \sim \begin{cases} r^h & \text{if } \underline{x} \in S \\ 0 & \text{otherwise} \end{cases} \qquad (3.6)$$

with $h = \frac{D-2}{3}$. Since at scale r there is only a fraction $\sim r^{3-D}$ occupied by the "active" eddies, we have in the inertial range the following behaviour for the structure functions

$$\langle |\Delta V(r)|^p \rangle \sim r^{hp}\, r^{3-D} = r^{\zeta(p)}$$

$$\zeta(p) = \frac{D-2}{3} \cdot p + (3-D) \qquad (3.7)$$

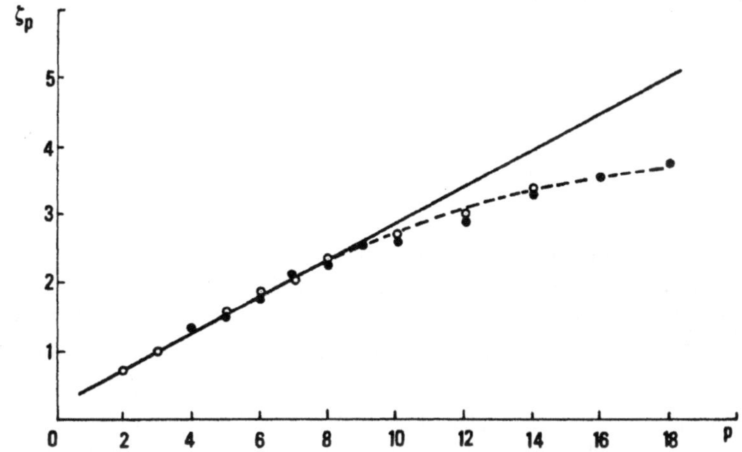

Fig. 3. $\zeta(p)$ vs p. Dots and circles are experimental data (Anselmet at al. 1984) the full line is the β-model result (3.7) with D = 2.83 and the dashed line is the random β-model result (3.16) using the distribution (3.22) with x = 0.125.

In the limit D=3, we recover the K41 results. In this approach D is a free parameter and cannot be obtained with simple arguments. Let us stress that $\varepsilon(\underline{x})$ is not distributed over all the fluid as in K41, since by (3.5b) one sees that $\varepsilon(\underline{x})$ has a singular structure. We shall discuss again this model in the following. In fig. 3 we report the experimental data (Anselmet at 1984) of $\zeta(p)$ vs p and the implications of the homogeneous fractal model (eq. 3.7). A linear fit leads to a good agreement with the experimental data for $p < 7$, while for larger values of p one observes a nonlinear behaviour.

The hypothesis of the existence of a whole spectrum of singularities allows to justify the non linearity of $\zeta(p)$. The model can be improved by considering the set on which the energy dissipation is concentrated as a multifractal set. Let us namely define S(h) as the set of point for which in the inertial range

$$\Delta_{\underline{x}} V(r) \sim r^h$$

indicating with d(h) the fractal dimension of S (h). It is easy to computer $\zeta(p)$ noting that the fraction of cubes with edge r in the set S(h) is proportional to $\frac{r^{-d(h)}}{r^{-3}} = r^{3-d(h)}$. Therefore one gets

$$< | \Delta V(r) |^p > \sim \int d\rho(h)\, r^{ph}\, r^{3-d(h)} \sim r^{\zeta(p)} \tag{3.8}$$

and by the steepest descent method:

$$\zeta(p) = \min_h \{ p\, h + 3 - d(h) \} \tag{3.9}$$

Eq. (3.9) shows that at a given value of p, $\zeta(p)$ depends on a particular value of h. Hence the kind of instabilities needed to set up the sets S(h) are picked up by different moments. We have worked out the multifractal approach in term of singularities of $\Delta \underline{V}_x(r)$ only because in the literature of turbulence the moments $< |\Delta \underline{V}(r)|^p >$ are usually involved. However it is simple to emphasize the correspondence with the multifractal language if one consider the scaling laws of energy dissipation. Let us note that

$$\int_{\Delta \underline{V}(r)} \varepsilon(\underline{y})\, d^3(\underline{y}) \sim r^3\, \tilde{\varepsilon}_{\underline{x}}(r) \sim r^{3h+2} \tag{3.10}$$

so that the analogous of the exponent α and $f(\alpha)$ are 3h+2 and d(3h+2) (for a general review on multifractal objects see Paladin and Vulpiani (1987)).

The homogeneous fractal case is the limit of the multifractal one when d(h) is defined only for $h = \frac{D-2}{3}$ and $d(h) = D$. Up to now we have remained at a rather descriptive level in the problem of intermittency. d(h) contains all the relevant features, but cannot be obtained by a first principle calculation based on the N-S equation singularities.

A pictorial scenario of the energy cascade can be given in terms of multiplicative processes (absolute and weighted curdling). We think that the details of the model (Frisch at al. 1978) and of the random β model (Benzi at al 1984) are useful to give a more direct idea of the fragmentation processes in turbulence. We want here remind that all "modern" fractal and multifractal cascade approaches have been originated by ad hoc models involving particular structures, as vortex sheets or vortex tubes, for the region containing the energy dissipation (Saffman 1970). The explicit idea of the β-model is due to Novikov and Stewart (1964) and to Kraichnan (1974).

Let us consider the scales $l_n = 2^{-n} l_o$, where $l_o = L$ is the scale at which energy is injected and the scaling factor 2 between l_n and l_{n+1} is conventional. Let us call $V_n = \Delta V(l_n)$ the typical velocity difference across a distance l_n in an active eddy. In order to take into account the intermittency Frisch et al. (1978) introduced the coefficient $\beta = 2^{D-3}$ equal to the fraction between the volume of the daugthers eddies at scale l_{n+1} and the volume of the mother eddy at scale l_n. The transfer energy from the eddy at scale l_n to that at scale l_{n+1} is

$$\varepsilon_n \sim \frac{V_n^3}{l_n}$$

Since the energy transfer rate is constant in the cascade process one has

$$\varepsilon_n = \beta\, \varepsilon_{n+1}, \quad \frac{V_n^3}{l_n} = \beta \frac{V_{n+1}^{\,3}}{l_{n+1}} \tag{3.11}$$

Iterating (3.11) one then obtains

$$V_n \sim l_n^{1/3} \left(\frac{l_n}{l_o} \right)^{(D-3)/3} \tag{3.12}$$

i.e. the eq. (3.6) with $h = \frac{D-2}{3}$.

In the previous model one essentially has a two values multiplicative process: each eddy at scale l_n is divided into eddies of scale l_{n+1}, in such a way that the energy transfer for a fractions β of eddies increases by a factor 1/β while it becames zero for the other ones.

Let us generalize the β-model. We namely assume that at scale ln there are N_n active eddies, each eddy l_n (k) (k labels the "mother" eddy and k=1,..., N_n) generates active eddies covering a fraction of volume $\beta_{n+1}(k)$. Since the rate of energy transfer is constant among and daughters, we get:

$$\frac{V_n(k)^3}{l_n} = \beta_{n+1}(k) \frac{V_{n+1}(k)^3}{l_{n+1}} \tag{3.13}$$

The iteration of (3.13) gives for V_n in an eddy generated by a particular "history" of fragmentations $[\beta_1 .... \beta_n]$:

$$V_n \sim l_n^{1/3} \left(\prod_{i=1}^{n} \beta_i \right)^{-1/3} \tag{3.14}$$

Let us remark that the fraction of volume occupied by an eddy generated by $[\beta_1,..,\beta_n]$ is $\prod_{i=1}^{n} \beta_i$., so from eq. (3.14) it follows

$$< | \Delta V(l_n)|^p > \sim l_n^{p/3} \int \prod_{i=1}^{n} d\beta_i\, \beta_i^{(1-p/3)}\, P(\beta_1 ... \beta_n) \tag{3.15}$$

Assuming no correlation among different steps of the fragmentation, i.e. $P(\beta_1,..,\beta_n) = \prod_{i=1}^{n} P(\beta_i)$, one obtains for $\zeta(p)$

$$\zeta(p) = \frac{p}{3} - \ln_2 \{\beta^{(1-p/3)}\} \tag{3.16}$$

where $\{\cdot\}$ stands for the average over the distribution $P(\beta)$. If β_n is a constant $(= 2^{(D-3)})$ one recovers the results of the β-model. The knowledge of the probability distribution $P(\beta)$ is related to the understanding of the nature of the N-S equation singularities. However this problem is far to be solved at present. The fractal object generated by random β-model (or more general a multifractal object) has no more global dilatation invariant properties; even if, one can still compute the fractal dimension D as:

$$\overline{N_n} \sim l_n^{-D} \tag{3.17}$$

where N_n is the number of active eddies at the n-th step uf the fragmentation and $\overline{(\cdot)}$ is an average over an ensemble of cascades. It is easy to show that

$$D = 3 - \zeta(0) \tag{3.18}$$

which in the random β-model is given by:

$$D = 3 + \ln_2 \{\beta\} \tag{3.19}$$

Moreover the analogous of correlation dimension in the chaotic dynamics (Grassberger and Procaccia 1983) d_2 is D^* defined by:

$$D^* = 1 + \zeta(6) \tag{3.20}$$

and in terms of the random β-model

$$D^* = 3 - \ln_2 \{\beta^{-1}\} \tag{3.21}$$

Let us recall that D^* is related to the scaling of energy dissipation density correlation (Frisch et al, 1978),

$$<\varepsilon(\underline{x} + \underline{r})\, \varepsilon(x)> \sim r^{(3-D^*)}$$

and that in the experimental literature the fractal dimension is usually estimated by D^* even if in general $D>D^*$. $D=D^*$ actually holds only for homogeneous fractals. A simple fit of the experimental data chosing for $P(\beta)$ the form

$$P(\beta) = x\, \delta(\beta - 0.5) + (1-x)\, \delta(\beta - 1) \tag{3.22}$$

and $x = .125$ gives a good agreement with the experimental data (see fig.3). There is no deep reason to choose the form (3.22); we have simply followed some phenomenological ideas considering two possible kinds of fragmentation: an active eddy can generate either vorticity sheets (β= .5) or space filling Kolmogorov-like eddies (β=1). With the fit (3.22) we get D = 2.91 and D* = 2.83, with a small but significative difference. There exist some physical arguments to give a bound to the values of h.

In set S(h) the local Reybolds number at scale r is $R_e\,(r,h)=\frac{r\cdot r^h}{\nu}\sim r^{1+h}$. Therefore in order to stop the turbulent cascade one must require that R_e (r,h) decreases with r implying h >-1. Let us not however, that it is reasonble to assume $h \geq 0$ because for negative h one could have points for which $|\Delta V(r)|$ increases when r decreases and this seems quite unrealistic.Note that in the distribution (3.22) we have taken h_{min}= 0 (corrresponding to β_{min}=1/2).

The shape of d(h) obtained with the eq.(3.22) is shown in fig. (4).

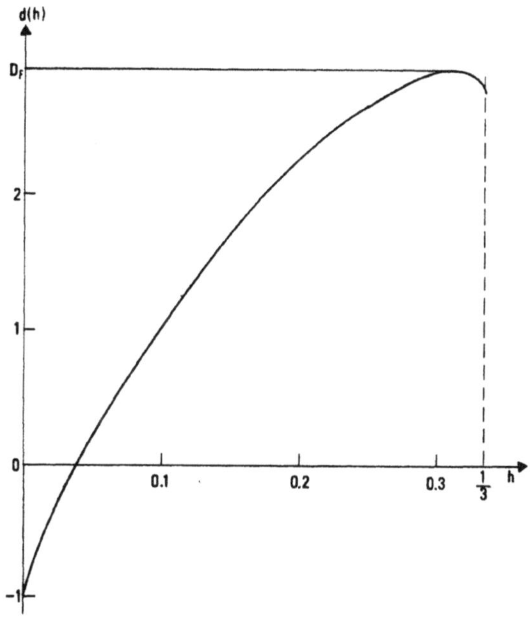

Fig.4. d(h) vs h given by the Legendre transform of (3.16) using the fit (3.22) with x=0.125.

We recall that the β-model (and random β-model) are just the simplest phenomenological description of the fractal (multifractal) nature of the distribution of singularities of the velocity field. Recentely Siebesma et al (1988) have introduced a version of the random β-model in which the boundary condition fluctuations directly effect the fragmentation spectrum.

Some other non fractal models for the description of intermittency have been proposed (Nakano and Nelkin 1985, Nakano 1986). They are alternative to the scenario of this section. We do not discuss them, but we want just to note that they imply $\zeta(p)$=p/3 for $p<p_c = 5\div 6$. We think that this is in strong disagreement with all experimental results. Even if one could think that for large values of p(>8) the experimental data for $\zeta(p)$ are not enough accurate in order to prefer definitively a model or another, all the recent experiments nevertheless give values for $\zeta(2)$ and $\zeta(4)$ respectively larger and smaller than 2/3 and 4/3 obtained by the K41 (e.g. $\zeta(2) = 0.70 \pm 0.01$).

4. REMARKS AND CONSEQUENCES OF MULTIFRACTALITY IN TURBULENCE

The concept of "multifractality" is related to the properties of the distribution of mass (in turbulence the density of energy dissipation) and not to "geometrical" properties. This implies that for certain feature the multifractality do not imply an anomalous scaling.

Let us now show why the multifractal structure is not relevant for the relative diffusion of particles pairs [Crisanti et al. 1987]. Indeed, the growth of the moments of the relative distance R between a pair of particles which scales with time as:

$$\overline{R^{2a}} \sim t^{2q\nu(q)} \tag{4.1}$$

$\overline{(\,)}$ is now an average over a large number of pairs. We find that for each q, $\nu(q) = \nu$ and ν is only related to the exponent $\zeta(1)$:

$$\nu = \frac{1}{1-\zeta(1)} \tag{4.2}$$

Let us consider M>>1 pairs of particles at positions $\underline{r}_i(1)$ and $\underline{r}_i(2)$ (i=1,...,M). The interparticle distance is $\underline{R}_i = (\underline{r}_i(1) - \underline{r}_i(2))$ and the relative velocity $\delta\underline{V}_i = \frac{d}{dt}\underline{R}_i$.

Let us compute the time derivative of $\overline{R}^2$:

$$\frac{d}{dt}\overline{R}^2 = 2 \lim_{M\to\infty} \frac{1}{M}\sum_{i=1}^{M} \delta\,\underline{V}_i\,(\underline{R}_i)\cdot\underline{R}_i =$$

$$= 2 \lim_{M\to\infty} \frac{1}{M}\sum_{i=1}^{M} \delta\,V_i\,(\underline{R}_i)\,R_i \cos\theta_i \tag{4.3}$$

where θ_i, is the angle between $\underline{R}_i$ and $\delta\,\underline{V}_i\,(\underline{R}_i)$. In the case of isotropic turbulence $\overline{\cos\theta_i}$ is positive and does not depend on R[Cocke 1969]. Therefore one has

$$\frac{d\overline{R}^2}{dt} = 2\,\overline{(\cos\theta)}\;\overline{\delta V(\underline{R})R} \tag{4.4}$$

In order to compute $M^{-1}\sum_{i=1}^{M}\delta V_i\,(\underline{R}_i)\,R_i$ we group together all the n (α) pairs with the same value R(α) of the interparticles distance in such a way that one obtains:

$$\sum_{i=1}^{M} \delta\,V_i\,(R_i)\,R_i = \sum_{\alpha}\Big[\frac{1}{n(\alpha)}\sum_k \delta V_k\Big]\,R\,(\alpha) \tag{4.5}$$

The sum Σ_α, is over the set of different values of $R(\alpha)$ and Σ_k is over the $n(\alpha)$ pairs with $R_k = R(\alpha)$. Note that for large M (and $n(\alpha)$)

$$\frac{1}{n(\alpha)} \sum_k \delta V_k \simeq \langle|\Delta(VR(\alpha))|\rangle \sim R(\alpha)^{\zeta(1)} \tag{4.6}$$

therefore

$$\frac{d\,\overline{R^2}}{dt} \sim \overline{R^{1+\zeta(1)}} \tag{4.7}$$

It is trivial to repeat the same computations of $\overline{R^{2q}}$:

$$\frac{d\,\overline{R^{2q}}}{dt} \sim \overline{R^{2q+\zeta(1)-1}} \tag{4.8}$$

Now it is easy to see that $\nu(q)$, as defined in (4.4), must be constant. In fact by (4.8) and (4.1) one has

$$2q\,\nu(q) - 1 = (2q-1+\zeta(1)) \cdot \nu\left(\frac{2q-1+\zeta(1)}{2}\right) ;$$

moreover $\nu(q)$ does not increase when q increases [Feller 1971], therefore one obtaines:

$$\nu(q) = \nu = \frac{1}{1-\zeta(1)}, \ \forall q \ .$$

Let us remark that the multifractal structure induces only a (slight) correction to the Richardson law $\nu = 3/2$ [Richardson 1926] and in the diffusion process there is no anomalous scaling. The scaling laws (4.1) are parametrized by a single exponent $\zeta(1)$; the same result holds for a homogeneous fractal [Hentschel and Procaccia 1983] (with $\zeta(1) = \frac{7-2D}{3}$) or a multifractal.

Let us now consider the problem of the number of degrees of freeedom of the turbulence. It is clear that a satisfactory description of turbulent fluids needs a resolution up to scale of same order of the dissipative Kolmogorov length η at which the molecular friction is able to compete with the non linear transfer. One has:

$$\eta = (\nu^3/\varepsilon)^{1/4} \tag{4.9}$$

where ε is the rate of the energy dissipation for unit mass and time (assumed to be constant in K41).

If L is the system characteristic length at which the external energy imput is pumped then the adimensional ratio $R_e = (\varepsilon L^4)^{1/3}/\nu$ is the Reynolds number. The number of grid points for unit volume necessary to obtain a resolution up to η is thus

$$N(R_e) \sim (L/\eta)^3 \sim R_e^{9/4} \qquad (4.10)$$

This argument (due to Landau and Lifchitz (1971)) hides the central assumption that all the fluid is "active", i.e. that energy dissipation density fields is smoothly distributed on a three dimensional region.

Kraichnan (1985) has repeated the Landau-Lifshitz argument by making the hypothesis that the energy dissipation $\varepsilon(\underline{x})$ is concentrated on a homogeneous fractal with non integer dimension $D < 3$. The dissipation scale η can be now determined by imposing that the Reynolds number related to an eddy of length scale η is of order one:

$$\frac{\eta\, \Delta V(\eta)}{\nu} \sim O(1) \qquad (4.11)$$

This is equivalent to require that the dissipative (linear) term of the N.-S. equations is able to compete with the non linear transfer term.

Inserting eq. (3.6) in eq. (4.11) we obtain

$$\eta \sim \frac{L}{R_e^{1/(1+h)}} \qquad (4.12)$$

It follows that:

$$N(R_e) \sim \left(\frac{L}{\eta}\right)^D \sim R_e^{3D/(1+D)} \qquad (4.13)$$

Let us remark that some other variables are also necessary for describing the non active regions of the fluid but their number does not depend on R_e. If the β-model assumptions were correct, eq. (4.13) would give (in principle) the scaling law for $N(R_e)$. The number of degrees of freedom necessary for describing the multifractal structure of turbulence must be defined with much more carefulness (Paladin and Vulpiani 1987a). In fact, for each singularity h a different dissipative length $\eta(h)$ is picked up by condition (4.12): $\eta(h) \sim R_e^{-1/(1+h)}$.

Since the number of eddies at scale l with singularity h is proportional to $l^{-d(h)}$, one deduces that the number of grid points which have to be considered for resolving the set S(h) is

$$N_h(R_e) \sim \left(\frac{L}{\eta(h)}\right)^{d(h)} \sim R_e^{d(h)/(1+h)} \qquad (4.14)$$

We thus get the total number of degrees of freedom by integrating (4.14) over h:

$$N(R_e) = \int d\rho(h)\, N_h(R_e) \sim R_e^{\delta} \qquad (4.15)$$

where δ can be estimated by the steepest descent method in the limit of large R_e.

$$\delta = \max_{h} [d(h)/(1+h)] \qquad (4.16)$$

A fit of the experimental data (Anselmet et al 1984) gives the value $\delta \simeq 2.2$ which is close to the value given by eq. (4.13). The results (4.13) and (4.14,16) are nevertheless quite different from a conceptual point of view.

We must stress that the estimate (4.15,16) has just a theoretical relevance since it is rather difficult in a computer simulation to locate the grid points on the sets S(h) (which also evolves in time). Indeed one usually works with a fixed grid or with a pseudospectral method (Patterson and S.Orszag 1971). It follows that the only relevant parameter is the minimal scale l_{min} considered which is bounded from below by the dissipative length related to the strongest singularity:

$$l_{min} \sim \eta\ (h_{min}) \sim R^{-1/(1+h_{min})} \qquad (4.17)$$

The estimate $l_{min} = \eta\ (h_{min})$ assures that all the sets S(h) (i.e. even very improbable events) are taken into account.

The number of equations which allows to get such a fully accurate description is thus:

$$N_T^* \sim \left(\frac{L}{l_{min}}\right)^3 \sim R_e^{3/(1+h_{min})} \qquad (4.18)$$

Eq. (4.18) is in agreement with rigorous bounds (Ruelle 1982 and Constatin et al 1985) On the other hand, if one decides to neglect the rare events it is sufficient a resolution $\tilde{l} >> l_{min}$ on which just the relevant features of turbulence are reproduced loosing some details. In this case the number of equations is reduced to

$$\tilde{N}^* \sim (L/\tilde{l})^3$$

This scale $\tilde{l}$ can be estimated by the dissipative length $\eta(\tilde{h})$ related to an effective singularity $\tilde{h}$.

Let us define an "effective" mass dimension $\tilde{D}$ of the object on which the energy dissipation is concentrated by:

$$\tilde{h} = \frac{\tilde{D}-2}{3}$$

Mandelbrot (1976) has e.g. assumed $\tilde{D}$ = the information dimension and from the data (Anselmet et al 1984) one has $\tilde{D} \simeq 2.87$. This assumption corresponds to select a $\tilde{h} = d\zeta(p)/dp|_{p=3} \simeq 0.29$ and, roughly speaking, $\tilde{l}$ is thus the smallest scale on which in average active eddies are still present.

On the other hand, some heuristic arguments (see sect. 3) as well as the fit of experimental data shown in figure (3) indicate h_{min}=0. It follows that:

$$N_T^* \sim R_e^3 \quad \text{and} \quad \tilde{N}^* \sim R_e^{3/(1+\tilde{h})} \sim R_e^{2.3} .$$

Let us emphasize that N_T^* is much greater than $\tilde{N}^*$ which is close to the estimate of the number of degrees of freedom obtained respectively in the K41, in the β-model and in the framework of the multifractal approach.

5. TWO-DIMENSIONAL TURBULENCE

The physics of two dimensional flows is somehow different from the three dimensional case. For the inviscid two dimensional case a global regularity theorem has been proved together with the uniqueness and existence theorem. Thus no singularity of the velocity field can develop in a finite time (see for example Rose and Sulem 1978). Moreover, beside energy, any function of vorticity, like enstrophy, is conserved. It follows that energy cannot be transferred from large to small scales in two dimensional turbulence. Yet, in analogy with the three dimensional case, we expect that for two dimensional turbulence there exists an inertial range where enstrophy is cascading from large to small scale (Kraichnan 1967, Batchelor 1969). Former theories pointed out the existence of two inertial ranges: a k^{-3} enstrophy cascading range for the small scales and a $k^{-5/3}$ reverse energy cascading range for the large scales. On the other hand numerical simulations (Basdevant et. al. 1981, Mc Williams 1984) with both forcing and decaying systems show an enstrophy cascading range with a spectral slope $-4\div-6$ much steeper than -3. Basdevant et. al. (1981) argued that this difference between theoretical prediction and numerical result is due to both spatial and temporal intermittency: enstrophy dissipation is a highly fluctuating quantity whose statistical properties affect significantly the energy spectrum at small scales. Moreover as noted by Basdevant et al. (1981), and Mc Williams (1984) two dimensional turbulence is characterized by the existence of coherent structures, namely vortices, with a lifetime much longer than their characteristic eddy turnover time.

Naively one could think that in two dimensional turbulence all the previous arguments can be repeated simply considering an enstrophy cascade instead of an energy cascade. This is not possible because in two dimensional Navier-Stokes equations there are no singularities in the velocity field. Indeed it is well known for two dimensional Euler equaiton that the following inequality holds for any time (see for example Rose and Sulem 1978):

$$\Delta V(r) \leq \text{const}\ r\,|\ln r| \tag{5.1}$$

This is a consequence of vorticity conservation for each fluid particle. Inequality (5.1) holds also in the Navier-Stokes equations and implies:

$$\zeta(p) \geq p \tag{5.2}$$

Moreover, for a general theorem of probability theory (Feller 1971), $\zeta(p)$ must be a convex function of p. Assuming $\zeta(3) = 3$ (i.e. a constant forward enstrophy cascade) (5.2) and convexity of $\zeta(p)$ one obtains (apart logarithmic corrections) the result:

$$\zeta(p) = p \tag{5.3}$$

Thus we obtain the apparently surprising result tha tin two dimensional turbulence the Kolmogorov scaling law (5.3) holds also in presence of intermittency. Note that, except the

Kolmogorov law ($\beta_n = 1$) any random β-model gives wrong results in two dimensional turbulence. Indeed we can repeat the considerations done for the three dimensional case using the assumption of constant enstrophy transfer rate. In this case equation (3.13) becomes:

$$\frac{V_n^3(k)}{l_n^3} = \beta_{n+1} \frac{V_{n+1}^3(k)}{l_{n+1}^3} \tag{5.4}$$

By (5.4) we obtain for $\zeta(p)$ a convex function with $\zeta(3) = 3$ and consequently inequality (5.2) is broken by the singularities bearing in the fragmentation mechanism. We remark that this undesired result (i.e. the appearing of singularities of the velocity field) is due to the fact that in the fragmentation process β_n is independent of β_{n-1} i.e to the bernoullian nature of the random β-model. Let us consider a simple modification to the cascade model in order to satisfy (5.1). We still consider a constant enstrophy transfer rate i.e. (5.4) but with the further constraint:

$$\beta_{n+1}^{(k)} = 1 \quad if \ \frac{V_n^3}{l_n^3} \geq \eta_{max} \tag{5.5}$$

where η_{max} is a bound to the enstrophy transfer which reflects the constraint (2.10)

With the (5.6) the fragmentation process has now a markovian nature because the steps of the cascade depend on the previous ones. We think that constraint (5.6) is the simplest way, at least in fragmentation models, to avoid singularities. It is easy to see that with this model we obtain $\zeta(p) = p$. Indeed the regions where enstrophy dissipation is concentrated have fractal dimension equal to 2, i.e. they occupy an area non decreasing for decreasing scale length. Roughly speaking, we have no more a multifractal but a "checkers"-like structures, at least at very small scales. We remark that, unlike three dimensional turbulence, in the two dimensional case it is not possible to get information on the behavior of the energy spectrum E(k) from the knowledge of $\zeta(p)$. With naive dimensional arguments one could conclude that $E(k) \sim k^{-(1+\zeta(2))}$ but this conclusion is wrong if $\zeta(2) \geq 2$ (see for example Babiano et al 1984b). Therefore the only result from the bound (5.1) is

$$E(k) \sim K^{-\alpha} \quad \text{with } \alpha \geq 3. \tag{5.6}$$

therefore, neither the α value nor the structure functions (since $\zeta(p) = p$) give us information about the "intermittency" in two dimensional turbulence. Numerical experiments (Benzi et al 1986) confirm that the fragmentation is space filling on the small scales (but larger than the viscosity dissipation ones). The intermittency should be regarded as a somewhat "macroscopic" phenomena related to coherent structures. The enstrophy cascade indeed seems to be inhibited in some highly organized structures which dominate the energy spectrum. Moreover the turbulent field seems to be decomposed in two parts: a background with an energy spectrum k^{-3} in the inertial range and a finite number of vortices (coherent structures) which advect the background field.

ACKNOWLEDGMENTS

I enjoyed many exchanges of ideas with A.Crisanti, M.Falcioni and G.Paladin.

REFERENCES

F.Anselmet, Y.Gagne, E.J.Hopfinger and A.R. Antonia 1984, J. Fluid. Mech. 140, 63.

A.Babiano, C.Basdevant ard R.Sadourny 1984, C.R.Acad. Sci. Paris B299, 495.

C.Basdevant, B.Legras, R.Sadourny and M.Beland 1981, J.Atoms. Sci. 38, 2305.

G.K.Batchelor and A.A.Townsend 1949, Proc. Roy. Soc. A199, 238.

G.K.Batchelor 1969, Phys. Fluids 12, S233.

R.Benzi, G.Paladin, G.Parisi and A.Vulpiani 1984, J.Phys. A17, 3521.

R.Benzi, G.Paladin, S.Patarnello, P.Santangelo and A. Vulpiani 1986, J.Phys. A19, 3771.

A.Crisanti, G.Paladin and A.Vulpiani 1987, Phys.Lett. A126, 120.

W.J.Cocke 1969, Phys. Fluids 12, 2488.

P.Constantin, C.Foias, O.P.Manley and R.Teman 1985, J.Fluid Mech. 150, 427.

M.Falcioni, G.Paladin and A.Vulpiani 1988, J.Phys. A21, 3451.

W.Feller 1971, "An Introduction to probability theory and its applications" vol. 2 (New York, Wiley).

U.Frisch and G.Parisi 1985, in "Turbulence and predictability of geophysical flows and climatic dynamics" ed. N.Ghil, R.Benzi and G.Parisi (North Holland).

U.Frisch, P.Sulem and M.Nelkin 1987, J.Fluid, Mech. 87, 719.

P.Grassberger and I.Procaccia 1983, Phys.Rev.Lett. 50, 346.

M.Henon 1966, C.R.Acad. Sci, Paris A262, 312.

K.Huang 1987, "Statistical mechanics" (Wiley N.Y.).

H.G.E.Hentschel and I.Procaccia 1983, Phys. Rev. A27, 1266.

A.N.Kolmogorov 1941, Dokl, Akad, Naukk SSSR 30, 299.

A.N.Kolmogorov 1962, J.Fluid Mech 13, 82.

R.H.Kraichnan 1967, Phys. Fluid 10, 1417.

R.H.Kraichnan 1974, J.Fluid Mech. 63, 305

R.H.Kraichnan 1985, Phys. Fluids 28, 10.

A.Y.Kuo and S.Corrsin 1971, J.Fluid Mech 50, 285.

A.Y.Kuo and S.Corrsin 1972, J.Fluid Mech. 56, 447.

D.Landau and L.Lifschitz 1971, "Mecanique des fluides" (MIR ed. Moscow).

D.C.Leslie 1973, "Developments in the theory of turbulence" (Clarendon Press, Oxford).

B.B.Mandelbrot 1972, in "Statistical models and turbulence" pag.333 eds. M.Rosenblatt and C.Van Atta, Lectures Notes in Physics 12 (Springer, Berlin).

B.B.Mandelbrot 1974, J.Fluid. Mech. 62, 331.

B.B.Mandelbrot 1976, in "Turbulence and Navier-Stokes equation" pag. 121 ed. R.Teman, Lectures Notes in Mathematics 565 (Springer, Berlin).

J.C.McWilliams 1984, J.Fluid Mech. 146, 21.

T.Nakano and M.Nelkin 1985, Phys. Rev. 31A, 1980.

T.Nakano 1986, Progr. Theor. Phys. 75, 1295.

A.A.Novikov and R.W.Stewart 1964, Izv. Akad. Nauk SSSR, Ser. Geofiz. 3, 408.

A.M.Obukhov 1962, J.Fluid Mech 13, 77.

G.Paladin and A.Vulpiani 1987a, Phys, Rev. A35, 1971.

G.Paladin and A.Vulpiani 1987b, Phys, Rep. 156, 147.

G.S.Patterson and S.Orszag 1971, Phys. Fluids 14, 2538.
L.F.Richardson 1922, "Weather prediction by numerical process", (Cambridge Un. Press).
L.F.Richardson 1926, Pr. of the Royal Society of London A110, 709.
H.A.Rose and P.L.Sulem 1978, J.Physique 39, 441.
D.Ruelle 1982, Comm.Math.Phys. 87, 287.
P.G.Saffman 1970, Phys. Fluids 13, 2193.
A.P.Siebesma, R.R.Tremblay, A.Erzan and L.Pietronero 1988, Preprint.
E.D.Siggia 1981, J.Fluid Mech. 107, 375.
A.M.Yaglom 1966, Dokl. Akad. Nauk, SSSR 166, 49.

NONLINEAR VARIABILITY IN GEOPHYSICS: MULTIFRACTAL SIMULATIONS AND ANALYSIS

Daniel Schertzer* and Shaun Lovejoy**

*EERM/CRMD, Météorologie Nationale
Paris, France

**PhysicsDept., McGill University
Montréal, Canada

ABSTRACT

Many geophysical fields show extreme variability over wide ranges of scale. We review and develop theoretical insights and empirical evidence concerning the multiple scaling/multifractal behavior of these fields. We emphasize the very singular behavior of geophysical observables, usually obtained by space-time averaging over scales much greater than that of the homogeneity. On the one hand we render more direct the link between statistical singularities (divergence of high order statistical moments) and singularities per realization (small scale divergence of densities). We recall also that in order to deal with the strong (but scaling) anisotropy of these fields we must generalize the idea of scale invariance beyond the familiar self-similar (or even self-affine) notions. On the other hand we examine the conditions of the existence of two-parameter universality classes of the generic multifractal processes. These have many important theoretical and practical consequences: infinite hierarchies of dimensions depending only on two parameters, the five main subclasses are determined. These facts greatly facilitate both the empirical characterization of multifractals, as well as their numerical simulation.

INTRODUCTION

A central and common feature of geophysical phenomena and processes is their extreme variability over wide ranges of scale, whose ratios easily reach nine orders of magnitude (earth radius scale/ centimeter scale). Recently it has been increasingly recognized that this feature provides a powerful unifying *problematic* of Geophysics whose advance constitutes key steps both in increasing fundamental knowledge in Geophysics (especially turbulence), as well as in many practical applications (especially remote sensing techniques). More precisely the question of *scaling* behavior -i.e. a common behavior at different scales- became central simply because this (scale) *symmetry assumption is not only the simplest but also the only assumption acceptable in the absence of more information or knowledge*. Since this behavior is the result of nonlinear interactions -leading to nonlinear (i.e. non-proportional) response to a given excitation- between different scales (and/or processes), there arises the general question of *scaling nonlinear variability in Geophysics*. Mushrooming interest in geophysical applications of such nonlinear variability has lead to two workshops on the theme "Scaling, fractals and Nonlinear Variability in Geophysics 1, 2" in August 1986 at McGill University (Lovejoy and Schertzer 1988, Schertzer and Lovejoy 1989), and at the former Ecole Polytechnique in Paris France, in June 1988. There was also a session on "Chaos, Turbulence and Nonlinear variability in geophysics" at the March 1989 European Geophysical Society meeting where many of these questions were discussed.

Fractals' Physical Origin and Properties
Edited by L. Pietronero
Plenum Press, New York

We will argue that a general consequence of scaling nonlinear variability is that the notion of observables (roughly speaking: what we can observe or measure) is far from being trivial, mainly due to the fact that the details of the process may be overwhelmingly important (due to small scale or high frequency "ultraviolet" divergences, and unfortunately our observations and measurements are nearly always restricted to resolutions much higher than the scale of the smallest detail (i.e. the inner scale of the process or the scale of homogeneity which is typically of the order of millimeter or less). Note that full knowledge down to this inner scale is usually out of our scope due to large number of degrees of freedom involved. When we are speaking of large numbers, we of course refer to the *physicists' infinity* such as the Avogadro's number (10^{23}): indeed the number of mm^3 involved in the atmosphere is of order[1] $10^{10}x10^{10}x10^7= 10^{27}$

Let us briefly note that this question of the "details" has a rather long history, as is testified by the introduction of Perrin in his edited thesis (1913) and especially his valuable quotation of E. Borel about abstract vs. "real world" measures. We may also note the permanent question of fine graining vs. coarse graining , or the question of "homogeneization", "renormalization" (how to define smooth macroscopic "effective" fields from irregular microscopic ones), the above quoted question of "ultra violet divergences". Concerning fluid dynamics, the question of the singularities became more precise with the works of Leray (1934), and in Von Neuman's review on turbulence (Von Neuman (1963), but also in the debate between Richarson[2] and Bjkernes: is the characterization of a few large scale singularities (the meteorological fronts) sufficient to forecast the evolution of the weather? The present day debate could be much more precise dealing with characterization of hierarchies of scaling singularities. In the following we hope to give more easier insights into this fundamental question with the help of seemingly (at first glance) simple models (phenomenological models or "mock geophysics"), which nevertheless possess surprising properties which we argue to be quite general.

Let us also emphasize that the (nonlinear!) path historically followed to explore nonlinear variability crossed the geometrical world and was maintained in its restrictive frontiers for too long a period. This period created some unfortunate consequences and attempted to bypass some fundamental problems. Indeed, the development of concrete analytical methods has tended to show that geometrical frameworks can often be misleading and fractal notions have been most fruitful when divorced from geometry. In particular, the abandonment of the dogma of the uniqueness of fractal dimension (Grassberger (1983), Hentschel and Proccacia (1983), Schertzer and Lovejoy (1983,1984) Frisch and Parisi (1985), Halsey et al. (1986), Pietronero and Siebesma (1986), Bialas and Peschanski (1986), Stanley and Meakin (1988), Levich and Shtilman (1989)...) in favour of hierarchies of dimensions and singularities with their non-geometric generators has been one of the most important recent advances.

These new ideas involve both the possibility of very general anisotropic types of scaling (necessary, for example to deal with rotation, stratification or "texture"), as well as "multiple scaling" or "multifractality" associated with highly intermittent processes in which the weak and intense regions have different scaling behavior. In a general manner, a system may be said to be scaling (or scale invariant) over a range if the small and large scale structures are related by a scale changing operation involving only the scale ratio. Hence, scale invariance is not restricted to the familiar self-similar (or even self-affine) notions and we outline the necessary formalism (generalized scale invariance discussed by Schertzer and Lovejoy 1985, 1987a-b).

---

[1] Considering the scale of homogeneity of the order of the millimeter, and the (outer) vertical scale of the order of ten kilometers and the horizontal scale of the order of ten thousand kilometers. In a similar manner the Reynolds number of atmospheric turbulence is usually estimated as $\approx 10^{12}$, taking the ratio of injection (1000 km)/dissipation (1mm) (horizontal) scales as 10^9, since it is the 4/3 power of this ratio.

[2] Recall that Richardson (1926) didn't hesitate to raise the (sacrilegious?) question "does the wind have a velocity?" (i.e. are the time derivatives regular?). Indeed, he pointed out the very irregular Weierstrass function as a counter example.

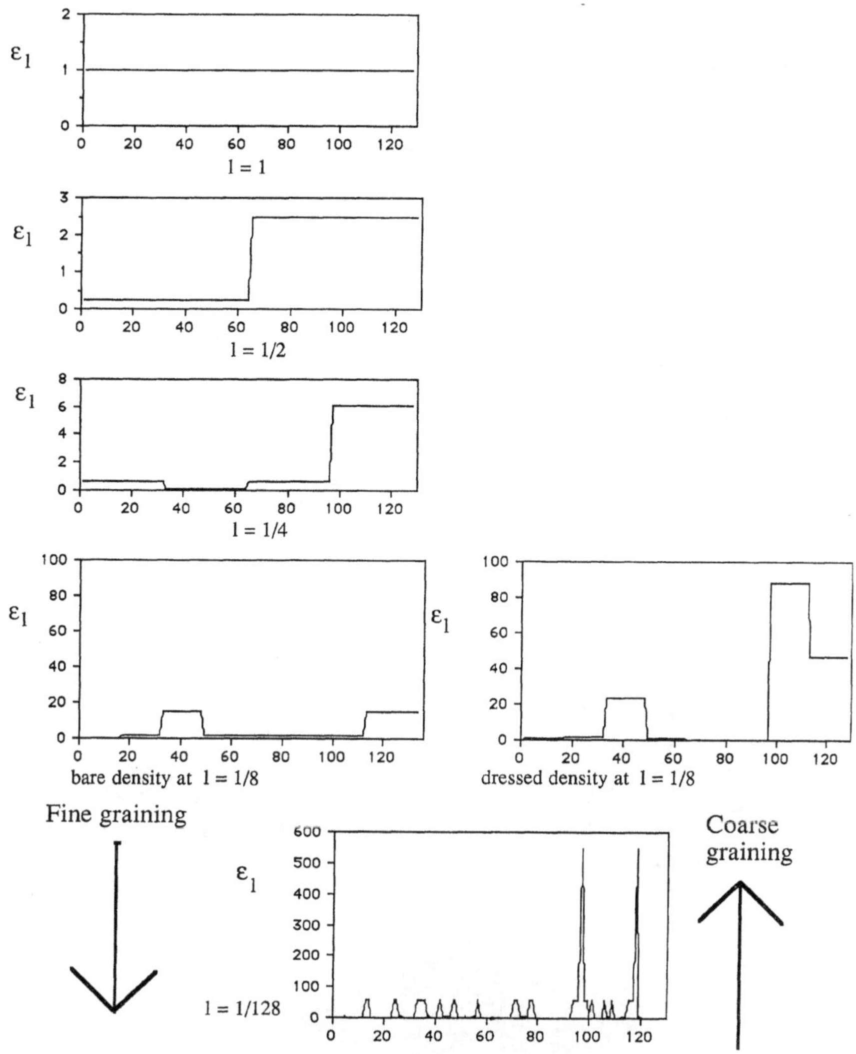

Fig. 1a . Illustration of the "bare"and "dressed" energy flux densities. The left hand side shows the construction step by step of the bare field produced by a multifractal cascade process (the α-model, discussed below) starting with an initially uniform unit density. At each step the homogeneity scale is divided by a constant ratio λ=2 From top to bottom, the number of cascade steps takes the following values n = 0, 1, 2, 3 and 7, with the corresponding length scale values l = 1, 1/2, 1/4, 1/8, 1/128. When the number of steps n increases, some rare regions of high intensities ("singularities") appear, most of the space becomes inactive. At l =1/8, n=3, one may compare the rather more intense dressed density with the bare density. The sharp contrast arise from the smaller scales singularities, as seen on step n=7, which contribute to high fluctuations of the dressed density.

As we will insist that it is now rather obvious that multiple dimensions and singularities are the rule rather than the exception for fields. However, as we will discuss after having left the uniqueness for infinity, the important question of existence of universality classes gives credence to returning to two fundamental parameters!

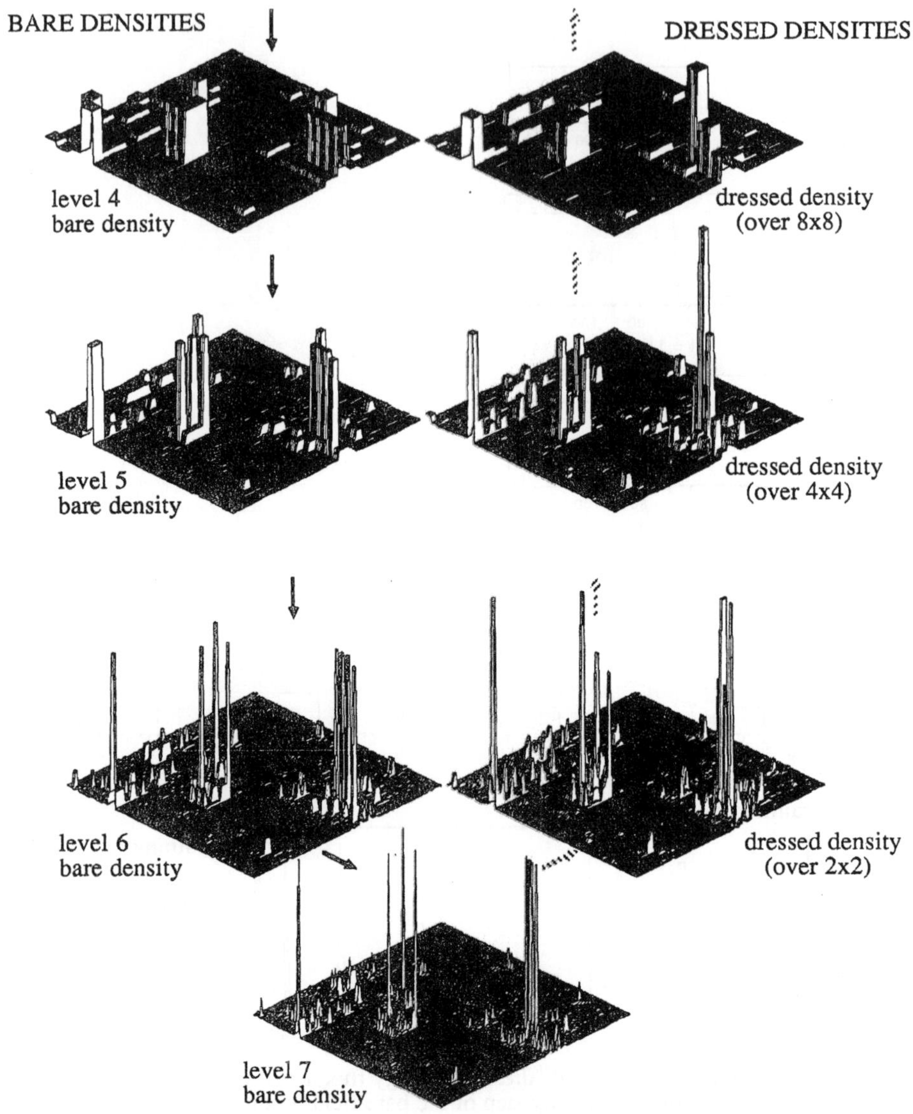

Fig. 1b . as in Figure 1a, illustration of the "bare"and "dressed" energy flux densities, but on a 2 dimensional space. The dressed energy flux densities, obtained by averaging, are presented on the right hand side of the figure. At intermediate scales, level 3 or 4, one may still note the important contributions from smaller scales singularities to high fluctuations of the dressed density.

On the other hand, the breathtaking pictures of (geometrical) fractal objects often inclined us not to explore the rather immediate question: how will we be able to see them due to the limited resolution of our eyes if the computing process goes down to a much smaller scale? In other words, we must explore the fundamental *symmetry breaking caused by the observation* at a given scale. This is the reason why we will insist on the fundamental difference between *"bare" and "dressed" properties* at a given (non-zero) scale i.e. the important differences between a process with a cut-off of small scale interactions and one with these interactions restored (cf. Fig. 1a-b for illustrations)

The bare properties are related to fine graining (e.g. developing a cascade...) and are the properties of the process with nonlinear interactions at scales smaller than the observation scale being filtered out (i.e. truncation of the process at the scale of observation). The dressed properties are related to coarse graining and are the observed properties at a given scale of resolution (i.e. linear or nonlinear averaging on the observation scale over the smaller details of the same process but with all interactions: the process fully developed down to the smallest scale). In other words, only half the problem has been explored (and even a smaller fraction of the real problem): the "dressed" truth is the one which counts! The terms "bare" and "dressed" are borrowed from renormalization jargon, but here due to the extreme variability, they will become quite different; not only by a renormalizing factor but by different statistical behavior, thus the overwhelmingly important question of singular statistics (divergences of statistical moments, Schertzer and Lovejoy 1987a-b) linked to multiple ultraviolet divergences.

PIXEL WORLDS AND "MOCK GEOPHYSICS"

On the one hand geophysical phenomena (especially when remotely sensed) are more and more often represented with the help of digitized "images", pixel sets. On the other hand the "theoretical" representations of the same phenomena are still believed to be of a certain continuous type. Such continuous representations are thought to be rather obvious limits of the pixel representation when the resolution (scale of observation) goes to zero. In particular one usually would associate with such an image, a function, a "density", and the digitized field corresponding to averages on a pixel of this density. Hence, from a very rough knowledge of the pixel values, one "naturally" tries to associate a hypothetical function. Such a "natural" hypothesis is far from being physically obvious: it requires ample (mathematical) regularity constraints which are the opposite of the observed strong variability down to smaller scales. Mathematically, it corresponds to very particular measurable properties: one considers only regular measures with respect to the usual line, surface, volume measures, i.e. Lebesgue measures. Indeed, the simplest illustration of scaling and scale invariance is to consider the (apparently "metric" in fact "measure") idea of dimension of a set of points as it often occurs in geophysics. The intuitive (and essentially correct) definition is that the "size" of the set n(L) at scale L is given by:

$$n(L) \propto L^D \tag{1}$$

where D is the dimension (e.g the length of a line $\propto$ L, the area of a plane, $\propto L^2$...or the number of in situ meteorological measuring stations on the earth in a circle radius L $\propto L^{1.75}$ (Lovejoy et al , 1986a,b), the distribution of raindrops on a piece of blotting paper $\propto L^{1.83}$ (Lovejoy and Schertzer , 1989a) and the occurrence of rain during a time period T $\propto T^{0.8}$ (Hubert and Carbonnel (1988), Tessier et al. (1989)) .... The "volume" (actually the measure of the set) is therefore a simple scaling (power law) function, and the dimension is important precisely because it is scale invariant (independent of L). We recall that the Hausdorff dimension D(A) of a (compact) set A may be defined by generalization to non-integer D of the divergence rule "the length of a surface is infinite, its volume is zero..."

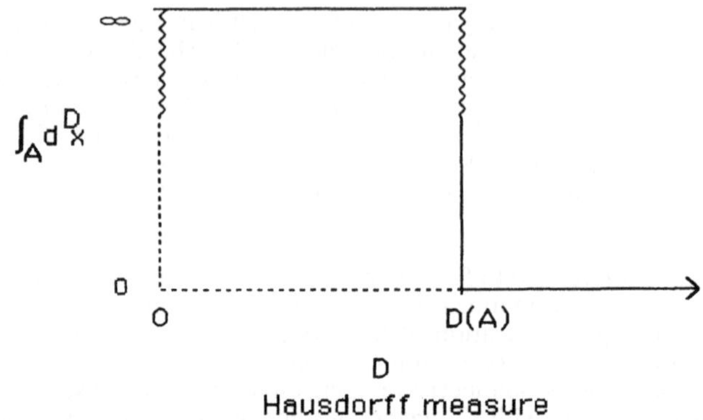

Fig. 2. Illustration of the divergence rule for Hausdorff measures, generalizing the divergence rule "the length of a surface is infinite, its volume is zero...". The transition at D=D(A), from infinity to zero, defines the Hausdorff dimension of the set A.

with the rather straightforward extensions (to non-integer D) of the d-Lebesgue measure (defined for integer d) to the D-dimensional Hausdorff measure. Thus we use the notation $\int_A d^D x$ for the D-dimensional Hausdorff measure of a (compact) set A and the Hausdorff dimension D(A) of A is hence defined by the divergence rule [1] (see Fig. 2):

$$\int_A d^D x = \infty, \text{ for } D<D(A); \int_A d^D x = 0 \text{ for } D>D(A) \tag{2}$$

One may note that the D(A)-measure of A is not necessarily finite and non-zero: some logarithmic corrections (exponents Δ_i on the i-th iterate of the logarithm[2], are "sub-dimensions") may be needed to obtain fineness and precise determination of the Hausdorff dimension (they may give rise to the appearance of 'lacunarity', eg. Smith et al. (1986)).

In other words, the "natural" framework for fields is not functional analysis (nor geometry...!), but (mathematical) measures. Indeed, the use of functions rather than the (more general) measures is often purely a mathematical artifact. It is unnecessarily stringent since really what we can empirically measure or describe is not in fact a value at a (geometrical) point, but rather a value on "nearly any" (small) set surrounding this point . Such considerations are at the basis of (mathematical) measure theory which renders quite precise the notion of "nearly any" set [3]. Thus geophysics seems more and more associated with singular measures with respect to Lebesgue measures[4]. Going a step further we will be interested in (random) *linear operators acting on measures*, as fundamental tools to study nonlinear variability. Such apparently abstract questions can be concretely addressed by apparently simple-minded geophysical models, but with rather general non-trivial consequences and properties corresponding to the more abstract tools mentioned above. In fact we will try to give two approaches to the same problem: one which is constructivist (the multiplicative processes) and the other one which is non-constructivist ("flux dynamics").

---

[1] It is easy to check that Eq. 1 is consistent with this divergence rule. Indeed, interpreting Eq. 1 as the fact that the number of cubes of size $l = L/\lambda$ needed to cover the fractal set will be of the order λ^D and since the D'-volume of an elementary cube is $l^{D'}$, it follows that the sum of their D'-volumes -of the order of the D-Hausdorff measure- will follow the indicated divergence rule.

[2] The volume of an elementary cube (l^D) is now 'corrected' by factors of the type $[\mathrm{Log}_i (1/l)]^{\Delta_i}$; where Log_i is the i-th iterate of the logarithm.

[3] It needs to be member of the "tribe", usually the borelian tribe...

[4] Regular (respectively singular) measures with respect to Lebesgue measures means that (almost everywhere) they correspond to a product of a density (a function) and a Lebesgue measure (resp. they don't).

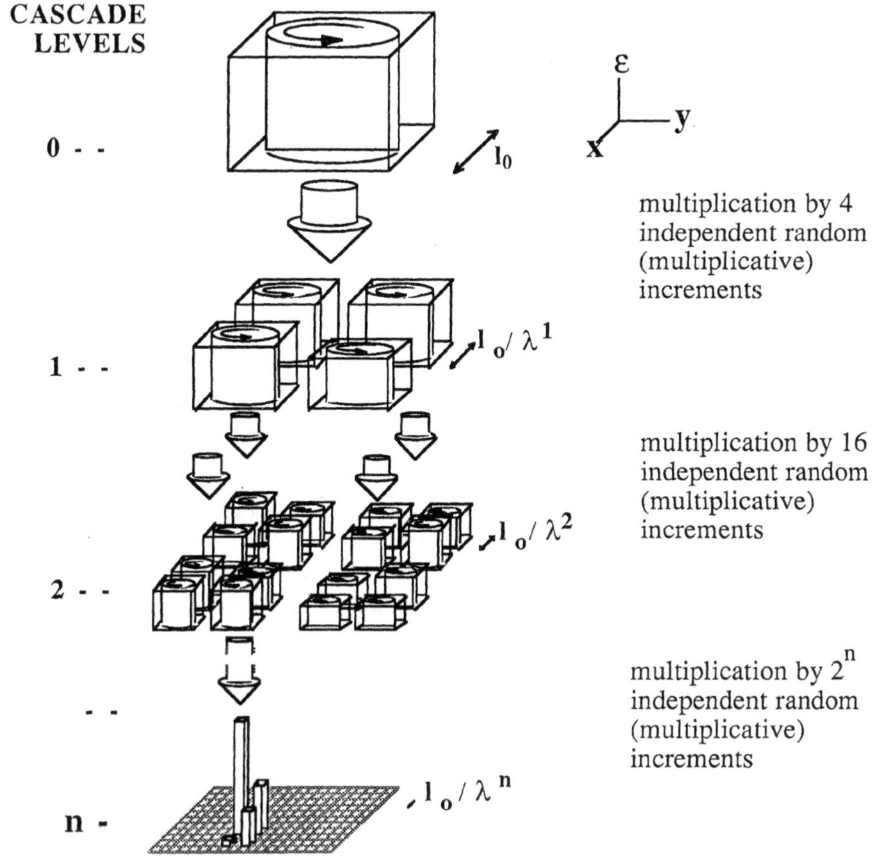

Fig. 3. A schematic diagram showing few steps of a discrete multiplicative cascade.process, here the "α-model" with two pure singularity orders γ^- (>-∞) and γ^+ (corresponding to the two values taken by the independent random increments, $\lambda^{\gamma^-}<1$ and $\lambda^{\gamma^+}>1$) leading to the appearance of mixed singularity orders γ ($\gamma^- \leq \gamma \leq \gamma^+$).

In both cases, the abstract object studied remains the scale invariant group of geodynamical equations (e. g. Navier-Stokes equations for flows).

The problematic of nonlinear variability, over wide range of scale, has been considered for a long time with respect to the mysterious turbulent behavior of fluid dynamics, especially their asymptotic (and universal) behavior when the dissipation length goes to zero (fully developed turbulence). Conceptual advances occurred using apparently simple models of self-similar cascades, as opposed to the frustratingly tedious developments of renormalization techniques... which still fail to grasp the intermittency problem. From very general considerations (going back to the famous poem of Richardson (1922)), the phenomenological models of turbulence have become more and more explicit (to quote a few: Novikov and Stewart (1964), Yaglom (1966), Mandelbrot (1974), Frisch et al. (1978)...; see for review Monin and Yaglom (1975)), sometimes in an overly restrictive manner. However their common theme -how does the energy flux spreads into smaller scales in successive steps while respecting a scale invariant conservation principle- is far from being restricted to turbulence since spreading into small scales is a general theme in Geophysics (from concentration of (passive) substances/scalar fields to the spreading of points on a strange attractor). Note that the notion of flux here is linked to flux through a scale, e.g. in Fourier space through the surface of a sphere of radius roughly proportional to this scale. In this sense we can speak of probability flux of points on a strange attractor, e.g. the flux of points flowing to smaller scales on this strange attractor, hence this generality of "flux dynamics" we will discuss, paralleling the classical thermodynamics, but with very strong divergences.... Note the basic fluxes will respect important scale conservation properties (e.g. the ensemble average of the energy flux ...) as some corresponding basic quantities (e. g. ensemble average of the energy) in the framework of thermodynamics... We will also discuss the related fields which are not constrained to such scale conservation (such as scalar concentration, velocity field...).

MULTIPLICATIVE PROCESSES AND FLUX DYNAMICS

The key assumption in phenomenological models of turbulence (which has recently became more explicit) is that successive steps define (independently) the fraction of the flux of energy distributed over smaller scales. Note that it is clear that the small scales cannot be perceived as adding some energy but can only (multiplicatively) modulate the energy passed down from larger scales (hence the lack of relevance of additive processes which nevertheless have been sometimes used to simulate such fields (e.g. Voss 1983)). Hence bare densities ε_λ, resulting from cascade processes from outer scale l_0 (which will be assumed equal to 1, without loss of generality) to l (the homogeneity scale)$=l_0/\lambda$ are multiplicatively defined (see Fig. 3 for illustration):

$$\varepsilon_{\lambda\lambda'} = T_\lambda\,(\varepsilon_{\lambda'})\;\varepsilon_\lambda \tag{3}$$

T_λ denotes a spatial contraction of ratio λ (>1). In the isotropic case, for any point $\underline{x}$; $T_\lambda\,\underline{x} = \underline{x}/\lambda$; for any set A: $T_\lambda(A)= \{T_\lambda\,\underline{x}\,/\underline{x}\in A\}$; for any function f :$T_\lambda\,[f(\underline{x})] = f(\lambda\underline{x})$; for any measure μ and any set A $\int_A d[T_\lambda\,(\mu)] = \int_{T_\lambda(A)} d\mu$ and more generally for any function f (i.e. not only for 1_A, the indicator function of the set A): $\int f d[T_\lambda\,(\mu)] = \int T_\lambda(f)d\mu$.

In case of (scaling) anisotropy, more involved contractions of space are required (see Schertzer and Lovejoy 1989b for a review). For instance, in order to avoid the classical but untenable 2D/3D dichotomy between large and small scale atmospheric dynamics, we have proposed an anisotropic scaling model of atmospheric dynamics (Schertzer and Lovejoy (1983, 1984, 1985a,b, 1987a,b), Lovejoy and Schertzer (1985), Levich and Tzvetkov[1] (1985)). In this model, the anisotropy introduced by gravity via the buoyancy force results in a differential stratification and a consequent modification of the effective dimension of space, involving a new "elliptical" dimension (d_{el}, see below), with resulting anisotropic shears. In isotropy, $d_{el}=3$, while in completely flat (stratified) flows, $d_{el}=2$. Empirical and theoretical evidence were given indicating d_{el} is rather the intermediate value $d_{el}\approx 23/9=2.5555...$ Indeed, the requisite scale changes T_λ can be far more general than simple magnifications or reductions. It turns out that practically the only restrictions on T_λ are that it has group properties, viz: $T_\lambda = \lambda^G$ where G is a the generator of the group of scale changing operations, and that the balls $E_\lambda=T_\lambda(S_1)$ (S_1 being the unit sphere) decreasing with λ,. In this "Generalized Scale Invariance" ("GSI"), G can be either a matrix -"linear GSI" (Schertzer and Lovejoy 1983, 1984) E_λ are self-affine ellipsoids rather than the self-similar spheres of the isotropic case (G=identity)-, or even a non-linear operator (see Schertzer and Lovejoy 1987b,

[1] They also pointed out the possible breaking of mirror symmetry for atmospheric dynamics, hence the importance of the associated helicity.

1989b for examples). In fact, (generalized) scale invariance allows a tremendous variety of behavior, since the only constraint on G turn out to be that every (generalized) eigenvalue of G has a non-negative real part[1] (Schertzer and Lovejoy 1985b): anisotropic ("elliptical") scale ϕ_{el}. is then defined by the volume of the E_λ (hence is a measurable property, rather than a metric property) This anisotropic framework allows rather straightforward extensions of Hausdorff measures and dimensions, still based on the divergence rule (Eq. 2), and the effective dimension of the space, the "elliptical" dimension d_{el} of the space, is simply the trace of G[2]: $d_{el}=Tr(G)$

Leaving additive (stochastic) processes (which had been used on purely geometrical grounds, e.g. fractional brownian motions -for modelling landscapes etc...- of the fractal geometry) to multiplicative processes, one encounters surprising properties: multiplicity of singularities, scaling and dimensions, rather than uniqueness. Let us discuss these properties briefly: a priori a fairly direct consequence of Eq. 3 is the existence of a generator for the one parameter multiplicative (semi-) group of the bare densities:

$$\varepsilon_\lambda = e^{\Gamma_\lambda} \tag{4}$$

where Γ_λ is its generator, still with the homogeneity scale $l = l_0/\lambda$. Γ_λ is a certain operator whose main properties (especially its asymptotic behavior, l going to 0 or λ going to ∞) we will analyze. Γ_λ should in *some sense* (see below) become independent of λ, i.e. approach its limit Γ as the homogeneity scale approaches zero. For positive values γ of Γ_λ, divergence of ε_λ occurs as λ tends to ∞, hence such values correspond to (algebraic) orders (γ) of singularity. Conversely negative values correspond rather to (algebraic) orders of regularity. Nevertheless for brevity, we will keep frequently the expression singularity (instead of regularity) in both cases to shorten the expressions. As soon as this generator does not reduce (Schertzer and Lovejoy 1983 and 1984) to only two values $\gamma^+>0$ and $\gamma^- = -\infty$ (the once celebrated "β-model" (Novikov and Stewart 1964, Mandelbrot 1974, Frisch et al. 1978) corresponding to the alternative of dead ($\lambda^{\gamma^-}=0$) or alive (and $\lambda^{\gamma^+}>1$) sub-eddies, the *pure singularity orders* γ^- and γ^+ lead to the appearance of *mixed singularity orders*. In particular, as soon as $\gamma^- > -\infty$ (the "α-model"), mixed singularities of different orders γ, are built up step by step (cf. Fig. 3) and bounded by γ^- and γ^+ ($\gamma^- \leq \gamma \leq \gamma^+$, γ^- and γ^+ corresponding then to the alternative of weak ($1>\lambda^{\gamma^-}>0$) or strong ($\lambda^{\gamma^+}>1$) sub-eddies). In other words, as pointed out by Schertzer and Lovejoy (1983), leaving the far too simple alternative dead or alive ("β-model") to weak or strong ("α-model") leads to the appearance of a full hierarchy of levels of survival, hence the possibility of a hierarchy of dimensions of the set of survivors for these different levels. In this α-model (as in more elaborate ones) the different orders of singularities (or survival levels) define the multiple scaling of the (one-point) probability distribution [3]:

$$\Pr(\varepsilon_\lambda \geq \lambda^\gamma) \approx N_\lambda(\gamma)/N_\lambda \approx \lambda^{-c(\gamma)} \tag{5}$$

where $N_\lambda(\gamma)$ is the number of occurrences of singularity order greater than γ, N_λ is the total number of events examined. We temporarily postpone discussion on the accuracy of the

---

1 i.e. inf Re $\sigma(G)\geq 0$; $\sigma(G)$ being the (generalized) spectrum of G (acting on $\Re^d$): $\sigma(G)= \{\mu \in C \mid G-\mu 1$ non-invertible on $C X \Re^d\}$.

2 However, G needs to be correctly normalized as discussed by Schertzer and Lovejoy 1987b.

3 Note we are studying a whole family of measures defined by just one density, this the reason why our notation can't reduce to the very specialized notation (α, $f(\alpha)$) introduced by Halsey et al. (1986), since they refer at one dimension (the dimension d of the embedding space) and the corresponding specialized measure. Hence, $\alpha = d-\gamma$ as singularity of the d-dimensional Lebesgue measure, and $f(\alpha))=d-c(\gamma)$.

approximations indicated in Eq. 5 -e. g. the sub-multiplicity problem already pointed out by Schertzer and Lovejoy (1987a-b), and presentation of a more general and rigorous definition of multiple scaling (which is not restricted to one-point distributions, the latter being of course incomplete statistical descriptors of a field)- and rather convenient empirical analysis technique to test the the probability distribution multiple scaling (PDMS, introduced by Lavallée et al 1989) and to determine $c(\gamma)$. For the moment, we would like to insist on the interest of such a formula in gaining insights in different fundamental aspects of multiple scaling.

Obviously singularities will prevent convergence in the usual sense, i.e. even if the ε_λ are rather smooth functions (for a given λ), they do not admit a function as their limit. Indeed, their limit will be rather defined by the limit of the fluxes (i.e. integrals of the density) over differents sets. One may note also that N_λ will be proportional to λ^d -the number of boxes, size λ^{-1}, required to cover the relevant region of the embedding space (which can be fractal...) of dimension d (integer or not)- multiplied by the number (N_i) of realizations (e.g. images) examined. Hence, when $c(\gamma)$ is smaller than d it has a rather immediate meaning of a codimension[1] = $d\text{-}d(\gamma)$; $N_\lambda(\gamma) \approx \lambda^{d(\gamma)}$, where $d(\gamma)$ (>0) is the dimension of the fraction of the space occupied by the singularities of order greater than γ on "nearly" each realization. Larger values of $c(\gamma)$, which have often been disregarded, correspond to more rare events: singularities of orders which "nearly" never appear on a realization. At first glance they seem to correspond to negative dimensions, sometimes mysteriously called "latent dimensions". However, there is no mystery at all, since $c(\gamma)$ still has a meaning of a codimension: no any longer in an individual realization, but in the subspace of the (infinite dimensional) probability/state space that our finite sample size enables us to explore by a cut of finite dimension. Indeed the dimension of this subspace can be estimated as $d + d_s$, where d_s - termed as the "sampling dimension" (at scale λ^{-1})- is estimated by writing the number of images (or realizations) N_i as λ^{d_s}. Indeed when $c(\gamma)$ is smaller than $d + d_s$, γ occupies a fraction of the accessible subspace having dimension $d(\gamma) = d + d_s - c(\gamma)$. Of course, increasing the number of images, hence the sampling dimension, allows us to encounter more easily higher singularities occupying a fraction of the accessible subspace, with well defined dimension ($d(\gamma) = d + d_s - c(\gamma) > 0$). The corresponding mathematical subtlety underneath the important difference between cases $c(\gamma)<d$ and $c(\gamma)>d$, is the "almost surely" or not properties, the latter do correspond to extremely rare events.

However, these extremely rare events are in fact of overwhelming importance since they imply divergence of statistical moments, i.e.these singularities prevent convergence of all statistical orders: by integrating the density over a set A with dimension D (to obtain the flux through A), the resulting smoothing may be sufficient so that convergence is obtained for low order statistics, but not for orders higher than a critical order h_D of divergence. Indeed, let us point out this rather immediate consequence of Eq. 5, by introducing first the trace (paralleling the definition of the trace of the density operator in Quantum Statistical Mechanics, see below) of the hth power of the flux Π_λ over an (averaging) set A of dimension D (integration performed with resolution λ^{-1} on A_λ, A measured with the same resolution):

$$\mathrm{tr}_{A_\lambda}\, \varepsilon_\lambda^{\,h} = \int_{A_\lambda} \varepsilon_\lambda^{\,h}\, d^{hD}x$$

$$\approx \sum_{A_\lambda} \varepsilon_\lambda^{\,h}\, \lambda^{-hD} \qquad (6)$$

[1] In particular, in the case of the β-model there is a unique codimension c, characterizing the fraction of the space occupied by alive sub-eddies. The parameter β is λ^{-c}.

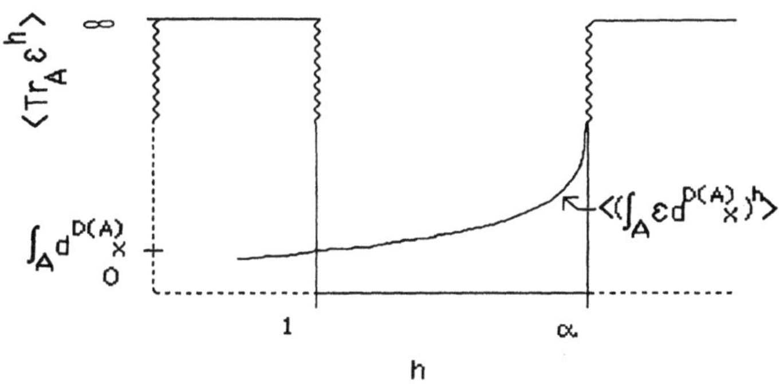

Fig. 4. the twin divergence of trace-moments.

a-priori any singularity of order higher than D, may create divergences of the trace but are extremely rare (since their frequency of occurrence tends to zero as $\lambda^{-c(\gamma)}$). One may evaluate the importance of these by considering their statistics (trace-moments introduced by Schertzer and Lovejoy 1987 a-b) for an arbitrary singularity of order γ:

$$Tr_{A_\lambda} \varepsilon_\lambda^h = \langle tr_{A_\lambda} \varepsilon_\lambda^h \rangle \geq N_\lambda(\gamma)\, \lambda^{h\gamma} \lambda^{-hD} = \lambda^{[h\gamma - c(\gamma)]-(h-1)D} \quad (7)$$

thus diverges, for some orders of singularity, as soon as:

$$K(h) \geq (h-1)D \quad (8)$$

where:

$$K(h) \equiv \sup_\gamma[h\gamma - c(\gamma)] \quad \{\text{hence: } c(\gamma) \equiv \sup_h[h\gamma - K(h)]\}$$
$$\text{or: } h = dc(\gamma)/d\gamma,\ K(h) = h\gamma - c(\gamma) \quad \{\gamma = dK(h)/dh,\ c(\gamma) = h\gamma - K(h)\} \quad (9)$$

On the one hand, Eq. 9 corresponds to the Legendre transform of $c(\gamma)$ as pointed out by Frisch and Parisi (1985), Halsey et al. (1986) and as the resulting K(h) does correspond -by the method of steepest descent to the exponent of the moment of the density of the flux (at least to first order, i.e. omitting logarithmic corrections):

$$\langle \varepsilon_\lambda^h \rangle = \lambda^{K(h)} \langle \varepsilon_1^h \rangle = e^{K(h)\mathrm{Log}(\lambda)} \langle \varepsilon_1^h \rangle \quad (10)$$

the Legendre transform establishes a well defined relation between orders of singularities and orders of moments. Note that conservation in ensemble average of the flux requires conservation of densities ($\langle \varepsilon_\lambda \rangle = \langle \varepsilon_1 \rangle$) thus K(1)=0. On the other hand, as pointed out by Schertzer and Lovejoy 1983, the divergence rule, Eq. 8, introduces a hierarchy of critical codimensions C(h), simply defined as:

$$C(h)\,(h-1) = K(h) \quad (11)$$

since the former divergence rule (Eq. 8) can be rewritten ($\lambda \to \infty$, $\varepsilon_\lambda \to \varepsilon$):

$$Tr_A\, \varepsilon^h = \infty,\ D < C(h),\ \text{i. e. } h > h_D,\ C(h_D) = D \quad \{\gamma_D = dK(h)/dh|_{h_D}\} \quad (12)$$

where h_D is the critical moment order, and γ_D the critical singularity order, at which divergence of trace moments of the flux on the set A of dimension D occurs. For $h_D>1$ it does imply the divergence of the usual statistical moments, since:

$$Tr_{A\lambda}\, \varepsilon_\lambda^{h} \leq \langle \Pi_\lambda^{h}(A) \rangle \text{ any } h\geq 1 \tag{13}$$

Conversely, as discussed more thoroughly by Schertzer and Lovejoy 1987b, convergence of statistical moment of order h (h>1) is assured by the convergence of the hth trace moment ; for h<1 divergence of the trace moment implies degeneracy of the flux (the set A has a so small dimension ($D<C_1\equiv C(1)$) that almost surely the flux is null). We thus obtain a twin divergence rule for the trace moments (represented in Fig. 4) implying non-degeneracy of the flux ($h\leq 1$) and divergence of the flux ($h\geq h_D>1$). Note that non-degeneracy of the flux implies conservation of the ensemble average flux[1]:

$$\langle\varepsilon_\lambda\rangle = \langle\varepsilon_1\rangle = 1 \text{ and } D>C_1\ (\equiv C(1)) \Rightarrow \langle\Pi_\lambda(A)\rangle = \langle\Pi_1(A)\rangle\ (\equiv \int_A d^D x\,) \tag{14}$$

Note that C_1 ($\equiv C(1) = K'(1)$, due to Eq. 11) is at same time the codimension of singularities contributing to the average (h=1) and the order of these singularities, since by virtue of Legendre transform it is the fixed point of $c(\gamma)$:

$$c(\gamma) = \gamma \Rightarrow \gamma = C_1\ (\equiv C(1) \equiv K'(1)) \tag{15}$$

Multiple scaling (for the statistical moments) corresponds to the fact K(h) is no longer linear ($= C_1(h-1)$) as in the β-model but depends on a whole hierarchy of codimensions C(h) ($\neq C_1$, for $h\neq 1$). As the first characteristic function (or moment generating function) $Z_\lambda(h)$ and second characteristic function (or cumulant generating function) $K_\lambda(h)$ of the generator Γ_λ, are by definition:

$$Z_\lambda(h) = e^{K_\lambda(h)} = \langle e^{h\Gamma_\lambda}\rangle \quad (\equiv \langle\varepsilon_\lambda^{h}\rangle) \tag{16}$$

multiple scaling corresponds to algebraic divergence ($\lambda\rightarrow\infty$) of $Z_\lambda(h)$ and thus to logarithmic divergence of $K_\lambda(h)$ (see Eq. 10), a fundamental property we will exploit below. Note here, we are dealing with characteristic functions in the Laplace sense, since $Z_\lambda(h)$ is obtained by Laplace transform (instead of Fourier transform) of the probability distribution. In order to make some crude connections with statistical physics, Γ_λ can be considered as the negative of a pseudo-hamiltonian ($-H_\lambda=\Gamma_\lambda$), with h as the inverse of temperature (h=1/T, the Boltzmann constant being set equal to 1), Z_λ is called a partition function and the "free-energy" (F_λ) would correspond to $K_\lambda(h)/h$. More generally (in statistical Quantum Mechanics), the "density operators" $\rho_\lambda = e^{-H_\lambda/T}$ (corresponding to $\varepsilon_\lambda^{h} = e^{h\Gamma_\lambda}$) are considered along with their trace over different sub-spaces of states, each trace corresponding to a partition function. The densities ρ_λ and ε_λ are both defined on a fairly abstract space [eg. in quantum mechanics the space of wave functions]. The trace moments correspond to the trace of the density operator but here on the space of the measures of (compact) supports (the different sets A, used for averaging). Finally, as $c(\gamma)$ characterize the logarithm of the probability distribution of Γ_λ, they correspond to entropies (S_λ) (of the state γ), and indeed the Legendre duality between $K_\lambda(h)$ and $c(\gamma)$ does correspond to the same duality between $F_\lambda(T)/T$ and $S_\lambda(E)$ (the conjugate variables being 1/T and the energy E). Let us emphasize that in both cases, this property simply results from the fact that the Laplace transform of the

---

[1] As it corresponds to a "martingale "property, it assures a "weak measurable' convergence of the process (see Schertzer and Lovejoy 1987b for discussion).

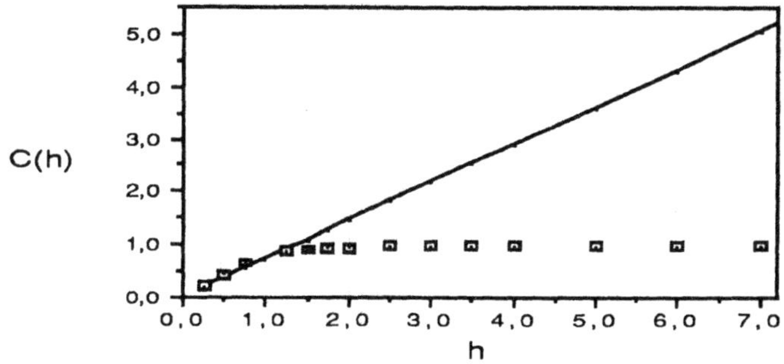

Fig. 5. Spurious scaling obtained with a Gaussian generator, the theoretical line is the solid line $C(h) \propto h$, squares are observed points and lead to the spurious appearance of bounded $C(h)<C_\infty<\infty$!

probability distribution[1] (or conversely of the partition function) reduces to Legendre transform of the exponents. In order to develop a nonconstructive approach, which can be called "fluxdynamics", considering ε *per se* (the limit ε of the ε_λ, at zero homogeneity scale, λ going to infinity) as a linear operator on the measures (converting the D-volume, D being the dimension of A, integer or not, into the flux over the set A) we need to investigate some basic properties of this limit and its generator.

WILD/SMOOTH MULTIFRACTALITY AND CANONICAL/MICRO-CANONICAL CONSERVATION

In this section we emphasize the consequences of divergence of moments before proceeding to characterizing the generator. Divergence of moments is a wild statistical behavior very far from gaussianity (or quasi-gaussianity), and is due to "hyperbolic" (algebraic) fall-off of the probability distribution:

$$\Pr(|X|\geq s) \approx s^{-\alpha}\ (s>>1) \Rightarrow \text{any } h\geq\alpha : \langle|X|^h\rangle=\infty \qquad (17)$$

It turns out, that among these "hyperbolic" random variables some are rather well defined, since they are mostly (but surprising!) generalizations of gaussian laws. These are the Lévy stable random variables ($0<\alpha<2$) satisfying "generalized central limit theorems", hence intervening in additive processes as discussed in subsequent sections and especially with the help of Appendix A dealing with a particular type of them. However we (Schertzer and Lovejoy 1985) already used the expression "hyperbolic intermittency" to describe the effect of this strong variability for a wider range of α (i.e. $\alpha\geq2$), as we pointed out this divergence as a general consequence of multiplicative processes and that the corresponding critical order of divergence $\alpha = h_D$ (theoretically, determined by Eq. 12) has no absolute bound. Waymire and Gupta (1985) have used the expression "fat-tailed" for such (asymptotically algebraic) distributions, and "long-tailed" for the log-normal law, to distinguish these distributions from standard exponential "thin-tailed" distributions. In the preceding section we showed that hyperbolic behavior is expected from averaging a multifractal field on a set of too small dimension D. It has been empirically estimated in a variety of meteorological fields: $h_D\approx5$, for temperature (Lovejoy and Schertzer 1986a,b, Ladoy et al 1986), $h_D\approx 1.66$ in changes in storm integrated rainrates (Lovejoy 1981), $h_D\approx1.06$ in radar reflectivity factors of rain (Schertzer and Lovejoy 1987), and respectively

[1] It implies also the convexity of K(h) (or F((T)/T), hence of $c(\gamma)$ (or S(E)).

$h_D \approx 5$ and 3.33 for wind speed and potential temperatures, $h_D \approx 1$ for the Richardson number (Schertzer and Lovejoy 1985)... An important consequence of the divergence of statistical moments is that the usual estimation procedures no longer work efficiently, but rather exhibit spurious (or pseudo) scaling exponents. Indeed, these methods are based extensively on the law of large numbers which blows up due to the statistical divergences. Fig. 5 shows how misleading can be the appearance of spurious scaling, on a well known simulated field: classical estimation will lead to bounded codimensions C(h)... even though the true C(h) increases linearly with h! Conversely, clear understanding of spurious scaling can be used to explain most of the behavior of certain data. For instance we argue (Schertzer and Lovejoy 1983,1984, 1985, Lovejoy,and Schertzer, 1986a) that the presumed critical moment order $h_D \approx 5$ for wind speed, may well explain the overall behavior of the observed scalings exponents of the structure functions of the velocity field collected by Anselmet et al. (1984)!

A direct consequence of the hyperbolic behavior of the dressed densities $\varepsilon_{\lambda, D}$ (obtained by D-dimensional averaging, at scale λ^{-1}) is that their singularity codimensions $c_D(\gamma)$ are quite different from their bare counterparts $c(\gamma)$, since they become linear for orders greater than the critical singularity order γ_D:

$$c_D(\gamma) \approx h_D(\gamma - \gamma_D),\ \gamma \geq \gamma_D \tag{18}$$

this is an immediate consequence of hyperbolic behavior as described by Eq. 17, as well as from the corresponding divergence of characteristic function ($K_{\lambda, D}(h)=\infty$, $h \geq h_D$) and the fact that Legendre transform breaks down[1] for linear functions. Conversely, for the same reasons, K(h) becomes linear as soon as there is an upper bound (γ_0) of the singularity order:

$$c(\gamma) \rightarrow \infty, \text{ when } \gamma \rightarrow \gamma_0 \Leftrightarrow K(h) \approx \gamma_0 h\ (h>>1), \text{ hence } C_\infty = \gamma_0. \tag{19}$$

However, the hyperbolic behavior is expected only for singularities of order greater than the dimension of the averaging set A. It obviously can't occur if we are imposing a much more strict conservation than conservation in ensemble average i.e. a strict conservation on A of the flux in each realization, since we have in the latter case:

$$\varepsilon_\lambda\, \lambda^{-D} \leq \Pi_\lambda(A) = \Pi_1(A) \tag{20}$$

Paralleling, once again classical thermodynamics, one can speak respectively of canonical conservation (or cascade) in the former case, and micro-canonical conservation (or cascade) in the latter (see for instance[2] Benzi et al. (1984) Pietronero and Siebesma (1986), Sreenivasan et Meneveau (1988)). Micro-canonical conservation assumption has many defects: not only we are usually dealing with open systems (as in thermodynamics), but this assumption turns out to be quite demanding. Indeed it requires in fact conservation at every scale, so we can even speak of "*pico-canonical*" assumption: strict conservation is implied not only on the largest scale of A, but on the smallest scale due to scaling behavior of the consider process! Hence, we have rather sharp distinctions[3] between wild multifractality associated with canonical conservation on the one hand, and smooth multifractality associated with micro- (in fact pico-) canonical conservation.

---

[1] A rather direct consequence of the geometrical interpretation of the Legendre transform as the envelope of the tangencies.

[2] In fact a micro-canonical version of the α–model is often called a "random β–model". The latter expression (trying to designate that the fraction of the space occupied active sub-eddies is randomly chosen) is somewhat misleading, since the "β–model" is already a random model...

[3] On the other hand, one may note that micro-canonical conservation refers to a given set and dimension: it no longer holds on sets of smaller dimensions. Hence, micro-canonical conservation is at the same time too precise and too vague...

CHARACTERIZATION OF THE GENERATOR AND UNIVERSALITY CLASSES

Since a (multiplicative) one-parameter group is involved, the characterization of its generator Γ -the limit of the Γ_λ - is fundamental. Corresponding to the definition of the Γ_λ (Eq. 4), we have, at least formally:

$$\varepsilon \equiv \text{limit}_{\lambda \to \infty}(\varepsilon_\lambda) = e^{\Gamma} \tag{21}$$

One may note also we have (corresponding to Eq. 4) the following "dynamical" (and somewhat formal) equation for the ε_λ:

$$\partial\varepsilon_\lambda/\partial\lambda = \gamma_\lambda\, \varepsilon_\lambda \;\; ; \gamma_\lambda = \partial\Gamma_\lambda/\partial\lambda \tag{22}$$

where γ_λ is the infinitesimal generator. This equation gives the cascade dynamical sense when we are studying a cascade on a space-time domain[1]. As discused by Schertzer and Lovejoy (1987a-b, 1989a), the generator must satisfy four main properties:

i) Γ is a random noise,with infinite band-width $[1, \infty]$. The bare or (finite resolution) generator Γ_λ are rather to be understood as the corresponding filtered noises restricted to the wave number band $[1, \lambda]$.

ii) the second characteristic function (or cumulant generating function) $K_\lambda(h)$ of the bare generator Γ_λ has a logarithmic divergence ($\lambda \to 0$) in order to assure multiple scaling, i.e.:

$$K_\lambda(h) \approx \text{Log}(\lambda)\; K(h). \tag{23}$$

iii) in order to have some finite moments of positive orders ($Z_\lambda(h)$ and $K_\lambda(h) < \infty$ for $h > 0$), the probability distribution of positive fluctuations of the bare generators Γ_λ must fall off more quickly than exponentially.

iv) the generator needs to be normalized ($K_\lambda(1)=0$) in order to assure (canonical) conservation of the flux.

It turns out that properties i) and ii) correspond (Schertzer and Lovejoy 1987b) to the fact that the (generalized) spectrum $E_\Gamma(k)$ of the generator should be then proportional to the inverse of the wave-number:

$$E_\Gamma(k) \propto k^{-1} \tag{24}$$

since the characteristic function will correspond to its integral. Such noises are often called "1/f noises" or "pink noises". Usually, one considers only gaussian noises or quasi-gaussian noises. We have already indicated that there is no fundamental reason to restrict our attention to quasi-gaussianity, and thus consider hyperbolic noises. Indeed, among the hyperbolic noises, Lévy stable noises ($0<\alpha<2$) are particularly important, since they define a family of universal generators as we will discuss latter. However, the third property indicated, which is due to the fact the moments of ε_λ, are Laplace transforms of the probability density of Γ_λ, lead us to restrict our attention to extremely unsymmetric hyperbolic noises, since we can accept a hyperbolic fall-off of the probability distribution only for the negative fluctuation of Γ_λ. Considering Lévy stable noises (or hyperbolic noises $0<\alpha<2$), one has to generalize the notion of spectrum (the usual one diverges, since it corresponds to a second order moment) as discussed by Schertzer and Lovejoy (1987a-b, 1989). The fourth property is easy to satisfy since if Γ'_λ is not yet normalized, we can deduce a normalized generator Γ_λ by:

$$e^{\Gamma_\lambda} = e^{\Gamma'_\lambda} / \langle e^{\Gamma'_\lambda} \rangle \tag{25}$$

[1] The scaling is usually then strongly anisotropic on the space time domain.

however, as we will insist latter this not the unique way to normalize a generator, since a fractional integration may achieve the same normalization.

Note that the properties of the generator stressed above are on the one hand quite different from the usual properties of (pseudo-) Hamiltonians, especially their scale dependency[1]. On the other hand, they give a precise definition of multiple scaling, especially by requisite properties of the second characteristic functional or of the (more or less) equivalent of the free energy (which might be called "free flux"?).

As in additive processes, one may look for universality classes in the sense that for whatever generator is used (here the flux generator, the infinitesimal increment in the additive ones) under repeated iteration -through (renormalized) multiplication or addition- it may converge to a well defined limit which depends on relatively few of its characteristics. Appendix A first recalls the classical (but not well enough known) results for additive processes associated with generalized central limit theorem, here the classes and "basins of attraction" are primarily[2] defined by the Levy index α, the critical moment order (i.e. higher order moments diverge) of the increments

One has to be careful about the definitions of convergence and universality, since it has been obscured by some misplaced claims (Mandelbrot, 1989)that such universality cannot exist in multifractal processes. Indeed, it is easy to check that repeated multiplications corresponding to a process with fixed discretization (i.e. a fixed elementary ratio of scale $\lambda_0>1$) fails to create a simplifying convergence to universal generators (eg. the α-model remains an α-model), and it seems that this is the reason why Kolmogorov (1962) postulated a lognormal behavior, without postulating convergence[3] to it . However, if we are discussing continuous cascade processes, i. e. processes which have an infinite number of cascade steps over any *finite* range of scales (i.e. elementary ratio of scale $\lambda_0 \to 1_+$), we are facing quite a different problem. Indeed, such processes may be obtain from a discrete model (finite number of discrete steps over the given ratio of scales) by introducing more and more steps up to an infinity of infinitesimal ones and keeping some properties (e.g. the variance of the generator on this given scale ratio). Obviously while such properties are best mathematically studied directly on the generator, we should also establish the physical relevance of doing so. Indeed, -generalizing the test field method introduced in homogeneous turbulence by Kraichnan (1971)- we may introduce new intermediate scales first as rather passive components, advected by the others, and then include them in the whole set of "active" scales. In this respect, the passive scalar example studied by Schertzer and Lovejoy 1987a is illustrative: the density of the flux (φ) controlling the passive scalar diffusion is a product powers of densities the energy flux (ε) and the scalar scalar variance flux (χ) -mainly from dimensional arguments, we have: $\varphi=\chi^{3/2}\varepsilon^{-1/2}$. In the first step, χ and ε can be considered as rather independent, then in the second step considered of the same type, and identify φ as a more complete ε. Hence, we are multiplying densities by densities, or simply adding generators to generators...

Now, we have to investigate which classes of generator are stable and attractive under addition and such that for the corresponding density ε_λ will at least converge for some positive order moments (i. e. the probability density of the generator admits a Laplace transform as already discussed). Either we examine those Levy stables -usually studied in a Fourier framework (e.g. Lévy (1924, 1925, 1954), Gnedenko and Kolmogorov (1954), Gnedenko (1969), Feller (1971), Zolotarev (1986)- which also satisfy a Laplace transform or

---

1 However, the related log divergence may be loosely understood as a phase transition at low temperature (i.e. considering the h Log(λ) as the inverse of the temperature 1/T.

2 There are two subsidiary parameters which are fixed in our case: the 'location parameter' (fixed by the normalization constraint) and the 'skewness' (set to its extremal value -1 by the condition iii, as explained below). The third subsidiary parameter, the 'scale parameter' is defined by C_1.

3 Yaglom (1966) seems to be less cautious on that point.

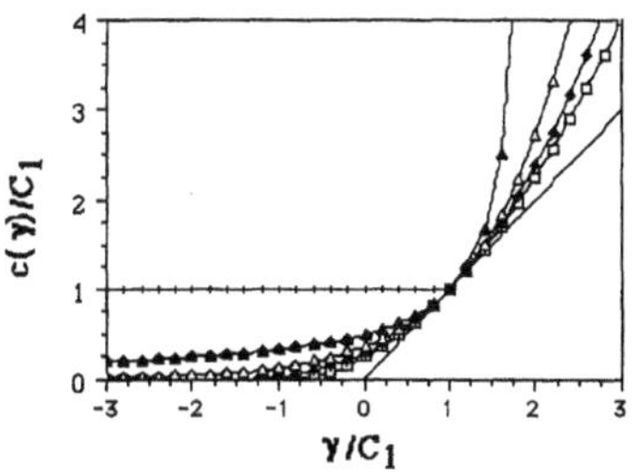

α=2 (–□–), α=1.5 (–◆–), α=1 (–△–), α= .5(–▲–), α=0 (—)

Fig. 6a. universal (bare) singularities codimension $c(\gamma)/C_1$ corresponding to the five classes; here α=2, 1.5, 1, .5, 0.

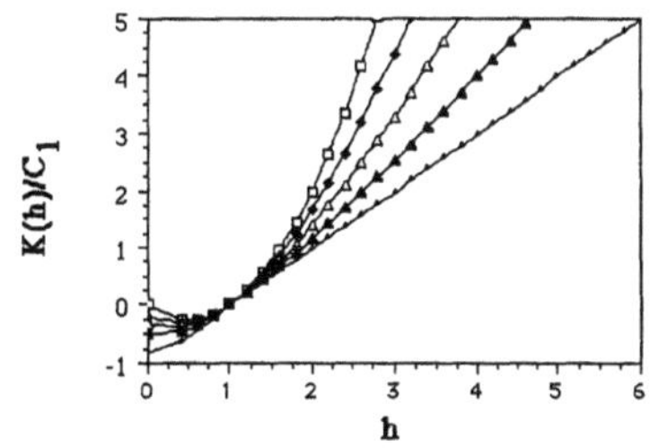

α=2 (–□–), α=1.5 (–◆–), α=1 (–△–), α= .5(–▲–), α=0 (—)

Fig. 6b. universal (bare) second characteristic function $K(h)/C_1$ ($\equiv h.F(h)/C_1$, F(h) being the "free energy"), corresponding to the five classes; here α=2, 1.5, 1, .5, 0.

we directly study the generalized central limit theorem in the Laplace framework, as done in Appendix A[1]. In any case, it is immediately clear that the restriction imposed by Laplace transform is that we need (as condition iii) already discussed) a steeper than an algebraic fall-off of the probability distribution for the (positive) orders of singularities, hence with the exception of the Gaussian case (α=2), we have to employ strongly asymmetric, "extremal" Levy laws. In our case, we are not considering random variables but noises, however the same characterization are relevant (characteristic functionals intervene instead of characteristic functions).

Let us examine the universal generator classes (from α =2 down to α =0), recalling that the corresponding characteristic function K(h) and codimension functions $c(\gamma)$ estimated by Legendre transform, are (Schertzer and Lovejoy, 1987a-b, 1989a) since h^{α}/α and $\gamma^{\alpha'}/\alpha'$ are Legendre dual ($0\leq\alpha\leq 2$, $1/\alpha+1/\alpha'=1$):

$$\alpha\neq 1:\ K(h) = \frac{C_1\alpha'}{\alpha}(h^{\alpha}-h) \qquad \text{(only for } h\geq 0 \text{ when } \alpha<2;\ =\infty \text{ for } h<0); \tag{26}$$

$$\alpha=1:\ K(h)= C_1\, h\, \mathrm{Log}(h) \tag{27}$$

and (restricted to increasing branches when $\alpha<2$, since $dc/d\gamma \equiv h$):

$$\alpha\neq 1: \quad c(\gamma) = C_1\left(\frac{\gamma}{C_1\alpha'} + \frac{1}{\alpha}\right)^{\alpha'} \qquad (dc/d\gamma>0 \text{ when } \alpha<2) \tag{28}$$

$$\alpha=1: \quad c(\gamma)= C_1 \exp\left(\frac{\gamma}{C_1}-1\right) \tag{29}$$

We recall that C1 ($\equiv C(1) = K'(1)$) is the fixed point of $c(\gamma)$, being at same time the codimension of singularities contributing to the average and the order of these singularities (see Eq. 15). We may introduce another convenient characteristic order of singularity :

$$\gamma_0 = -\frac{C_1\alpha'}{\alpha} \tag{30}$$

---

[1] One may note that only the case $0<\alpha<1$ is classically treated by Laplace transform, Appendix A extends the result for $1\leq\alpha\leq 2$.

γ_0[1] is either the lower bound (α>1, α'>2) of fractal singularities ($c(\gamma)=0$, i.e. singularities occupying all the space) or (α<1, α'<0) the upper bound of singularities ($c(\gamma)=\infty$, i.e. unreachable singularities). It is then also the slope of the tangent at the origin of K(h) ($\gamma_0=K'(0)$; $\alpha>1$) or of the asymptote ($\gamma_0=K'(\infty)$; $\alpha<1$) We may then rewrite Eq. 28 ($\gamma\geq\gamma_0$ when $2\geq\alpha>1$; $\gamma<\gamma_0$ when $\alpha<1$) as:

$$\alpha\neq1,\ \gamma_0=-\frac{C_1\alpha'}{\alpha},\ c_0=c(\gamma):\ c(\gamma)=c_0\left(1-\frac{\gamma}{\gamma_0}\right)^{\alpha'} \tag{31}$$

One may note that the $c(\gamma)$ introduced here corresponds rather to the probability density, instead of the probability distribution. Both are equal when $c(\gamma)$ is increasing (eg. for extreme singularities: $\gamma>>0$), but obviously decreasing $c(\gamma)$ (eg. for extreme regularities: $\gamma<<0$) of the probability is offset for the probability distribution by its minimum value (see below the role of γ_0 for the gaussian case). On the other hand, the $c(\gamma)$ don't coincide with the log of the probability density due to (at least!) some logarithmic terms (corresponding to sub-codimensions) which are missed by the Legendre transform, but are of no fundamental importance (as easily seen by considering the exact log of the probability density).

Let us review briefly the main properties of the five classes (α going from 2 to 0, hence α' going from 2 to ∞, then from $-\infty$ to 0), from the gaussian generator to the β-model, crossing three Levy cases (see the corresponding Fig. 6a and Fig. 6b):

i) $\alpha=\alpha'=2$: the Gaussian generator is almost everywhere (almost surely) continuous. K(h) and $c(\gamma)$ are parabolae, $c(\gamma)$ is tangent on the γ axis at $\gamma_0=-C_1$, C(h) is linear (= C1 h). The corresponding $c(\gamma)$ of the probability distribution, will remain on the γ axis for $\gamma\leq\gamma_0$.

ii) $2>\alpha>1$ ($2<\alpha'<\infty$): the Lévy generator is almost everywhere (almost surely) discontinuous and is extremely asymmetric. The lower bound γ_0 (=-C1 a'/α) of fractal singularities is decreasing from $-C_1$ to $-\infty$, as α decreases from 2 to 1. $c(\gamma)$ will remain on the γ axis for $\gamma\leq\gamma_0$ and is thus strongly asymmetric (even for the probability density, since $K_\lambda(h)=\infty$ for h<0), the large orders of singularities order give rise to a steeper algebraic branch than before ($c(\gamma)\propto\gamma^{\alpha'}$, $\alpha'>2$).

iii) $1>\alpha>0$ ($-\infty<\alpha'<0$) the generator is everywhere (almost surely) discontinuous, and is obtained in fact by a one-sided unnormalized generator hence the orders of singularities are bounded by γ_0 (thus decreasing, with α, from $-\infty$ to C_1), which defines thus a vertical asymptote, and now the algebraic asymptote intervenes for the large orders of regularity ($\gamma\to-\infty$, $c(\gamma)\propto\gamma^{-|\alpha'|}$). As the singularities are bounded, the same occurs for the hierarchy of critical codimension C(h) of the different moments, since we can now smooth out the highest singularity on a set A of high enough dimension D. Indeed γ_0 bounds also C(h) (see Eq. 19), hence to obtain convergence of every (positive order) moment of the flux it suffices that: $D>C_\infty=\gamma_0=\frac{C_1|\alpha'|}{\alpha}$.

iv) $\alpha=1$ ($\alpha'=\pm\infty$!): it is the special in-between case, associated with the ambiguity on α' (note the opposite occurs to $\gamma_0=\pm-\infty$), this corresponds in fact to a special case of quasi-stability (or not strict stability) briefly outlined in Appendix A. Note that the curves K(h) and $c(\gamma)$ are nevertheless the limits ($\alpha\to1\pm$, $\alpha'\to\pm-\infty$) of the two preceding cases, especially

[1] This is the negative of the former γ_0 introduced by Schertzer and Lovejoy 1987a-b. The change of sign is required to obtain directly the bounds of singularities/regularities as explained.

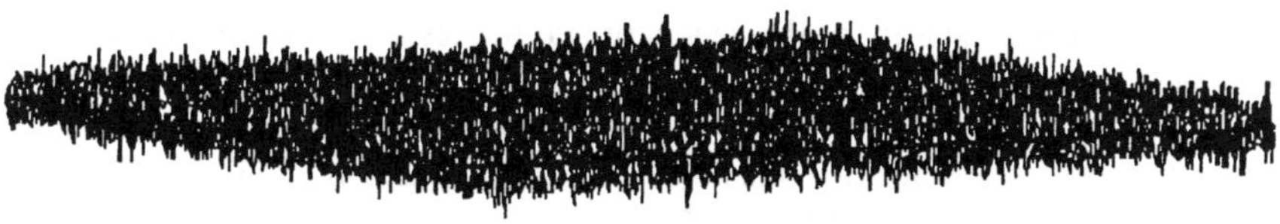

Fig. 7a. a gaussian white-noise (α=2), fluctuations are symmetric.

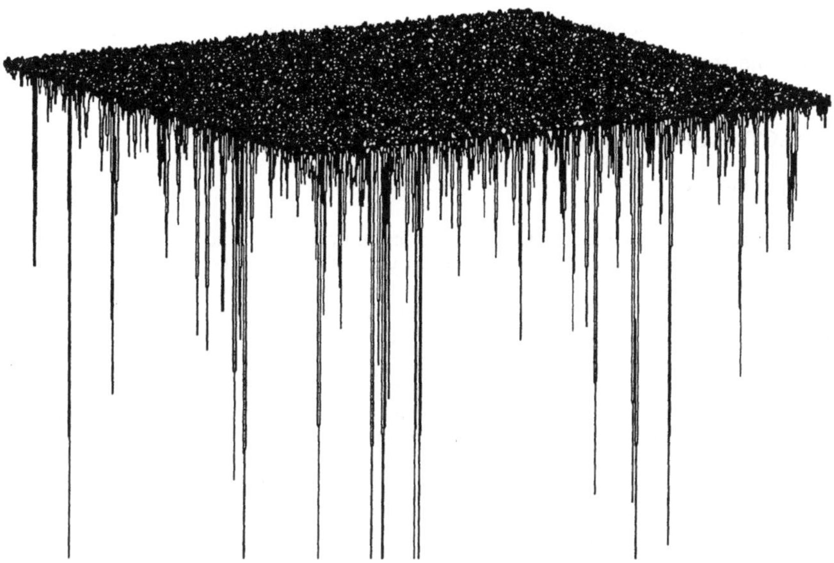

Fig. 7b. an extremal Lévy white-noise (α=1.5), fluctuations are extremely asymmetric: only *negative* hyperbolic jumps are allowed for the generator, "digging" wild regularities ("holes")

the former algebraic asymptotes of $c(\gamma)$ tend to exponential behavior since: $(x/\alpha'+1)^{\alpha'} \rightarrow e^x$ when $\alpha' \rightarrow \infty$.

v)$\underline{\alpha=0+}$ $\underline{(\alpha'=0\text{-}1)}$: this limiting case corresponds to divergence of every statistical moment of the generator and seems at first glance very strange, but one of its representations is none other than the once celebrated β-model ($\gamma^-=-\infty$, $\gamma^+=C_1$ =limit $_{\alpha\rightarrow 0+}(\gamma_0)$)! This fact, in turn, shows clearly the peculiarities of the β-model, once thought to be a more or less crude approximation of intermittency...

Let us point out briefly some consequences:

- the Levy cases fill the gap between the two more or less classical cases the so-called lognormal (α=2) and the β-model, which now represent just two extremes of the whole spectrum of universal generators.
- the very symmetric gaussian case is the exception which assures the existence of negative order moments, on the contrary the asymmetric "extremal" character of Levy case corresponds to the fact that we are "digging" wild regularities ("holes") with the algebraic extremes of the Levy generator which preventing convergence of any negative order moment. (see the relevant Fig. 7a-b).

- the links between regularity of the generator and the resulting flux are at first glance somewhat paradoxical since as α decreases the generator is more and more wild but the resulting fluxes more easily have all finite positive order moments since the upper bound C_∞ of C(h) ($\equiv\infty$ for $\alpha\geq1$; $\equiv\gamma_0<\infty$ for $\alpha<1$) is decreasing with α, leading to the finiteness of all moments for set A of dimension D>.C_∞ . However, it is merely due to the fact that the wild behavior of the generator is restricted to regularities (hence the particular problem of negative order moments since they interchange regularities with singularities and conversely. The β-model yields the extreme regularity since: $C_\infty= C_1=C(h)$, any set A where the process is not degenerate,will have regular flux at all positive orders (but still none at negative orders!).

One may note that exact mathematical results have been obtained on the case $\alpha=2$ (Kahane 1985, 1987) and $\alpha<1$ (Fan, 1989).

MULTIFRACTAL SIMULATIONS AND ANALYSIS

Stochastic simulations

Although concentrating their attention on a particular problem, the advection of passive scalar field (eg. concentration of a passive substance) by a turbulent velocity field, Schertzer and Lovejoy (1987), Wilson et al. (1989) show a rather general procedure for simulation of multifractal fields. Indeed, we may first readily produce conserved fluxes. Indeed, due to the existence of universality classes, a Gauss or Lévy generator is rather easily obtained by "coloring", via fractional integration, a corresponding Gauss or Lévy white-noise (represented in Fig. 7a-b in order to obtain a desired Gauss or Lévy pink-noise (most of the details are given by Wilson et al. (1989), especially the Fourier techniques needed). From these fluxes, we may build up others by taking products of them or raising them to different powers. We may even fractionally integrate over them, which is especially desirable when we want to obtain for instance the concentration field itself, rather than the flux of the scalar variance. However, doing so, we will fundamentally add only an extra parameter (the order of fractional integration) to our two basic C_1 and α. Indeed, a fractional integration (order -b) on a power (a) of a conserved flux.corresponds (as pointed out by Schertzer and Lovejoy (1987a)) to an affine transformation on the orders of singularity (leaving $c(\gamma)$ invariant):

$$\gamma'=a\gamma+b;\ h'=h/a;\ K'(h')= K(h) +bh';\ c'(\gamma')=c(\gamma) \tag{32}$$

staying in the same type of universality (same α). We could mainly restrict our attention to transformation with a=1, since it corresponds, at least formally[1], to the result of a fractional integration of order -b'=-(b+K(a)) on a new conserved flux (obtained by power and fractional integration K(a)).

Fig. 8 shows the two main steps needed to obtain a concentration field over a 2^8x2^8 pixel grid simulated (a=-b=1/3) on a personal computer, Fig. 8a shows the corresponding conserved flux (identified to ε), then the resulting concentration field after fractional integration. Larger simulations are expected to be quite useful in studying radiative transfer in highly inhomogeneous (i.e. multifractal) clouds, which could be notably important to developing remote sensing techniques (cf. Gabriel et al. (1988)). See also Fig. 9a-b

Probability Distribution Multiple Scaling (PDMS)

In analyzing empirical data of a field f known at a given resolution ($\Lambda=L/l$, L being the larger scale of the sample, eg. the size of a satellite image, l being the smaller scale , eg. the size of a pixel), we seek, as proposed by by Lavallée et al. (1989), to directly apply Eq. 5 to

[1] Indeed there is no equivalence between the different ways of maintaining conservation of fluxes.

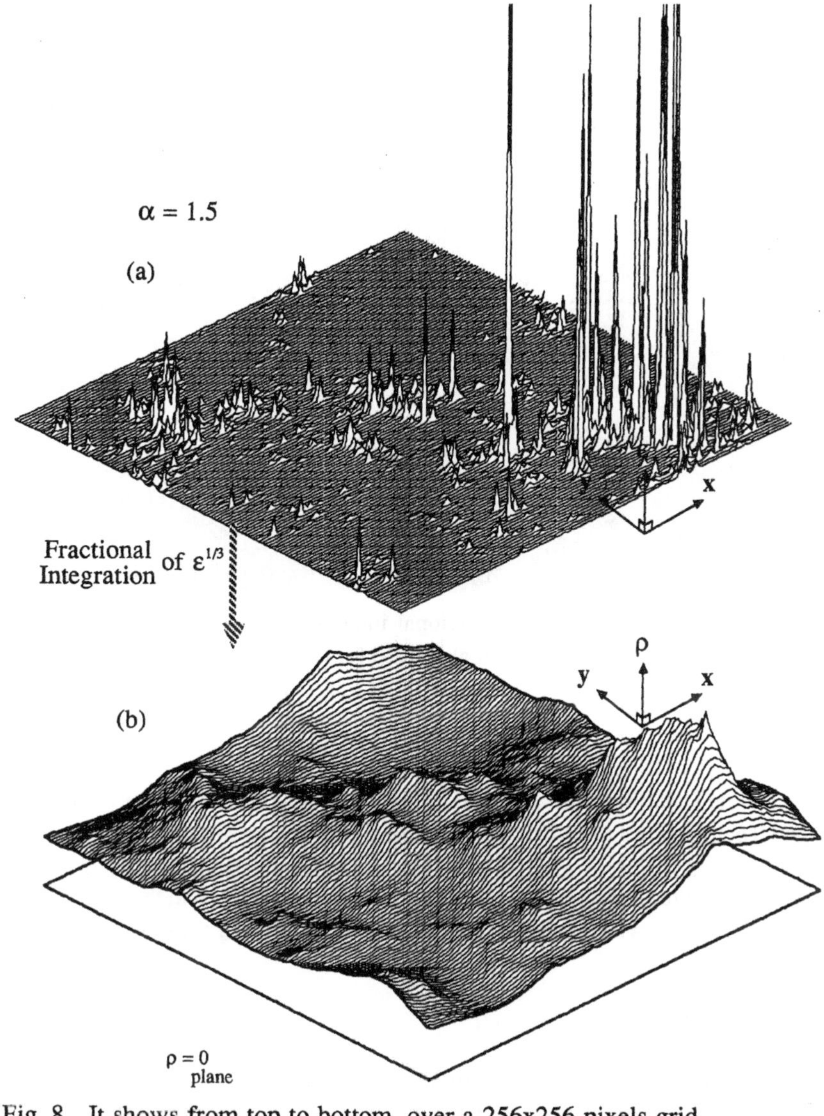

Fig. 8 . It shows from top to bottom, over a 256x256 pixels grid,
(a) the density of a conserved flux, obtained with a Lévy generator $\alpha = 1.5$
(b) the associated concentration field obtained by fractional integration (of order 1/3).

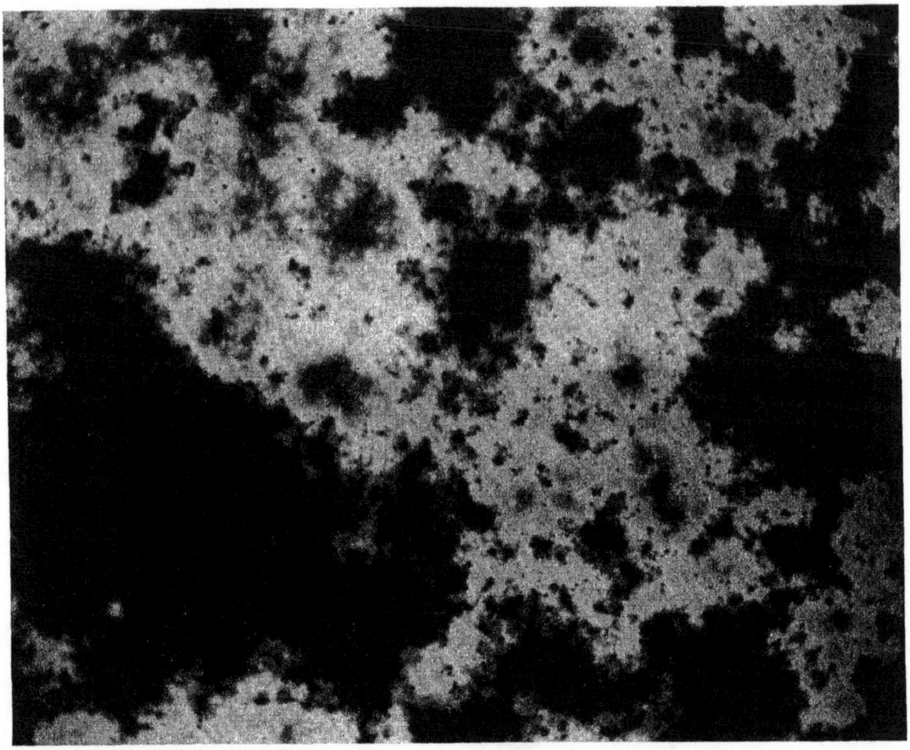

Fig. 9a. a cloud field obtained with a fractional integration (of order 1/3) and a Lévy generator (α=1.7). See Wilson et al. (1989) for more discussion.

determine the scale invariant probability distribution (characterized by the codimension function $c(\gamma)$). To do this, we must first estimate f at different intermediate scale ratios λ (f_λ; $\Lambda \geq \lambda \geq 1$) by coarse graining, eg. averaging on larger and larger pixels (successive factors of 2 can be easily implemented recursively until reaching the whole image) and the corresponding probabilities distributions with algebraic thresholds $\propto \lambda^\gamma$, estimating thus the codimensions of the singularities:

$$c(\gamma) \approx -\text{Log}_\lambda \Pr((\text{Log}_\lambda(f_\lambda) > \gamma) \qquad (33)$$

In order to avoid contributions given by different correcting terms (such as various logarithmic corrections...), it is often better to estimate $c(\gamma)$ as the slope of the probability distributions in Log-Log plots as discussed by Lavallée et al. (1989). This method can be called Probability Distribution Multiple Scaling (PDMS) and be tested on simulated fields whose codimension function is known. We can check also the validity of our assumptions on the limit of accuracy given by the sampling dimension we have introduced. Fig. 10 presents such a simulation, with a gaussian generator, which rather supports this method (cf. Lavallée et al.(1989) for more discussion).

Fig. 11a-b show the results when this technique is applied to 5 visible and 5 infra red GOES (Geostationary Operational Environment Satellite) pictures respectively over Montréal. The pictures were resampled on an 8X8km grid over a region of 1024X1024km. As can be

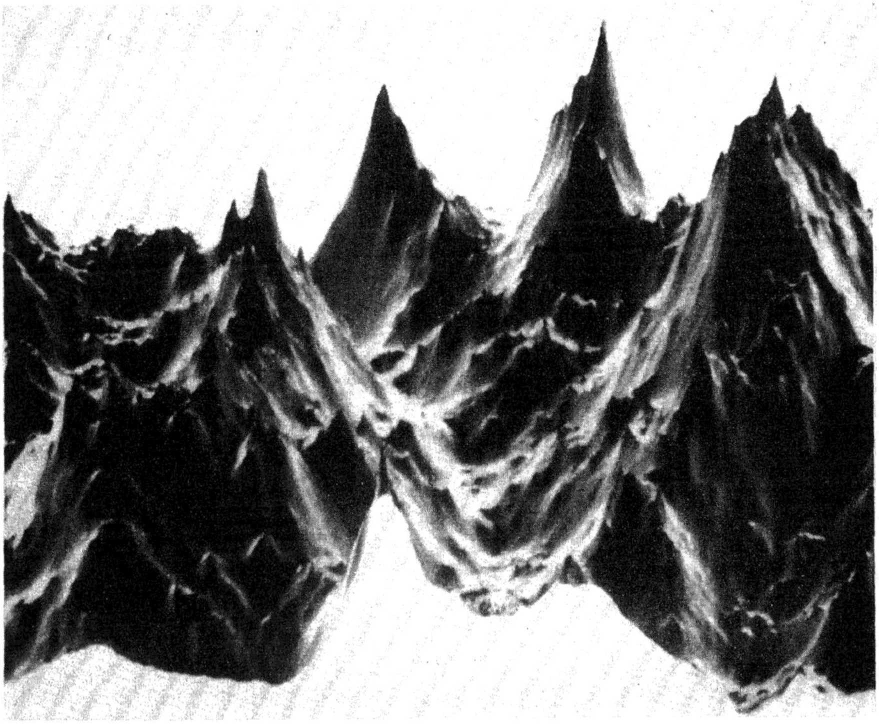

Fig. 9b. a landscape topography obtained with a fractional integration (of order 1/3) and a Gauss generator (α=2). See Sarma (1989) for more discussion.

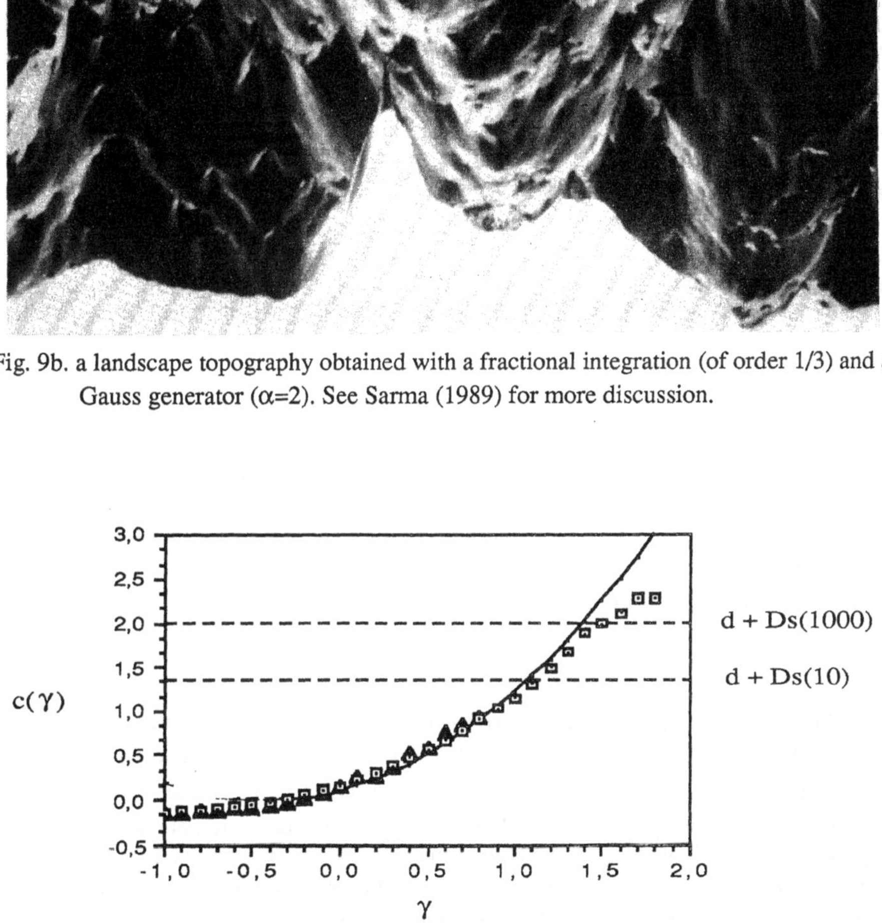

Fig. 10. Probability Distribution Multiple Scaling estimated on a multifractal field, generated by a gaussian generator. Solid line is the theoretical curve, for the probability density, black triangle are estimated codimensions of the probability distribution with a sampling dimension equals to 10 independent samples, open squares correspond to 1000 independent samples . Horizontal dashed lines, indicate the (estimated) upper limit of the validity of the estimations due to their limited sampling dimensions (resp. Ds(10) and Ds(1000). See Lavallée et al. (1989) for more discussion.

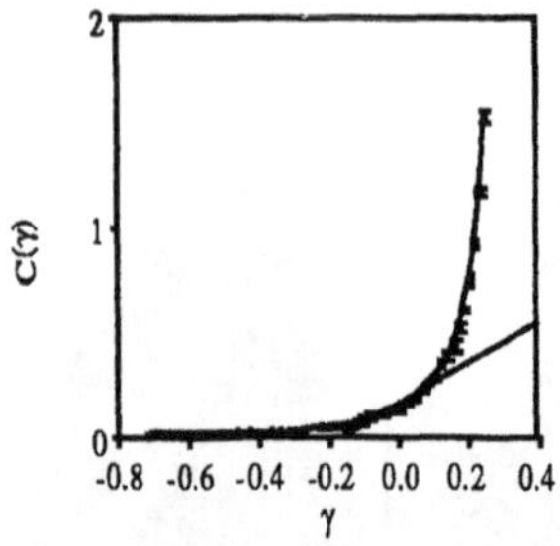

Fig. 11a PDMS estimates of the singularities codimension c(γ) from five visible GOES images over 1024x1024 km at 8, 16, 32, 64, 128, 256 km scales. The error bars indicate one standard deviation

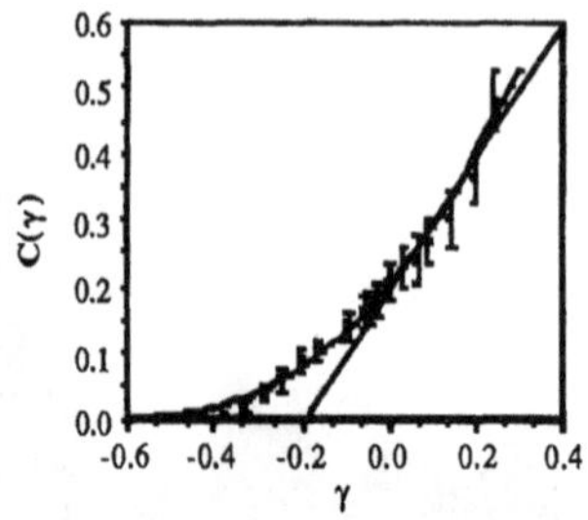

Fig. 11b PDMS estimates of the singularities codimension c(γ) from five infra-red GOES images with same range of scales. The error bars indicate one standard deviation. The mean standard error was ±.023, and the best regression to universal function (Eq. 31) yielded α'=2.52, α=1.66, with a standard error of the fit ±.015

seen, all the distributions are nearly coincident, in accord with the multifractal nature of the fields. To judge the closeness of the fits, we calculated the mean c(γ) curves as well as the standard deviations for 8, 16, 32, 64, 128, 256 km, finding that the variation is very small, being typically about ±0.02 in c(γ) which is appreciably more accurate than estimates obtained using functional box counting on very similar data (Gabriel et al 1988 found accuracies of ≈±0.05).

We have already argued that the resolution independent codimension function c(γ) is of considerably more interest than particular values of the function and may depend only on very few parameters due the universality classes we discussed: 2 in case of a conserved flux, mainly 3 in case of fractional integration (order -b) on a power (a) of a conserved flux. As discussed in the preceding sub-section, we may restrict our attention to a=1 and rewrite slightly differently this transformation, by introducing the empirically determined fixed point C_t (the subscript "t" indicates "tangent" to a line slope 1) of c(γ) and the corresponding translation γ_t necessary to reach it, i.e.

$$c(C_t - \gamma_t) = C_t \qquad [c'(C_t - \gamma_t) = 1] \qquad (34)$$

The difficulty in testing these ideas empirically is that the key parameter α' (recall 1/α'+1/α=1) characterizes the concavity of c(γ) which is only pronounced when γ and c(γ) vary over a substantial range. From the point of view of non-linear regression, to fit γ_t, C_t, α' to the data we find that C_t and α' are highly correlated and hence parameter estimates are not very sharp. In Gabriel et al 1988, functional box-counting was used yielding less accurate estimates of c(γ) than those obtained here. The issue was side-stepped by assuming α'=2 and testing the consistency of the data with that hypothesis.

Here we outline a very simple graphical method which proves quite accurate. The easiest parameter to estimate graphically is c_0=c(0), which yields c_0=0.16, 0.20 for visible and IR curves respectively. However, C_t, γ_t can also be found rather easily: a line slope 1 is tangent to c(γ) at the point c(γ)=C_t and will intersect the γ axis at the point γ= -γ_t. Note that all three parameters estimated this way depend on the values of the curve c(γ) in the statistically well defined region near $\gamma=0$, rather than on the large γ regime corresponding to extremely low probabilities, or the small negative γ regime which could easily be contaminated by noise. Using Eq. 31 we can obtain the estimates $\alpha \approx 0.65$, 1.7 for visible and IR respectively.

To improve on these results requires nonlinear regression (cf. discussion by Lovejoy and Schertzer (1989)). Here we determined α' by a least squares regression on the mean of the 8 to 256km curves in Fig. 11a-b. Maximum likelihood estimates for the parameter α were found to be: $\alpha=0.63\pm0.035$ and $\alpha=1.66\pm0.37$ for the visible and infra red data respectively. The large difference in the maximum likelihood errors cited here is due at least in part to the fact that we directly estimate α' and $\Delta\alpha=(1+\alpha)^2\Delta\alpha'$ hence this effect alone accounts for a factor 2.7 in difference. Fig. 11a-b shows the best fit and mean visible and infra red curves. The standard errors in the fit are ±0.011 and ±0.015 respectively. These results show the accuracy of the graphical method. We can also estimate the critical order of moments divergence h_D (cf. Eq. 11) and the corresponding critical order of singularity γ_D. We find, (using D=2) $h_D\approx13.80$, $\gamma_D\approx3.50$ for infra red images, but for the visible data (with $\alpha<1$, recall that the singularities are bounded) $C_\infty\approx0.42<2$, hence no divergence.

One may note also that, due to the fundamental discussion (Schertzer and Lovejoy, 1987b) on the method of elliptical dimensional sampling, the scaling anisotropy of the field can be investigated by this method in connection with PDMS, instead of the Functional Box Counting (as done earlier by Lovejoy et al. (1987)).

CONCLUSIONS

We sharpened the theoretical foundations of the singular statistics of multifractal fields, discussing in a rather general manner the conditions of their appearance, depending on the type of the process, as well as on the observation (scale and dimension). Thus we emphasized the non trivial behavior of geophysical observables. We clarified the fundamental difference between "bare" and "dressed" properties at a given (non-zero) scale i.e. the important differences between a process with a cut-off of small scale interactions and one with all these interactions. We point out also general properties of the generators of multifractal fields and their links with classical statistical physics notions, emphasizing their particularities.

We discussed in some detail the basic two-parameter (average singularities C_1, Lévy index α of the generator) family of universal (canonical) multifractal fields having strong attractive properties, with five important sub-classes: gaussian generator ($\alpha=2$), unbounded Lévy generator ($2>\alpha>1$), bounded Lévy generator ($1>\alpha>0$), a very special in-between case Lévy generator ($\alpha=1$)... as well as the once celebrated β-model ($\alpha=0$)! We also showed that multifractal fields not subject to some flux conservation will nevertheless depend primarily on only three parameters.

In our opinion, these findings may provide keys advances in Geophysics, especially in many practical applications (eg. remote sensing techniques) since they may well lead us to explore a hidden face of multifractality: bare universality under dressed pandemonium. We illustrated these ideas with passive cloud simulations and satellite data analysis.

ACKNOWLEDGMENTS

We thank D. Lavallée, G. Sarma, J. Wilson, for stimulating discussions and help preparing figures.
We also acknowledge discussions with, G.L. Austin, A. Davis, P. Gabriel, J.P. Kahane, P. Ladoy, E. Levich, A. Seed, G. Sèze, L. Smith, A.A. Tsonis.

REFERENCES

Anselmet, F., Y. Gagne, E.J. Hopfinger, and R. A. Antonia, 1984: High order velocity structure functions in turbulent shear flows, J. Fluid Mech., 140, 63-75.

Benzi, R., G. Paladin, G. Parisi, A. Vulpiani, 1984: J. Phys. A, 17, 3521.

Bialas, A., and R. Peschanski, 1986: Moments of rapidity distributions as a measure of short-range fluctuations in high-energy collisions, Nucl. Phys. B, B 273, 703-718.

Fan, A H., 1989: Chaos additif et multiplicatif de Lévy. C. R. Acad. Sci. Paris, 1, 308,151-154.

Feller, W. 1971: An introduction to probability theory and its applications. vol.2, Wiley, New-York.

Frisch, U., P. L. Sulem, and M. Nelkin,.1978: A simple dynamical model of intermittency in fully developed turbulence. J. Fluid Mech., 87, 719-724.

Frisch,U., G. Parisi, 1985: A multifractal model of intermittency, in Turbulence and predictability in geophysical fluid dynamics and climate dynamics, 84-88, Eds. Ghil, Benzi, Parisi, North-Holland.

Gabriel, P, S. Lovejoy, D. Schertzer, 1988a: Multifractal analysis of satellite resolution dependence. J.Geophys. Res. Lett. 1373-1376.

Gnedenko, B. and A. N. Kolmogorov, 1954: Limit distribution for sums of independent random variables. Addison-Wesley, Cambridge, Massachusetts.

Gnedenko, B. , 1969: The theory of probability. MIR, Moscow.

Grassberger, P., 1983: Generalized dimensions of strange attractors. Phys. Lett. A 97, 227.

Halsey, T.C., M.H. Jensen, L.P. Kadanoff, I. Procaccia, B. Shraiman, 1986: Fractal measures and their singularities: the characterization of strange sets. Phys. Rev. A 33, 1141-1151.

Hentschel, H.G.E., I. Proccacia, 1983: The infinite number of generalized dimensions of fractals and strange attractors, Physica 8D, 435-444.

Hubert P. and J. P. Carbonnel, 1988: Caractérisation fractale de la varaibilité et de l'anisotropie des précipitations tropicales. C. R. Acad. Sci. Paris, 2, 307, 909-914.

Kahane, J. P., , 1985: Sur le Chaos Multiplicatif, Ann. Sci. Math. Que., 9, 435-444.

Kahane, J. P., , 1987: Martingales and Random Measures, Chinese Ann. Math,.

Kolmogorov, A. N., 1949: Local structure of turbulence in an incompressible liquid for very large Reynolds numbers. Proc. Acad. Sci. USSR., Geochem. Sect., 30,299-303

Kolmogorov, A. N., 1962: A refinement of previous hypothesis concerning the local structure of turbulence in viscous incompressible fluid at high Reynolds number. J. Fluid Mech., 13, 82-85.

Kraichnan, R. H., 1971: An Almost-Markovian Galilean-invariant turbulence model. J. Fluid. Mech., 83, 349-367.

Ladoy, P., D. Schertzer, S. Lovejoy, 1986: Une étude d'invariance locale-regionale des temperatures, La Météorologie, 7, 23-34.

Lavallée, D. D. Schertzer, S. Lovejoy, 1988: On the determination of the codimension function. in Scaling, fractals and non-linear variability in geophysics I. D. Schertzer, S. Lovejoy eds., Kluwer, Dordrecht-Boston (in press).

Leray, J., 1934: Sur le mouvement d'un liquide visqueux emplisent l'espace. Acta Math., 63, 193-248.

Levich E., and E. Tzvetkov, 1985: Helical inverse cascade in three-dimensional turbulence as a fundamental dominant mechanism in meso-scale atmospheric phenomena, Phys. Rep., 128, 1-37.

Levich, E., and I Shtilman, 1989: Helicity fluctuations and coherence in developed turbulence, in Scaling, fractals and non-linear variability in geophysics I. D. Schertzer, S. Lovejoy eds., in press, Kluwer.

Lévy, P., 1924: Théorie des erreurs, la loi de Gauss et les lois exceptionnellles. Bull. Soc. Math., 52, 49-85.

Lévy, P., 1925: Calcul des Probabilités, Gauthier Villars, Paris.

Lévy, P., 1954: Théorie de l'addition des variables aleatoires, Gauthier Villars, Paris.

Lilly, D. K., 1983: Meso-scale variability of the atmosphere in Mesoscale Meteorology Theories, Observations and Models, edited by D. K. Lilly and T. Gal'Chen, pp.13-24, D.Reidel, Hingham, Mass..

Lovejoy, S., D. Schertzer, 1985: Generalized scale invariance in the atmosphere and fractal models of rain. Wat. Resour. Res 21, 1233-1250.

Lovejoy, S., D. Schertzer, 1986a: Scale invariance, symmetries fractals and stochastic simulation of atmospheric phenomena. Bull AMS 67, 21-32.
Lovejoy, S., D., Schertzer, 1989a: Multifractal analysis techniques and the rain and cloud fields from 10^{-3} to 10^{6}m, Scaling, fractals and non-linear variability in geophysics I. D. Schertzer, S. Lovejoy eds.,Kluwer, Dordrecht-Boston (in press).
Lovejoy, S., D., Schertzer, 1989b: Comment on "Are Rain Rate Processes Self-Similar?" by B.Kedem and L. S. Chiu. Wat. Resour. Res 25, 3,577-579.
Lovejoy, S., D., Schertzer, 1989c: Multifractal, universality classes, satellite and radar measurements of rain and clouds. J. Geophys. Res. (in press).
Lovejoy, S., D. Schertzer, A.A. Tsonis, 1987: Functional box-counting and multiple elliptical dimensions in rain. Science, 235, 1036-1038.
Mandelbrot, B., 1974: Intermittent turbulence in self-similar cascades: Divergence of high moments and dimension of the carrier. J. Fluid Mech., 62, 331-350.
Mandelbrot, B., 1989: An introduction to multifractal distribution functions. Fluctuations and Pattern Formation, Eds H. E. Stanley and N. Ostrowsky, Kluwer, Dordrecht-Boston (in press).
Meneveau, C. and K. R. Sreenivasan, 1987: Simple multifractal cascade model for fully developed turbulence. Phys. Rev.Lett., 59, 13, 1424-1427.
Monin, A.S.and A. M. Yaglom, 1975: Statistical Fluid Mechanics, vol 2, MIT Press, Boston.
Novikov, E. A., and R. Stewart, Intermittency of turbulence and spectrum of fluctuations in energy-dissipation, Izv. Akad. Nauk. SSSR, Ser. Geofiz. 3, 408-412, 1964.
Obukhov, A., 1949: Structure of the Temperature Field in a Turbulent Flow, Izv. Akad. Nauk. SSSR Ser. Geogr.I Jeofiz. 13, 55-69.
Obukhov, A., 1962: Some specific features of atmospheric turbulence. J. Geophys. Res.67, 3011-3014.
Perrin, J., 1913 (and 1948): Les Atomes, NRF-Gallimard, Paris.
Pietronero, L., and A.P. Siebesma 1986: Self-similarity of fluctuations in random multiplicative processes. Phys. Rev. Lett., 57, 1098-1101.
Richardson, L. F., 1926: Atmospheric diffusion shown on a distance neighbor graph. Proc. R. Soc., London, Sec. A, 110, 709-722.
Richardson, L. F., 1922, (Republished by Dover, New York,1965.): Weather prediction by numerical process, Cambridge U. Press.
Sarma, G., 1989: Analyses et simulations multifractales des champs de nuages, applications à la télédétection. Engineer's Thesis, Ecole Nationale Supérieure des Techniques Avancées, Paris.
Schertzer, D., S. Lovejoy 1983: On the dimension of atmospheric motions. Preprint Vol., IUTAM Symp on Turbulence and Chaotic Phenomena in Fluids, 141-144.
Schertzer, D., and S. Lovejoy, On the dimension of atmospheric motions in Turbulence and chaotic phenomena in fluids, edited by T. Tatsumi, pp.505-508, Elsevier North-Holland, New York, 1984.
Schertzer, D., S. Lovejoy, 1985a: The dimension and intermittency of atmospheric dynamics. Turbulent Shear Flow 4, 7-33, B. Launder ed., Springer, NY.
Schertzer, D., S. Lovejoy, 1985b: Generalized scale invariance in turbulent phenomena P.C.H. Journal, 6, 623-635.
Schertzer, D., S. Lovejoy, 1987a: Physically based rain and cloud modeling by anisotropic, multiplicative turbulent cascades. J. Geophys. Res. 92, 9693-9714.
Schertzer, D., S. Lovejoy, 1987b: Singularités anisotropes, et divergence de moments en cascades multiplicatifs. Annales Math. du Que. 11, 139-181.
Schertzer, D., S. Lovejoy, 1989a: Observables and universality classes for multifractal fields, in Scaling, fractals and non-linear variability in geophysics I. D. Schertzer, S. Lovejoy eds.,Kluwer, Dordrecht-Boston (in press).
Schertzer, D., S. Lovejoy 1989b: Generalized Scale invariance and multiplicative processes in the atmosphere. Pageoph. 130, 57-81.
Seed, A., D. Lavallée, S. Lovejoy, D. Schertzer, G.L. Austin, 1989: Multifractal analysis of radar rain measurements. (In preparation).
Smith, L A , J. D. Fournier, E. A. Spiegel , 1986: Lacunarity and interlittency in fluid turbulence. Phys. Lett. A, 8,9.
Stanley, H. E. P. , P. Meakin, 1988: Minireview on multifractals. Nature, 6, 116.

Tessier, Y., S. Lovejoy, D. Schertzer, 1989: Multifractal analysis of global rainfall from 1 day to 1 year. XXIV th. European Geophysical Society Assembly, Barcelonna.

Von Neumann, J., 1963: Recent theories in turbulence, in Collect. Works, 6, 437-450, Pergamon, New York.

Voss, R., 1983: Fourier Synthesis of gaussian fractals: 1/f noises, landscapes and flakes. Proceedings, Siggraph conf., Detroit, p1-21.

Waymire, E., and V.K. Gupta, 1981: The mathematical structure of rainfall representations, parts 1-3, Water Resour. Res., 17, 1261-1294.

Waymire, E., and V.K. Gupta, 1989: On scaling and log-normality in rainfall? in Scaling, fractals and non-linear variability in geophysics, edited by, D. Schertzer, and S. Lovejoy, Kluwer, Dordrecht-Boston (in press).

Wilson, J., S. Lovejoy, D. Schertzer, 1989: Physically based cloud modelling by scaling multiplicative cascade processes. Scaling, fractals and non-linear variability in geophysics, D. Schertzer, S. Lovejoy eds.,Kluwer, Dordrecht-Boston (in press).

Yaglom, A. M. 1966: The influence of the fluctuation in energy dissipation on the shape of turbulent characteristics in the inertial interval, Sov. Phys. Dokl., 2, 26-30 .

Zolotarev, V. M, 1986: One-dimensional stable distributions. Translations of Mathematical Monographs, Americ. Math. Soc., Providence, Rhode Island.

APPENDIX A

GENERALIZED CENTRAL THEOREM, EXTREMAL LEVY STABLE GENERATORS (in collaboration with R. Viswanathan[1])

Fixed points for sums of independent and identical distributed (i.i.d.) random variables and central limit theorems

In this sub-section we review briefly the classical features of Lévy stable variables, stressing that these variables emerge as generalizations of gaussian variables, which then are seen to be a very particular case of Lévy stable variable. Indeed, we are interested in the universal stable and attractive fixed points of renormalized sum of i. i. d variables, consider first the stable fixed points of renormalized sum ($\stackrel{d}{=}$ means equality in probability[2]):

$X_i \stackrel{d}{=} X_1 \quad i=1,n$ are stable points under renormalized sum iff (A1)
for any (integer) n ($\geq$2), ,there exists a (positive) b_n and a (real) a_n
$$\sum_{i=1,n} X_i \stackrel{d}{=} b_n X_1 + a_n$$

The well-known gaussian case corresponds to:

$$\langle X_1^2\rangle \leq \infty \Rightarrow b_n = n^{1/2},\ a_n = (n-1)\langle X_i\rangle \quad \text{(A2)}$$

hence the assumption of finite variance which has been considered as so "natural" that it has become a kind of dogma. The usual central limit theorem corresponds simply to the limit $n\to\infty$ in Eq. A1:

$$X = \lim_{n\to\infty} [(\sum_{i=1,n} X_i) - a_n]/b_n \quad \text{(A3)}$$

the X_i on the r.h.s. are not assumed to be gaussian but the X will be, hence the Gaussian law is attractive :

$$\langle X^2\rangle = \langle X_i^2\rangle \leq \infty \Rightarrow b_n = n^{1/2}, a_n = n\langle X_i\rangle - \langle X\rangle \quad \text{(A4)}$$

---

[1] Banque Indo-Suez, Paris, France.

[2], Note in order to be consistent, the use of this symbol requires that indicated variables should be mutually independent

one may note that the average $<X>$ can be arbitrary set set to 0, as usually done, due to the expression of the a_n.

Lévy (1925,1954) generalized the gaussian case by relaxing the hypothesis of finite variance for the X_i (which implies finiteness of every statistical moment for the limit itself) introducing on the contrary an order of divergence (α, $0<\alpha<2$) for the moments of the X_i (α is often called the Lévy index) which satisfies either A1 or A3:

$$h<\alpha \Rightarrow <|X_i|^h> < \infty \text{ and } h'\geq\alpha \Rightarrow <|X_i|^{h'}> = \infty \quad \text{i. e. : } Pr(|X_i|\geq s) \sim s^{-\alpha} \tag{A5}$$

$$\text{A1 or A3} \Leftrightarrow b_n = n^{1/\alpha} \quad (\text{and, if } \alpha>1;\ a_n = n<X_i> - <X>)$$

the variables X_i are very often termed "hyperbolic variables" (or even "hyperbolics") due the algebraic fall-off of their probability distribution tails, which are themselves sometimes termed "fat tail" due to their (unusually) important contribution. Hence, the Lévy stable variables are the stable and fixed points of (renormalized) sums of i. i. d. hyperbolic variables. Note that for $\alpha\leq1$, as the mathematical expectations of the X_i and their sums are divergent, the required recentring is a bit more involved than that indicated for $1<\alpha\leq2$ (subtracting out the averages) and will be only discussed later. The very special gaussian case appears as the (extreme) regular case $\alpha=2$, after a highly critical transition since for any $\alpha=2-\varepsilon$ (ε arbitrarily small) we have divergence of all orders greater than α whereas all divergences are suppressed for $\alpha=2$. One may note that the stable variables were introduced in a slightly different form (Lévy 1925, 1954) addressing the stability under any linear combination:

$X_i \stackrel{d}{=} X_2$ are said stable under linear combination iff (A6)
for any (positive) b_1 and b_2 , ,there exists (real) a and (positive)b, such that:
$b_1X_1+ b_2 X_2 \stackrel{d}{=} b\, X_1+a$

It is rather easy to check (by induction) that Eq. A1 and Eq. A6 are equivalent. One may furthermore note that "any n" in A1 can be equivalently reduced to "n=2,3" due essentially to the density of numbers $2^j\, 3^k$ among positive numbers, j and k being relative integers, (see for instance Zolotarev 1986).

Note that there exists a sub-class of stable variables which do not require recentring (i.e. $a\equiv0$, -it is rather obvious in the cases $1<\alpha\leq2$). These special cases (to which, Lévy (1925) restricted his study) are frequently called "strictly stable" (Feller 1971, Zolotarev 1986), more rarely the complementary cases (i.e. $a\neq0$) are called (Lévy 1954) "quasi-stable".

Characteristic functions of Levy laws

With the few notable exceptions $\alpha=2$, 1, 1/2 (and some further restrictions on the two latter cases, since they must be symmetric) the probability distributions of Levy stable variables are not expressible in a closed form. However, the second (Fourier or Laplace) characteristic function is easily expressible due to the basic properties of stability. K(h) is the logarithm of the first characteristic function Z(h), i.e. the (Fourier or Laplace) transform of the probability distribution dP(x)) and the argument h is purely imaginary in case of Fourier (h=ih'), real in case of Laplace (we will discuss later the restrictive conditions under which such a transform is possible) and a complex number (h+ih') in the case of Fourier-Laplace (or two-sided Laplace) transform:

$$e^{K(h)}= Z(h)= <e^{hX}> = \int e^{hx}\, dP(x) \tag{A7}$$

the fundamental property of the fixed point (Eq. A1) or the equivalent form (Eq. A6) are easily transposed for the characteristic functions: .

$X_i \stackrel{d}{=} X_1$ (i=1,n) of second characteristic function K(h) (A1') are stable points under renormalized sum iff. for any (integer) n ($\geq$2),there exists a (positive) b_n and a (real) such that: $a_n nK(h)= K(b_n h)+ a_n h$;

and:

$X_i =^d X_2$ of second characteristic function K(h) (A6')
are said stable under linear combination iff. for any (positive) b_1 and b_2
there exists a (real) a and a (positive)such that: $K(b_1 h)+ K(b_2 h) = K(bh) + ah$

the limit theorems correspond to (K_i second characteristic function of the X_i, K second characteristic function of X):

$$K(h) = \lim_{n\to\infty} n[K_i (h/b_n)- ha_n/nb_n] \qquad (A3')$$

We may infer, especially from A6', that these characteristic functions, up to the recentring term, should be of power law form whose exponent α is bounded above by 2 (the extreme regular gaussian case) and must of course be positive (to avoid divergence at h=0). It is obvious that the case α=1 is very special since this hyperbolic exponent becomes equal to the (linear) recentring term exponent, we may guess that conflict and compensation between the two terms will introduce logarithm corrections. For other values of α the (linear) recentring term has no importance and we can restrict our attention to strictly stable cases (a_n=0). As h^α (or h Log(h) for α= 1) is not analytical (except once again in the gaussian case α= 2) in the complex plane, we clearly expect on the one hand divergence of moments of order greater or equal to α, on the other hand that the inferred "power law form" may be rendered more precise in order to obtain a second characteristic function (e.g. Z(h) must be positive definite in case of Fourier transform (Bochner's theorem) or absolutely monotone in case of Laplace transform). Indeed, considering the symmetric (or symmetrized) probability distributions lead to the following law (partially known... since Cauchy 1853, but essentially obtained by Lévy (1925) of Fourier characteristic functions, since K(h) must be also symmetric:

$$K(ih') = -\lambda_\alpha |h'|^\alpha \qquad (A8)$$

with the obvious gaussian case when α=2, and Cauchy case when α=1. The λ_α characterizes the width of the probability distribution as in the gaussian case ($\lambda_2 = \sigma^2/2$) but doesn't correspond to the evaluation of an α-moment, since it diverges, but rather the rate of divergence of this moment.

Particular properties of extremal Levy laws

The symmetric case corresponds to limit sums of symmetric hyperbolics or mixing with equal probability (p=q=1/2) positive (with probability p) and negative (with probability q) one-sided hyperbolic distributions (concretely: just multiplying by a random sign positive one-sided hyperbolics) Asymmetric cases correspond to p$\neq$q. It is time to stress that if we want to have a Laplace transform. we can only consider extremal (asymmetric) hyperbolics, simply because algebraic fall-off could not tame an exponential divergence, hence we restrict here our attention to negative hyperbolics (p=0, q=1). However, note that the corresponding limits, the extremal Lévy stables, are not always one sided -precisely one sided probability distributions only occur for 0<α<1.

In order to assess different statements, it is interesting to consider the characteristic functions under their "canonical form" i. e:

$$K(h)= \int (e^{hx} -1 +hx)\, dF(x) \approx Z(h) -1+a'h \qquad (A9)$$

dF is often called the Lévy canonical measure or the spectral measure, which needs not be a probability measure. Indeed $\int dF(x)$ is not bounded, with the exception of the gaussian case, and we introduced a recentring term a' just to cancel the second term fo the exponential development (near h=0) when needed (for $1<\alpha<2$) . This form corresponds on the one hand to a first order term development of $\log[1+(Z(h)-1)]$, which is the only term kept in the limit theorem besides recentring and normalization of K(h) (i.e. K(0)=0 corresponding to $\int dP(x)=1$). On the other hand, it corresponds to the limit of (Poisson) random (renormalized) sums of i. i. d. variables, instead of uniform sums as discussed up to now. Indeed considering the characteristic function of the limit ($n\to\infty$) of the Poisson compound probability distribution generated by renormalized sum of n i. d. d. hyperbolic variables (as given by A1) lead us to a new version of the limit theorem (earlier stated under the forms A3 and A3') keeping in mind that the second characteristic function K(h) of the Poisson compound probability distribution is c(Z(h)-1), where c is the parameter of the Poisson process, Z(h) the first characteristic function of the generating probability distribution):

$$K(h) = \lim_{n\to\infty} K_n(h)$$
$$K_n(h)=n[Z_n(h) -1]$$
$$Z_n(h)= Z_i\,(h/b_n)\exp(- ha_n/nb_n) \qquad \text{(A3'')}$$

the "canonical form" (Eq. A9) is obtained by slightly recasting this equation to take directly into account arbitrary centering directly on K (no longer on Z_n or Z).

Let us consider the negative hyperbolic generation of extremal Lévy stable by negative hyperbolic, it suffices to put $dF(x) \propto 1_{x<0}x^{-\alpha}\,dx/x$ ($1_{x<0}$.being the indicator function of the negative x) and with repeated uses of the identity:

$$\Gamma(\beta)= z^{-\beta} \int_0^\infty e^{-zt}t^{\beta}dt/t \ ; \ \mathrm{Re}(z) \geq 0 \qquad \text{(A10)}$$

and integrations by parts, we obtain easily for $dF(x) = 1_{x<0}C(2-\alpha)\, x^{-\alpha}\, dx/x$:

$$\alpha\neq 1: K(h) =C\, h^{\alpha}\, \Gamma(3-\alpha)/\alpha(\alpha-1);\ \alpha\neq 1$$
$$\alpha=1:\ K(h) =C\, h\log(h) \qquad \text{(A11)}$$

one may note that the expressions for the corresponding Fourier transforms are a bit more complex (i.e. Fourier transforms, so convenient for symmetric laws, are inconvenient for extremal (and more generally for asymmetric laws), on the contrary Laplace is only fitted for the extremal, useless for the others):

$$\alpha\neq 1:$$
$$K(h)= |h|^{\alpha}\ C\, [\Gamma(3-\alpha)/\alpha(\alpha-1)]\ [\cos(\pi\alpha/2) + -i(\mathrm{sgn}(h)\ (p-q)\ \sin(\pi\alpha/2)]$$
$$\alpha=1:$$
$$K(h)= -|h|\ \ C\, [\pi/2 +i\ (\mathrm{sgn}(h)(p-q)\log|h|] \qquad \text{(A12)}$$

As a last general remark, one may note (from Eq. A11 or Eq. A12) it is only in the case of extremal stable distribution ($p-q=\pm 1$) that an analytic extension on the whole complex plane of K is possible (but with a cut along the ray $\arg(h)=-3\pi/4$), as it is for $\alpha=2$, or that the double-sided Laplace transform applies only to extremal stable variables.

Part 2

Fractal Properties of Critical Fluctuations and Polymers

FRACTAL CRITICAL PHENOMENA IN TWO DIMENSIONS AND CONFORMAL INVARIANCE

Bertrand Duplantier

Service de Physique Théorique de Saclay[†]
F-91191 Gif-sur-Yvette Cedex, France

ABSTRACT

The fractal properties of self-avoiding walks, percolation clusters, and also some non-trivial critical exponents or fractal dimensions associated with subsets of the planar Brownian motion are reviewed in two dimensions (2D). The conformal spectrum of these geometrical critical systems is made of an infinite discrete series of scaling dimensions. The latter are dimensions of critical geometrical systems in 2D like the $O(n)$ and Potts models within their loop expansions, and are calculated in the framework of Coulomb gas methods and conformal invariance. The statistical mechanics of the same critical models on a random 2D lattice (namely in presence of a critically fluctuating metric, in the so-called 2D quantum gravity) is also addressed, and the above critical geometrical systems are exactly solvable in this case. The new "gravitational" conformal spectrum so derived is found to satisfy a quadratic relation to the standard conformal spectrum in the plane, as predicted recently.

I. INTRODUCTION

We review the statistical mechanics of critical fractal objects in two-dimensions, like self-avoiding walks, percolation clusters or intersection of random walks. These systems are parts of critical geometrical models, where sets of lines (e.g. polymers or random walks) or sets of points (e.g. clusters) are fluctuating and characterized by infinite series of critical exponents or (fractal) Hausdorff dimensions. More generally, infinite sets of critical exponents are hidden in the geometrical versions of the $O(n)$ and Potts models, of which polymers and percolation are particular cases. The sets of new conformal dimensions correspond to specific geometric properties of the loop or polygon representations (i.e. high temperature expansions) of these models, and are obtained by branching and gluing together critical objects like several self-avoiding

[†] *Laboratoire de l'Institut de Recherche Fondamentale du Commissariat à l'Energie Atomique*

Fractals' Physical Origin and Properties
Edited by L. Pietronero
Plenum Press, New York

walks or several percolating clusters, etc... (Fig.1). In two dimensions (2D), in the plane, there exist some conformal operators $\phi_L\left(\vec{X}\right)$ source of L such objects at a point $\vec{X}$, with conformal dimensions $\Delta_L^{(0)}$, depending only on the universality class of the geometrical system under consideration. The values of the conformal dimensions $\Delta_L^{(0)}$ can be obtained in general by Coulomb gas techniques, starting from the lattice realization of the models. They fit into the classification scheme of 2D conformal field theories, based on the standard Virasoro algebra.

The geometric idea behind conformal invariance is a generalization of the standard scale invariance at a critical point. For infinite critical systems, where a length scale (the correlation length) has become infinite, the rotational and scale invariances should apply *locally* and one should be able to deform by local dilations and rotations the system without changing its statistics. This is expected to be valid for critical systems with short range interactions. The set of such local transformations is that of conformal mappings, which in two dimensions are any analytic transform. Actually this idea appeared explicitly as early as in Paul Lévy's work on Brownian motion[1], which is perhaps the simplest model of a conformally invariant process. The same idea in the more general framework of field theory was remarked by Polyakov[2], but the breakthrough occurred only in 1984 when it was applied to specific calculations[3] in field theory.

Here we shall concern ourselves with the obtention of geometrical scaling dimensions $x_L \equiv 2\,\Delta_L^{(0)}$, associated with the special vertices (point singularities), where infinite critical objects are fused together, like in Fig.1. From these scaling dimensions, one obtains all sorts of critical exponents and Hausdorff (fractal) dimensions, which provide an exact fractal critical 2D geometry, illustrating the general field of mathematical fractals[4].

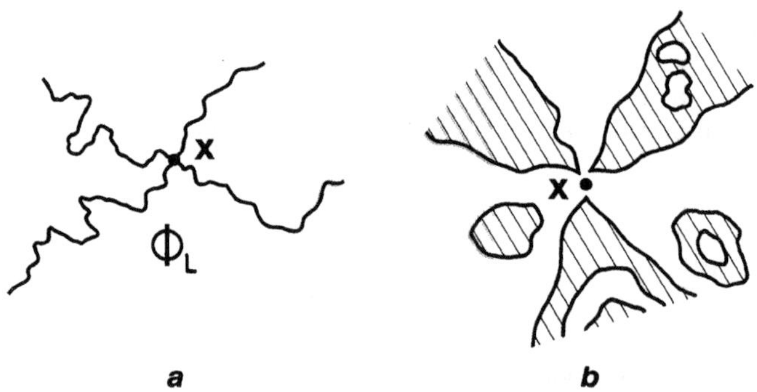

Fig.1. a) Branching of $L = 4$ self- and mutually-avoiding walks (polymers). A conformal operator ϕ_L is associated with this L−vertex. b) Similar branching of three percolating clusters at a point $\vec{X}$. The boundary lines form a 6-vertex.

For instance, the number of configurations $\mathcal{Z}_L$ of a self-avoiding star polymer (Fig.1), made of L arms of equal lengths S, scales as

$$\mathcal{Z}_L \underset{S\longrightarrow\infty}{\sim} \mu^{LS} S^{\gamma_L - 1} \tag{1.1}$$

where μ is the (nonuniversal) effective connectivity constant of the simple self-avoiding walk [e.g. $\mu = (2+\sqrt{2})^{1/2}$ on the 2D honeycomb lattice[5]], and γ_L an universal configuration exponent, which in 2D equals[6]

$$\gamma_L = \frac{68 + 9L(3-L)}{64} \tag{1.2}$$

For $L = 1,\ 2$ (linear SAW) one recovers the Nienhuis value[5] $\gamma = \frac{43}{32}$. Of course, the fractal dimension of each walk of the star is still[5]

$$D_F = 1/\nu = 4/3 \tag{1.3}$$

Notice that the fact that the polymer system embodies an infinite spectrum (1.2) due to the branching points should not be confused with the existence of a *multifractal* spectrum, and the comparison between conformal and multifractal spectra is an interesting problem[7].

Another case where an infinite spectrum of scaling dimensions appears, is provided by the topology of clusters in 2D percolation. We shall describe below how the probability of having a *pinching point* (Fig.1), where k *peninsulas* of the infinite incipient cluster join together, scales near the threshold p_c. One has[8]

$$P_k \sim (p-p_c)^{\beta_k}\,, \quad \beta_k = \frac{1}{9}\left(4k^2-1\right), \tag{1.4}$$

thus again an infinite set of independent critical exponents (with *no* gap scaling i.e. $\beta_k \neq k\ \beta_1$). The *fractal* dimensions are related to these exponents. For instance the *hull* fractal dimension is given by scaling arguments as[8]

$$D_H = 2 - \beta_1/\nu = \frac{7}{4}, \tag{1.5}$$

where $\nu = \frac{4}{3}$ is the standard thermal exponent of percolation. The fractal dimension of *red bonds* appears in this formalism as

$$D_{\text{red}} = 2 - \beta_2/\nu = \frac{3}{4} = 1/\nu \tag{1.6}$$

recovering a well-known result[9]. Notice that due to (1.4), higher pseudo-fractal dimensions $D_k \equiv 2 - \beta_k/\nu$ become negative, reflecting the low probability to find such high order pinching points in a percolating system. However, these dimensions are meaningful for the histogram of such points.

All of this applies to geometrical critical models embedded in the plane. Now, an extended type of fractal geometry is obtained by putting these critical systems on a random two-dimensional surface or lattice. For instance, instead of putting a SAW on a regular hexagonal lattice, one can place it on a disordered lattice, with the same connectivity (three) but where all lattice hexagons are distroyed and become arbitrary fluctuating polygons (Fig.2).

The disorder is here *annealed.* Thus the statistical system becomes coupled to the degrees of freedom of the internal metric, which freely fluctuates, like in Polyakov's string model (2D quantum gravity). A new type of conformal invariance then appears (discovered by Knizhnik, Polyakov and Zamolodchikov[10] (KPZ)) associated with a

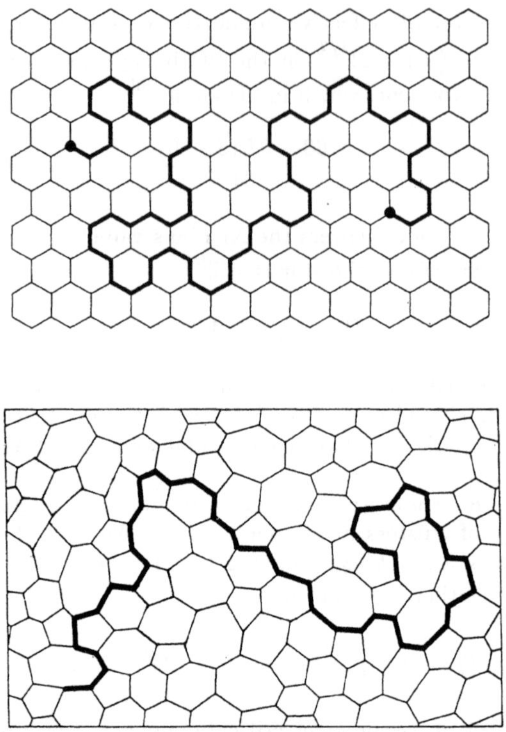

Fig.2. Self-avoiding walks on the honeycomb lattice or on a random φ^3–lattice made of three-leg vertices arbitrarily connected.

Kac-Moody algebra, where the critical properties of the statistical model and of the random surface have fused. It was shown recently by KPZ that the new conformal dimension Δ of any critical system on a random surface are actually *related* to the former ones $\Delta^{(0)}$ in the plane, the latter being quadratic forms of the Δ on the fluctuating surface.

Now, the same analysis of the geometrical models in terms of operators ϕ_L representing the branching of L fractal objects, here living on the fluctuating membrane, can be performed, and one expects new conformal dimensions Δ_L associated with them.

Then usual critical exponents, like the correlation length exponent ν, the fractal dimensions, etc... which are related to the conformal dimensions Δ_L, also change on the fluctuating membrane. For illustrating this phenomena, let us give some examples. Consider first a single self-avoiding walk. When embedded in the regular honeycomb lattice (Fig.2), it has asymptotically the fractal dimension (1.3) $D_F = 4/3$. Now, when living on the critically fluctuating lattice made of e.g. three-leg vertices arbitrarily connected, it acquires a new fractal dimension[11]

$$D'_F/D = 1/2 \tag{1.7}$$

where D is the (undetermined) fractal dimension of the fluctuating lattice. This *universal* relation (1.7) replaces the former

$$D_F/d = D_F/2 = 2/3$$

valid in the standard 2D plane. A new configuration exponent γ also appears for SAW in a fluctuating metric[11].

Similarly, one can consider *percolation* on a random 2D lattice, with annealed disorder. A new exact result is then for instance the fractal dimension of the hull on the fluctuating lattice

$$D'_H/D = 3/4, \tag{1.8}$$

which replaces the usual 2D result

$$D_H/2 = 7/8$$

We describe below how such results can be obtained from exact solutions. Indeed, the above geometrical critical systems (self-avoiding walks, $O(n)$ model...) appear to be *exactly* solvable on a *random* lattice, allowing a *direct* calculation of the dimensions Δ_L of the models, hence of all critical exponents. The Δ_L are furthermore shown to satisfy KPZ relation with those $\Delta_L^{(0)}$ of the plane, determined independently by Coulomb gas techniques. Thus this provides a cross check of conformal invariance principles in the Euclidean two-dimensional space and on a random surface, and of the remarkable relation between both. More technically, this allows also an indirect check of Coulomb gas techniques in the plane, and of the universal modelling of 2D quantum gravity by fluctuating lattices.

The organization is as follows. We first describe the general geometrical $O(n)$ and Potts models, of which particular cases will yield later polymers and percolation. In this rather abstract part, we describe the conformal dimensions associated with special geometrical critical objects. We briefly describe how their scaling dimensions are found by Coulomb gas techniques and fit (formally) in the conformal classification scheme.

We then review in a second part the new geometrical critical properties of systems like self-avoiding walks, percolation clusters, and intersections of random walks, obtained by considering fractal objects of more complex topologies like polymer networks, or pinching points of percolation clusters. In particular it is described how to built the representation of the latter in terms of basic conformal operators. A special section is devoted to recent conjectures about the non-intersection properties of random walks in two dimensions. In a last part, we study the same fractal geometry on a random lattice and show how the new dimensions can be determined, with emphasis on the relation to the planar theory.

II. GEOMETRICAL EXPONENTS IN O(n) AND POTTS MODELS

2.1 Watermelon Configurations

For definiteness we first consider the $O(n)$ model on the honeycomb two-dimensional lattice. Its partition function is defined as[12,13]

$$Z_{O(n)} = \int \prod_i \mathrm{d}\vec{S}_i \prod_{\langle i,j\rangle} \left(1 + K\ \vec{S}_i \cdot \vec{S}_j\right) \tag{2.1}$$

where the spin variables $\vec{S}_i$ are $n-$vectors with $S_i^2 = n$, and where $\langle i,j\rangle$ are nearest neighbour sites. One can show easily that on the honeycomb lattice $\mathcal{H}$ Eq.(2.1) reads

$$Z_{O(n)} = \sum_{\text{nonintersecting loops}} K^{\mathcal{N}_B} n^{\mathcal{N}_L} \tag{2.2}$$

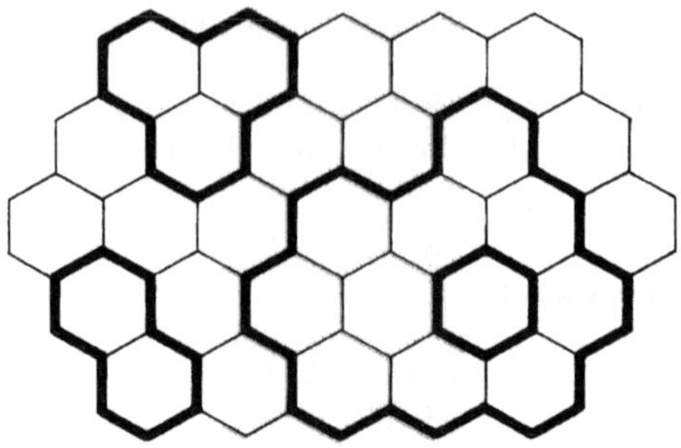

Fig.3. Loop representation of the $O(n)$ model on the honeycomb lattice (Eq.(22)).

where the sum runs on all configurations of closed and nonintersecting loops drawn on $\mathcal{H}$, with total numbers of bonds $\mathcal{N}_B$, and of loops $\mathcal{N}_L$ (Fig.3).

In this way, the high-temperature (i.e. small K) expansion of the $O(n)$ model gives a *geometrical loop model.* For a fixed value of $n \in [-2,2]$ there is a critical point $K_c = \left[2 + (2-n)^{1/2}\right]^{-1/2}$ (on the hexagonal lattice[5]) where the mean length $\langle \mathcal{N}_B \rangle \sim (K_c - K)^{-1}$ diverges. Geometrical correlation functions can be defined by considering *watermelon* configurations[14,15] on the lattice (Fig.4). One specifies to configurations $\mathcal{C}_L\left(\vec{X},\vec{Y}\right)$ such that L nonintersecting lines have a source point at $\vec{X}$ and a sink at $\vec{Y}$ where they all meet together, in a presence of vacuum loop of the $O(n)$ model. The associated correlator is defined as

$$G_L\left(\vec{X}-\vec{Y},K\right) = \sum_{\mathcal{C}_L(\vec{X},\vec{Y})} W(\mathcal{C}_L)/\, Z_{O(n)} \tag{2.3}$$

where the statistical weight of the configuration $\mathcal{C}_L$ (watermelon + vacuum loops) is

$$W(\mathcal{C}_L) = K^{\mathcal{N}_B} n^{\mathcal{N}_L}$$

where now $\mathcal{N}_B$ is the total length of the watermelon and loop lines. At K_c one expects a critical algebraic decay

$$\begin{aligned} G_L\left(\vec{X}-\vec{Y},K_c\right) &\equiv \left\langle \phi_L\left(\vec{X}\right)\phi_L\left(\vec{Y}\right)\right\rangle_c \\ &\sim \left|\vec{X}-\vec{Y}\right|^{-2x_L} \end{aligned} \tag{2.4}$$

where x_L is the scaling dimension of the (conformal) operator $\phi_L\left(\vec{X}\right)$ assumed to represent a source of L nonintersecting *infinite* lines at a point $\vec{X}$ (Fig.1). As we shall see these x_L are not linear in L (these is no gap exponent) and are independent of each other. Hence a new geometrical critical exponent x_L appears for each star-like critical object. It is also important to notice that in the $O(n)$ model, a second critical phase appears, the *dense* phase[13,16], for any value $K > K_c$. Geometrically, this corresponds to taking infinite loops or lines filling the lattice with a finite (non vanishing) density, even in the thermodynamic limit. The physical properties thus describe those of a loop melt in two-dimensions[16,17]. In this dense phase are associated other scaling dimensions x_L^D with each source operator ϕ_L.

2.2. Coulomb Gas Technique

It is known[13,14] that one can determine the geometrical exponents x_L by a Coulomb gas technique first devised in 1982[5] for obtaining the usual spin and energy exponents η and ν of the $O(n)$ model. As we shall see, the x_L also belong to the conformal Kac table of the (unitary) minimal theories with central charge $c \leq 1$. Lastly, let us mention that a derivation of the same dimensions is also possible through a Bethe Ansatz on the hexagonal lattice[18]. In the standard Coulomb gas technique[5,13], the $O(n)$ model can be transformed into a SOS model by orienting the loops and the watermelon lines and in the continuum critical limit, it renormalizes onto a Gaussian field with action $A = g/4\pi \int (\partial\varphi)^2 \, d^2x$, where g is the Coulomb gas coupling constant such that

$$n = -2 \cos \pi g \tag{2.5}$$

and $g \in [1,2]$ at K_c, while $g \in [0,1]$ in the *dense* phase[13].

Now, the watermelon correlation function generalized to the $O(n)$ model, can be associated in the SOS model with the existence of a dislocation. Indeed the L lines, once oriented, are interpreted as domain walls in a height model and a circuit around $\vec{X}$ or $\vec{Y}$ gives a height discontinuity depending on L (Fig.4).

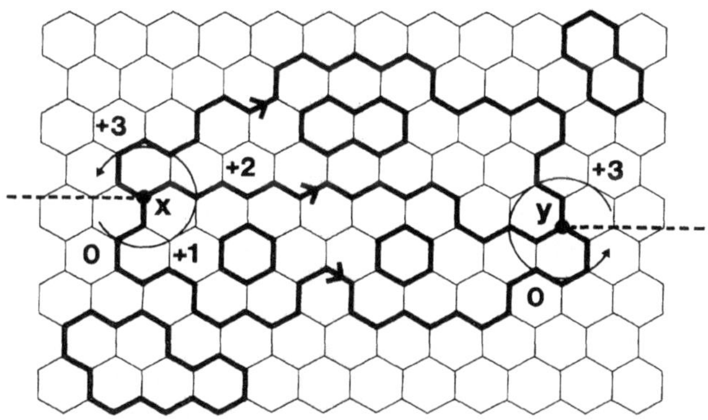

Fig.4. Watermelon configuration of $L = 3$ nonintersecting lines, in presence of vacuum loops of the $O(n)$ model. The integers indicate the heights on the equivalent SOS model, once the SAW are oriented and represent domain walls. The dotted lines represent dislocations associated with the watermelon.

As a result[13–15], the correlation function G_L (2.4) is simply a Coulomb gas correlator of two electromagnetic operators

$$G_L\left(\vec{X}-\vec{Y}\right) = \left\langle \mathcal{O}_{e_0,m'}\left(\vec{X}\right) \mathcal{O}_{e_0,-m'}\left(\vec{Y}\right)\right\rangle = \left|\vec{X}-\vec{Y}\right|^{-gm'^2+e_0^2/g} \tag{2.6}$$

where $e_0 = 1 - g$ is the standard floating electric charge[19] and m' the magnetic contribution coming from the L defect lines: $m' = L/2$. The name "Coulomb gas" is justified when one remarks that the correlator (2.6) reads also

$$e^{-(gm'^2 - e_0^2/g)\ell n|\vec{X}-\vec{Y}|}$$

i.e. is the *Gibbs weight* of pairs of magnetic and electric charges (m', e_0) and $(-m', e_0)$ located at $\vec{X}$ and $\vec{Y}$ respectively, and interacting via the Coulomb potential in 2D $\left(\ell n \left|\vec{X} - \vec{Y}\right|.\right)$ We refer the reader to Ref.[13-15] for precise geometric derivations of (2.6). Let us simply mention that the seemingly mysterious presence of the electric charge $e_0 = 1 - g$ is necessary for correcting curvature effects along the watermelon lines, which appear in the SOS model but not in the original $O(n)$ model, when the watermelon *winds* about one of its origins.

Hence the watermelon scaling dimension is finally

$$x_L = \frac{1}{2}\left(gm'^2 - \frac{e_0^2}{g}\right) = g\ L^2/8 - (1-g)^2/2g \tag{2.7}$$

for the $O(n)$ model where n is parametrized by (2.5).

Conformal invariance. These scaling dimensions can be rewritten as a Kac formula [20,3,21,22]

$$\begin{aligned} h_{p,q} &= \frac{[(m+1)p - mq]^2 - 1}{4m(m+1)}, \quad m \in \mathbf{N} \\ c &= 1 - 6/m(m+1) = 1 - 6(1-g)^2/g \\ x_L &= 2h_{L/2,0} \qquad \text{(dilute phase, } g \in [1,2]) \\ x_L^D &= 2h_{0,L/2} \qquad \text{(dense phase, } g \in [0,1]) \end{aligned} \tag{2.8}$$

The values of the conformal parameter m parametrizing the universality class are $m = \frac{1}{g-1} \in [1, \infty[$ for the dilute phase and $m = \frac{g}{1-g} \in [0, \infty[$ for the dense one. The $O(n = 2)$ model corresponds to the XY model at the Kosterlitz-Thouless transition point, for which $g = 1$, $m = \infty$, $c = 1$. The dilute and dense phases coincide there. Only this model and the $n = 1$ standard Ising model, for which $m = 3$, are unitary. The other $O(n)$ models (n continuous) are analytic extensions of the spin model (2.1) and have a purely geometrical interpretation (2.2) in terms of systems of nonintersecting loops. These values $h_{p,q}$ play a fundamental role in the representations of the conformal group. They are in a sense the *quantized* values allowed to the critical exponents, under the requirement that the critical system is *conformally* invariant (see Cardy[22]). This is very analogous to the quantification rules of angular momentum in quantum mechanics, which this time arises from the requirement of *rotational* invariance.

Polymers. When $n = 0$ in (2.2), all loops give a zero weight and only the empty graph contributes, leading to a trivial partition function $Z_{O(n=0)} = 1$. However, in the watermelon correlator (2.3), the L lines joining $\vec{X}$ to $\vec{Y}$ *survive* when $n \longrightarrow 0$, and describe in the continuum limit the correlation function of L self- and mutually-avoiding polymer lines, tied at their extremities $\vec{X}$ and $\vec{Y}$, and with *fluctuating* lengths $S_1, ..., S_L$

$$G_L\left(\vec{X} - \vec{Y}, K_c\right) = \int_0^\infty dS_1 ... dS_L\ K_c^{(S_1 + ... + S_L)} \mathcal{Z}_L\left(\vec{X} - \vec{Y}, S_1, ..., S_L\right) \tag{2.9}$$

where $\mathcal{Z}_L$ is the partition function of the watermelon, and K_c^{-1} is the usual effective connectivity constant. The expression (2.9) is written in the continuum limit where the sums over bond numbers $\mathcal{N}_B$ can be replaced by integrals over lengths $S_1, ..., S_L$.

The two possible phases for *polymers* ($n = 0$) correspond to $g = 3/2$ (dilute) or $g = 1/2$ (dense). Hence (2.7) (2.8) give the set of scaling dimensions:

$$\begin{array}{llll} x_L = \left(9L^2 - 4\right)/48, & c = 0, & g = 3/2, & m = 2 \text{ (dilute)} \\ x_L^D = \left(L^2 - 4\right)/16, & c = -2, & g = 1/2, & m = 1 \text{ (dense)} \end{array} \qquad (2.10)$$

It is interesting to remark that the usual conformal classification of "unitary" statistical systems started[21,22] with *integer values* $m \geq 3$ of the parameter m appearing in $h_{p,q}$ (2.8), $m = 3$ corresponding to the Ising model, and models with higher values of m being identified later[23]. The polymer case is special, since there is no symmetric transfer matrix, or equivalently it is an $n = 0$ vector model, and it is "non unitary". It fills then precisely the two missing values $m = 1, 2$ of Friedan, Qiu and Shenker classification[21]. Notice also that the interpretation of half-integer indices in $h_{p,q}$ is not yet clear. Formulas like (2.8) for the $O(n)$ model are thus to be interpreted as useful analytic continuations. The standard critical exponents ν and γ for SAW are obtained by scaling in terms of the first two x_L, namely

$$\nu^{-1} = 2 - x_2, \quad \eta = 2x_1, \quad \gamma = (2 - \eta)\,\nu$$

which, owing to (2.10), give Nienhuis values $\nu = 3/4$, $\gamma = 43/32$. Notice that the thermal exponent x_2 (2.10) was conjectured before (from the $O(n)$ model) by Cardy and Hamber[24]. For the dense phase of polymers, we find instead from (2.10)

$$\nu^D = \frac{1}{2}, \quad \gamma^D = \frac{19}{16}$$

The interpretation of $\nu^D = \frac{1}{2}$ is immediate: the fractal dimension is $D_F = 1/\nu^D = 2$, as expected for a dense walk filling the plane. The interpretation of the γ exponent is more subtle, and requires a careful analysis[16,17] of boundary conditions for dense SAW, since these conditions are able to add nonuniversal terms to γ^D.

Up to now we used only the first exponents x_1, x_2. The higher order ones x_L, $L \geq 3$ will play a fundamental role, described below (section 3), in the making of branched polymer networks.

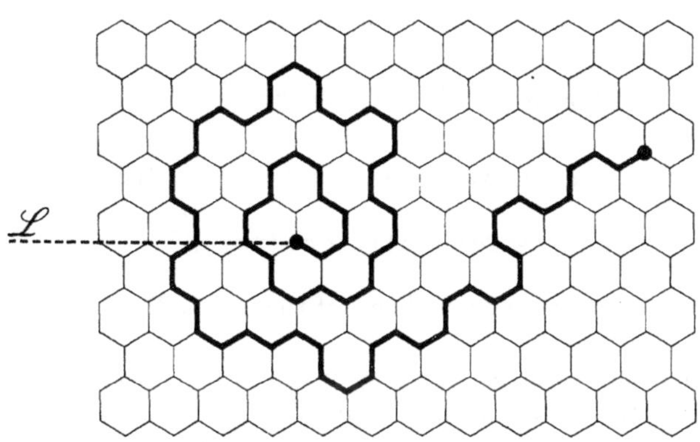

Fig.5. Winding of a self-avoiding walk about its origin. Asymptotically the winding angle is $\theta = 2\pi n_1$ where n_1 is the algebraic number of crossings with an infinite half-line $\mathcal{L}$.

Another interesting geometrical application of Coulomb gas methods in 2D is found in the problem of windings of a SAW about its extremities[25] (Fig.5). On e.g. the hexagonal 2D lattice the winding angle θ_1 of a self-avoiding walk around its extremity $\vec{X}$ is defined as $\theta_1 = 2\pi n_1$, where n_1 is the algebraic number of times the walk crosses a line joining $\vec{X}$ to infinity. A similar definition holds for the winding angle θ_2 around the other extremity $\vec{Y}$. One considers then the windings on presence of $O(n)$ loops, and shows[25] by a geometrical construction, involving the passage to the SOS model, that in Fourier space and at the critical point

$$\begin{aligned}\langle \exp\left[ie\pi\left(n_1 - n_2\right)\right]\rangle_{O(n)} &= \left|\vec{X} - \vec{Y}\right|^{-e^2/g} \\ &= \exp\left(-\frac{e^2}{g}\ell\mathrm{n}\left|\vec{X} - \vec{Y}\right|\right)\end{aligned}$$

where, as before g is the CG coupling constant such that $n = -2\cos\pi g$, and where the Fourier variable e is arbitrary. Hence the angular correlator appears as a Coulomb gas correlation function (2.6) of two electric charges e, $-e$ located at $\vec{X}$ and $\vec{Y}$ respectively. Since it is purely *Gaussian* in variable e, its inverse Fourier transform, i.e. the probability density of a relative angle $\hat{\theta} = 2\pi\left(n_1 - n_2\right)$ is also a Gaussian. Fourier inverting, going to finite chains of length S by scaling $\left|\vec{X} - \vec{Y}\right| \sim S^{\nu}$, and deconvoluting the single extremity winding distribution, one finds[25] for each angle $\theta = \theta_1$ or θ_2 *separately*

$$\underset{S \longrightarrow \infty}{P(\theta)} = \frac{1}{\sqrt{8\pi\nu g^{-1}\ell n\, S}} \exp\left(-\frac{g\theta^2}{8\nu\ell\mathrm{n}\, S}\right)$$

For polymers $n = 0$, $g = 3/2$, $\nu = 3/4$ and finally the winding probability distribution is the *universal* law in reduced units

$$\underset{S \longrightarrow \infty}{P_{\mathrm{SAW}}} \left(x = (4\ell\mathrm{n}\, S)^{-1/2}\,\theta\right) = \frac{1}{\sqrt{\pi}} e^{-x^2}$$

where S is the length of the SAW. The universal $\langle\theta^2\rangle = 2\ell\mathrm{n}\, S$ agrees well with earlier numerical results[26]. It is also interesting to compare $P_{\mathrm{SAW}}(x)$ to the Cauchy law for a planar Brownian path, derived by Spitzer[27] in 1958

$$P_{\mathrm{Brown}}\left(x = 2\theta/\ell\mathrm{n}\, S\right) = \frac{1}{\pi}\frac{1}{1 + x^2},$$

and to the result for 2D random walks, recently derived by Bélisle[28]

$$P_{\mathrm{RW}}\left(x = 2\theta/\ell\mathrm{n}\, S\right) = \left[2\ \mathrm{ch}\,(\pi x/2)\right]^{-1},$$

which coincides with that for "big windings" of the planar Brownian motion[29].

Percolation. Another interesting case is that of *percolation.* Let us considers the site percolation on the triangular lattice, dual of the hexagonal lattice (Fig. 6). The critical occupation probability is $p_c = \frac{1}{2}$. Then the internal and external perimeter lines surrounding clusters of occupied sites (Fig.6a) are configurations of the $O(n)$ – loop model for $n = 1$ and $K = 1$. Indeed there is an equal probability $\frac{1}{2}$ to occupy a site or not. One can draw freely with equal relative weight 1 any configurations of nonintersecting loops as cluster perimeters (up to the global choice empty versus occupied) and thus $n = 1$, $K = 1$ in Eq.(2.2). Since the Ising-like critical point of the $O(n=1)$ model is at $K_c(n=1) = 1/\sqrt{3} < 1$, the point $K_{\text{percolation}} = 1$ lies in the (low-temperature) *dense* phase of the $O(n=1)$ model. Hence the Coulomb gas coupling constant ($g \in [0,1]$) is $g = \frac{2}{3}$ and the scaling dimensions (2.7) of L lines are

$$x_L = \frac{L^2 - 1}{12}\,. \tag{2.11}$$

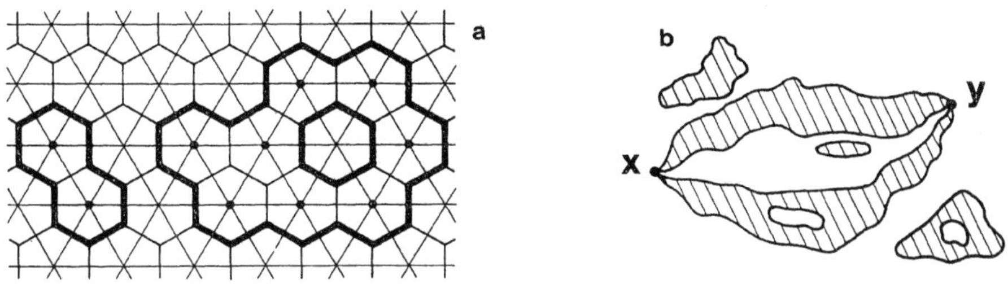

Fig.6. a) Site percolation on the triangular lattice, with hull perimeters drawn on the dual hexagonal lattice. b) $k = 2$ clusters joined together in a watermelon configuration.

We can now interpret them geometrically as the scaling dimensions associated with configurations of k clusters joining $\vec{X}$ to $\vec{Y}$ in the percolation problem (Fig.6b), if we simply remark that the $L = 2k$ external lines of these k clusters are describing all configurations $\mathcal{C}_{2k}\left(\vec{X}, \vec{Y}\right)$ of the $2k$–watermelon in presence of the loops of the $n = 1$, $K = 1$ model (i.e. the other cluster perimeters in percolation). Hence the end-to-end correlation function of k clusters at the percolation threshold decays as[8]

$$G_{2k}\left(\vec{X} - \vec{Y}\right) \sim \left|\vec{X} - \vec{Y}\right|^{-2x_{2k}}$$

$$x_{2k} = \frac{4k^2 - 1}{12} \tag{2.12}$$

The odd-L dimensions (2.11) have no obvious geometrical interpretation for percolation, but get one in terms of polymers at the tricritical Θ–point[30]. As a first application, let us remark that the hull of percolation clusters corresponds to the boundary-boundary correlation exponent x_2 of a $k = 1$ cluster. The hull fractal dimension is then given by scaling as [8]

$$D_H = 2 - x_2 = \frac{7}{4}, \tag{2.13}$$

a value which is checked numerically very well[31], and was also conjectured before from an analogy to diffusion fronts[32].

2.3 Surface Exponents

It is worth noting that all the previous discussion about the geometrical exponents x_L associated with the source of L lines in the $O(n)$ model can be generalized to *surface* geometrical phenomena[33,34]. One has simply to put the two extremities of the watermelon near the *boundary* of the half-plane. Then the correlator along the surface decays at criticality as[35]

$$G_L^S\left(\vec{X}-\vec{Y}\right) \sim \left|\vec{X}-\vec{Y}\right|^{-2x_L^S}$$

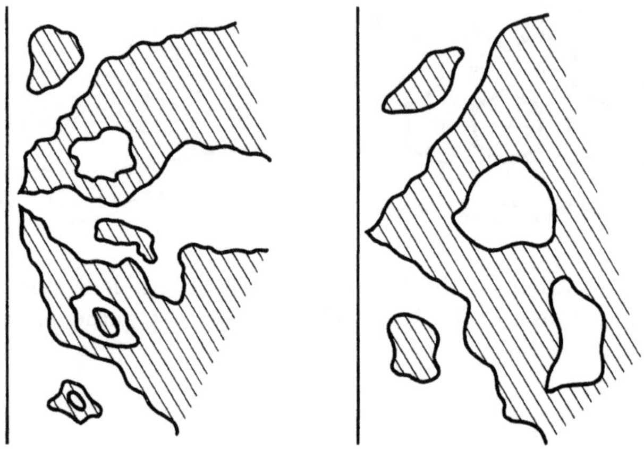

a b

Fig.7. a) A $L = 4$ line vertex near a surface line in the percolation problem (i.e. $k = 2$ clusters pinched at the surface); the scaling dimension is x_4^S (Eq.(2.14)). b) The hull near the boundary line has a new fractal dimension $D_H^S = 2/3$.

where the scaling dimension of a surface $L-$source operator is (Fig.7)

$$x_L^S = \frac{1}{4} g\, L^2 + \frac{1}{2} L\,(g-1) \tag{2.14}$$

In terms of the Kac formula these surface dimensions are expressed, using parametrization (2.8), as

$$\begin{aligned} x_L^S &= h_{L+1,1}\ , \quad \frac{m+1}{m} = g \qquad \text{(dilute phase)} \\ x_L^{S,D} &= h_{1,L+1}\ , \quad \frac{m}{m+1} = g \qquad \text{(dense phase)} \end{aligned} \tag{2.15}$$

An interesting application of these formula is the *fractal dimension of the loops of the $O(n)$ model at the boundary* (Fig.7):

$$D_F^S = 1 - x_2^S = 2\,(1-g)$$

These loops can be seen as hulls and for percolation ($n = 1$, $g = \frac{2}{3}$) we find the *new surface hull fractal dimension*

$$D_H^S = 2/3$$

Notice that this works for the dense phase of the $O(n)$ model (or the critical Potts model, as we shall see below) such that $g \in [0, 1]$. The *dilute* loops ($g \in [1, 2]$) are repelled from the boundary and one finds formally negative fractal dimensions, as expected. Up to now, the only geometrical constraint was that all elements end at the boundary line, corresponding to free boundary conditions, i.e. Dirichlet ones in the continuum limit[33], or in the terminology of critical phenomena, to the *ordinary surface transition.* Another case is the *special* surface transition were a supplementary attraction energy is given to any bond of the high-temperature loop expansion of the $O(n)$ model, which is near (or on) the surface line. At some special critical energy the loops just *adsorb.* Recent works[35,36], using numerical simulations, conformal invariance and Coulomb gas techniques indicate that the special surface dimensions for the watermelon are

$$x_L^{SP} = h_{L+1,3} = \frac{g}{4}(L+1)^2 - \frac{3}{2}(L+1) + \frac{9-(1-g)^2}{4g} \tag{2.16}$$

valid at the dilute critical point of the $O(n)$ model, $g \in [1, 2]$. The interpretation of this special transition for $1 \le n \le 2$, $g \in \left[\frac{4}{3}, 2\right]$ is subtle since no special magnetic transition is expected in 2D for $n \ge 1$; the surface line and the bulk should indeed order simultaneously, and it is well known that no transition takes place in 1D for $n \ge 1$. As an application to *fractal dimensions* let us consider again that of the points of the loops adsorbed at the boundary. We have

$$D_H^{SP} = 1 - x_2^{SP} = 5 - 2g - 2/g, \quad g \in [1, 2]$$

where this formula is restricted to the standard dilute critical point of the $O(n)$ model, hence $n = -2\cos\pi g$, $g \in [1, 2]$. For $g = 1$, $n = 2$ (XY model), $D_H^{SP} = 1$, the loops are filling the boundary line; for $g = 2$, $n = -2$, $D_H^{SP} = 0$, and the loops are completely repelled. For polymers ($g = 3/2$, $n = 0$) we find the new fractal dimension of the *adsorbed monomers*

$$D_H^{SP} = 2/3$$

Lastly, for *Ising clusters* ($n = 1$, $g = 4/3$), the adsorbed part of their hulls has a new fractal dimension

$$D_H^{SP} = 5/6$$

Before turning to some specific applications of the watermelon conformal spectrum, let us describe a useful geometrical equivalence to the Potts model.

2.4 Potts Model

The Q–state Potts model is defined by the Hamiltonian $\beta H = -\beta \sum_{\langle i,j \rangle} \delta_{\sigma_i \sigma_j}$ where the Potts variables can take Q values $\sigma_i = 1, ..., Q$, and where $\langle i, j \rangle$ are nearest neighbors on e.g. the square lattice $\mathcal{L}$. One can write the high-temperature expansion of the partition function as

$$Z_{\text{Potts}}(Q) = \sum_{\{\sigma\}} e^{-\beta H} = \sum_{\mathcal{C}} W(\mathcal{C}) \equiv \sum_{\mathcal{C}} \left(e^{\beta} - 1\right)^{\mathcal{N}_B} Q^{\mathcal{N}_C} \tag{2.17}$$

where the configurations $\mathcal{C}$ are those of spanning graphs made of bond clusters of connected sites on $\mathcal{L}$, $\mathcal{N}_B$ being the total number of bonds of $\mathcal{C}$, and $\mathcal{N}_C$ that of the connected components of $\mathcal{C}$, including all isolated sites (Fig.8). This expression now defines a model for any real Q; if $Q \longrightarrow 1$ one recovers bond percolation with occupancy probability $p = 1 - e^{-\beta}$. For $Q \in [0,4]$, there is a second-order phase transition, which can be studied with use of a Coulomb-gas mapping. First, a graph $\mathcal{C}$ on the original lattice $\mathcal{L}$ in the Potts model can be associated with a polygon decomposition of the surrounding lattice $\mathcal{S}$, here another square lattice, the sites of which are the mid-points of the edges of $\mathcal{L}$ (Fig.8). The rule is that some vertices of $\mathcal{S}$ are cut open to let the bonds of $\mathcal{L}$ go through unintersected. This also applies to the edges of the dual lattice $\mathcal{D}$ of $\mathcal{L}$. For a lattice $\mathcal{L}$ with a total number of sites S, one has (Euler's relation) $\mathcal{N}_L = \mathcal{N}_B + \mathcal{N}_C - \mathcal{N}_S$, where $\mathcal{N}_L$ is the number of loops within the clusters of the graph. On $\mathcal{S}$, the total number of polygons one can draw around each cluster and in each loop reads $\mathcal{N}_P = \mathcal{N}_L + \mathcal{N}_C$. Hence Z (2.17) can be rewritten as

$$Z_{\text{Potts}}(Q) = Q^{\mathcal{N}_S/2} \sum_{\mathcal{C}} \left[\left(e^{\beta} - 1\right) Q^{-1/2}\right]^{\mathcal{N}_B} Q^{\mathcal{N}_P/2} \tag{2.18}$$

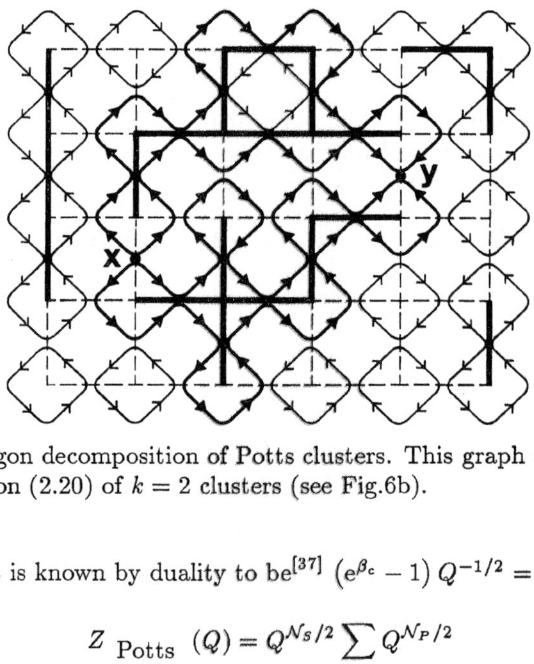

Fig.8. The polygon decomposition of Potts clusters. This graph contributes to the correlation function (2.20) of $k = 2$ clusters (see Fig.6b).

The critical point is known by duality to be[37] $\left(e^{\beta_c} - 1\right) Q^{-1/2} = 1$, hence

$$Z_{\substack{\text{Potts}\\ \text{critical}}}(Q) = Q^{\mathcal{N}_S/2} \sum_{\mathcal{C}} Q^{\mathcal{N}_P/2} \tag{2.19}$$

In this way, the *critical* Potts model appears simply as describing a dense geometrical set of nonintersecting polygons, filling the diagonal surrounding lattice, and with a weigth factor $\sqrt{Q}$ for each polygon. One guesses in this way that there should be a complete equivalence[15] to the *dense* phase of the $O(n)$ model, provided that $\sqrt{Q} = n$. This equivalence is checked by considering the watermelon scaling dimensions in the Potts model. One introduces correlation functions for the Potts model

$$G_k\left(\vec{X} - \vec{Y}\right) = \frac{1}{Z_{\text{Potts}}(Q)} \sum W(\mathcal{C}_k) \tag{2.20}$$

where the weight $W(\mathcal{C}_k)$ is defined in (2.17), and where the sum is taken over all graphs $\mathcal{C}_k$ of the surrounding lattice $\mathcal{S}$ formed by k polygons that join a neighborhood of a point $\vec{X}$ to a neighborhood of a point $\vec{Y}$ (the case $k=2$ is represented in Fig.8).

The polygon decomposition of the surrounding lattice $\mathcal{S}$ (Fig.8) allows one to consider $Z_{\text{Potts}}(Q)$ in (2.17) and (2.18) as the partition function of a special kind of six-vertex model or solid-on-solid (SOS) model. We state the facts we need here and refer the reader to previous works[8,15,38] for more details. The SOS model is driven by renormalization onto a critical Coulomb gas with a coupling constant g' given by

$$Q = 2 + 2\cos\frac{1}{2}\pi g', \quad g' \in [2,4], \quad Q \in [0,4], \tag{2.21}$$

Then G_k appears[8,15] as the correlation function of two combinations of vortex and spin wave with respective magnetic and electric charges $(m_X, e_X) = (k/2, g'/2-2)$ and $(m_Y, e_Y) = (-k/2, g'/2-2)$. It decays at criticality like

$$G_k\left(\vec{X}-\vec{Y}\right) = \left|\vec{X}-\vec{Y}\right|^{-2x'_k} \tag{2.22}$$

with a critical exponent given by the den Nijs-Nienhuis Coulomb gas formula[38,13]

$$x'_k = -\frac{g'}{2} m_X m_Y - \frac{1}{2g'} e_X e_Y = \frac{g'}{2}\left(\frac{k}{2}\right)^2 - \frac{(4-g')^2}{8g'} \tag{2.23}$$

This result is valid for any value of Q, $Q \in [0,4]$, with $g' \in [2,4]$ and thus gives the critical decay of the k-polygon correlation function (2.20).

Now we observe mathematically the complete equivalence between the geometrical exponents of the dense $O(n)$ model and the critical Potts model, which was anticipated from (2.19). The identity $\sqrt{Q} = n$, $Q \in [0,4]$, $n \in [0,2]$, is obtained for Coulomb gas coupling constants (2.5) and (2.21)

$$\begin{aligned} n &= \sqrt{Q} \in [0,2] \\ g\Big|_{\substack{O(n) \\ \text{low}-T}} &= \frac{1}{4} g'\Big|_{\substack{\text{Potts} \\ \text{critical}}} \in \left[\frac{1}{2}, 1\right] \end{aligned} \tag{2.24}$$

which implies in (2.7) and (2.23)

$$x_{L=2k} = x'_k \tag{2.25}$$

i.e. the scaling dimension of a watermelon with $L = 2k$ lines in the low-temperature phase of the $O(n)$ model is the same as that of a bundle of k polygons in the critical Potts model. These two critical phases thus belong to the same *geometrical universality class.* This has some interesting consequences. For instance the low $-\, T$ $n = 0$ model corresponds to dense SAW[16], while the $Q = 0$ Potts model is known to represent spanning trees[39] and Hamiltonian walks on the Manhattan lattice. This shows in particular that Hamiltonian walks (which are SAW visiting all lattice sites) are *universal* polymer melts[15,17]. Another expected application is found in percolation: we have seen above that *site* percolation corresponds to the low $-\, T$ phase of the $O(1)$ model. The $Q = 1$ Potts model is well known to describe *bond* percolation[39], and identity (2.25) shows that the critical geometrical properties of the multiple hulls of site and bond percolations are the same, as it must if one believes in universality of various percolation models. It is also worth noticing a *similar geometrical equivalence between the standard critical $O(n)$ model and the tricritical Potts model, still for $n = \sqrt{Q}$*. The tricritical Potts model (which is a diluted model with percolating vacancies[40]) is associated with the other analytic determination $g' \in [4,6]$ in (2.21). The relationship (2.24) (2.25) is then extended to

$$g = \frac{1}{4} g' \in \left[1, \frac{3}{2}\right]$$

$$x_{L=2k}\Big|_{\substack{O(n)\\ \text{critical}}} = x'_k\Big|_{\substack{\text{Potts}\\ \text{tricritical}}}, \quad n = \sqrt{Q} \tag{2.26}$$

and gives the same identity of watermelon exponents. An application of this is for instance the universality of SAW on the *Manhattan oriented square lattice.* This model can be transformed directly into a $Q = 0$ tricritical Potts model[41], following the same method as in Ref.[15]. Then (2.26) yields the identity to the standard $n = 0$ vector model, i.e. standard SAW on the hexagonal lattice, showing the irrelevance of orientations in a 2D Manhattan lattice.

Another application can be found in fractal dimensions associated with Potts clusters. The dimension $x'_{k=1}$ (2.23) gives the *fractal dimension of the perimeter* of a Potts cluster

$$D_H = 2 - x'_1 = 1 + 2/g' \tag{2.27}$$

where g' parametrizes $\sqrt{Q} = -2 \cos \frac{\pi}{4} g'$, $g' \in [2,4]$ for the standard critical Potts model, and $g' \in [4,6]$ for the tricritical one. For percolation $Q = 1$, $g' = \frac{8}{3}$ and we recover the standard hull fractal dimension $D_H = \frac{7}{4}$. If we want the *Ising hull fractal dimension* at the Onsager critical point we can take the equivalence to the $Q = 1$ Potts tricritical point and thus $g' = \frac{16}{3}$ giving

$$D_H\,(\text{Ising}) = \frac{11}{8} \tag{2.28}$$

The same fractal dimensions can be obtained from the standard $O(n)$ model in terms of the two-line vertex dimension x_2 (2.7)

$$D_H = 1 + \frac{1}{2g} \tag{2.29}$$

where $n = -2 \cos \pi g$, $g \in [0,1]$ for the low-temperature $O(n)$ model, and $g \in [1,2]$ at the critical point. Using the $O(n)$-Potts geometrical identification (2.24) (2.26) indeed gives the identity of the fractal dimensions (2.27) and (2.29) of the Potts hulls and of the $O(n)$ loops for $\sqrt{Q} = n$. Similar relationships exists for the fractal dimensions of Potts clusters. From den Nijs' work[38] one finds that the probability that two sites $\vec{X}$ and $\vec{Y}$ belong to the same Potts cluster scales as $P\left(\vec{X} - \vec{Y}\right) \sim \left|\vec{X} - \vec{Y}\right|^{-2x_M}$ where x_M is the magnetic exponent[38,13]

$$x_M = \frac{1}{2g'} - \frac{(4-g')^2}{8g'}$$

The fractal dimension of the cluster is then given by

$$D_c = 2 - x_M = 1 + \frac{g'}{8} + \frac{3}{2g'} \tag{2.30}$$

For percolation ($Q = 1$, $g' = \frac{8}{3}$) we recover the well-known result $D_c = \frac{91}{48}$. If we take spanning trees[15] ($Q = 0$, $g' = 2$) we find $D_c = 2$, as expected since the tree fills the space by definition. If we consider the $Q = 1$ *tricritical* Potts model, geometrically equivalent to the Ising model, we find ($g' = \frac{16}{3}$) $D_{\text{cluster}}\,(\text{Ising}) = \frac{187}{96}$, establishing[42] a result recently conjectured[43]. A direct derivation is also possible from the critical $O(n)$ model[42], where one finds $D_c = 1 + \frac{g}{2} + \frac{3}{8g}$, in agreement with (2.30) and the identification $g' = 4g$ (2.24) (2.26).

III. POLYMER AND PERCOLATION SYSTEMS OF HIGHER TOPOLOGY

3.1 Polymer Graphs

Consider a polymer graph $\mathcal{G}$ of arbitrary but fixed topology[6] (Fig.9), made of lines connected at some vertices i, $i = 1, ..., \mathcal{V}$, with L_i lines going out of vertex i.

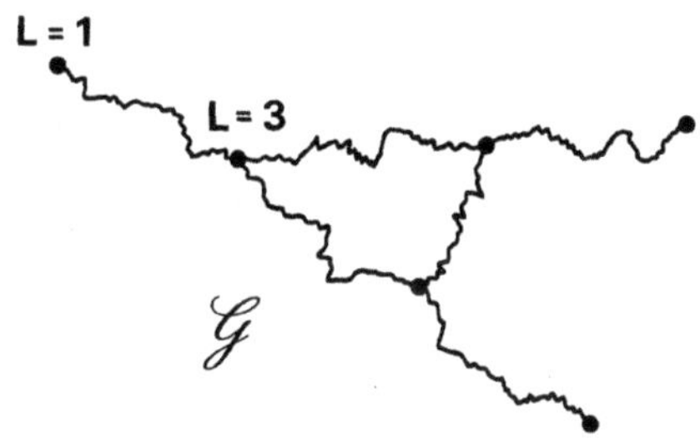

Fig.9. A polymer graph $\mathcal{G}$ or micronetwork, made of three $L = 3$ vertices and three $L = 1$ vertices (dangling ends). The total number of chains is $\mathcal{N} = 6$. The γ–configuration exponent of $\mathcal{G}$ is here $\gamma_{\mathcal{G}} = -\frac{43}{32}$ (Eq.(3.18)).

This graph represents physically a polymer micronetwork, floating in a solvent. If the solvent is good, the lines are self- and mutually avoiding because of the standard excluded volume effect. From a mathematical point of view, one can put the network on a 2D lattice and ask about the asymptotic number of configurations when the length of the lines diverge. One can distinsguish "monodisperse" networks where the lengths of the chains are all identical and equal to S, or scaling in the same way, from polydisperse networks where the lengths fluctuate with a fixed total length S. The first case is of course the experimental situation, while the second is mathematically suited for conformal field theory. Both numbers of configurations are trivially related by

$$\mathcal{Z}_{\mathcal{G}}^{\text{poly}} \sim S^{\mathcal{N}-1} \mathcal{Z}_{\mathcal{G}}^{\text{mono}} \tag{3.1}$$

where $\mathcal{N}$ is the total number of branches of $\mathcal{G}$, and where $S^{\mathcal{N}-1}$ is the "phase space" factor of the distribution of a total length S among $\mathcal{N}$ chains

$$S^{\mathcal{N}-1} \sim \int \delta\left(S - \sum_{\ell=1}^{\mathcal{N}} S_\ell\right) \mathrm{d}S_1 ... \mathrm{d}S_{\mathcal{N}}$$

For a monodisperse network $\mathcal{G}$, one expects the total number of configurations to scale as

$$\mathcal{Z}_{\mathcal{G}}^{\text{mono}} \underset{S \longrightarrow \infty}{\sim} \mu^{\mathcal{N}S} S^{\gamma_{\mathcal{G}}-1} \tag{3.2}$$

where $\mathcal{N}S$ is the total length of $\mathcal{G}$, μ is the entropy per monomer (an ultraviolet local and nonuniversal constant) and $\gamma_{\mathcal{G}}$ a universal configuration exponent. For a purely "Brownian" or "*phantom*" network on a $d-$ dimensional hypercubic lattice $\mathbf{Z}^d$ without self-avoidance one has for instance

$$\mathcal{Z}_{\mathcal{G}}^{\text{Brownian}} \sim (2d)^{\mathcal{N}S} S^{-\frac{d}{2}\mathcal{L}} \tag{3.3}$$

where $\mathcal{L}$ is the number of independent loops of the micronetwork $\mathcal{G}$, and $2d$ is the actual number of choices of a random walk at each step in $\mathbf{Z}^d$. When self-avoidance is present $\gamma_{\mathcal{G}}$ becomes a non trivial critical exponent depending on the topology of $\mathcal{G}$. We show now briefly how it can be expressed in terms of the watermelon exponents $\{x_L\}$, by decomposing the network $\mathcal{G}$ into its vertices[6].

One considers the multiple correlation function of the conformal operators ϕ_{L_i} associated with the vertices of $\mathcal{G}$,

$$G_{\mathcal{G}}\{z_i\} = \left\langle \prod_{i=1}^{\mathcal{V}} \phi_{L_i}(z_i) \right\rangle \tag{3.4}$$

where the $\{z_i\}$ denote the vertex positions in the plane. Dangling ends of $\mathcal{G}$ are to be included in the set of vertices I and are $L=1$ one-leg vertices. The above multiple correlator represents the Laplace transform of the partition function of the polydisperse network with respect to the lengths S_ℓ, $\ell = 1, ..., \mathcal{N}$ of the branches

$$G_{\mathcal{G}}\{z_i, K\} = \left\langle \prod_{i=1}^{\mathcal{V}} \phi_{L_i}(z_i) \right\rangle_K = \int_0^\infty \mathrm{d}S_1 ... \mathrm{d}S_{\mathcal{N}}\, K^{\sum_{\ell=1}^{\mathcal{N}} S_\ell} \mathcal{Z}_{\mathcal{G}}\{S_\ell, z_i\} \tag{3.5}$$

and become critical at $K_c = \mu^{-1}$ (see (2.9)). Now the scaling behavior (3.2) is easily derived by simple power counting. The polydisperse partition function is obtained by Laplace inverting (3.5) and integrating it over the positions of $\mathcal{V}-1$ vertices, keeping the last one fixed for eliminating the overall translational invariance. Hence

$$\mathcal{Z}_{\mathcal{G}}^{\text{poly.}}(S) = \int \prod_{i=1}^{\mathcal{V}-1} \mathrm{d}^2 z_i \oint \frac{d(K_c - K)}{2\pi i} K^{-S} \left\langle \prod_{i=1}^{\mathcal{V}} \phi_{L_i}(z_i) \right\rangle_K \tag{3.6}$$

where the contour of integration lies at the r.h.s. of singularities in the $K-$complex plane. Power counting implies that each conformal operator ϕ_{L_i} brings in a scaling power $[z]^{-x_{L_i}}$ is length unit (see Eq.(2.4)). So in the power counting or dimensional analysis sense

$$\mathcal{Z}_{\mathcal{G}}^{\text{poly.}}(S) \sim [z]^{2(\mathcal{V}-1)-\sum_{i=1}^{\mathcal{V}} x_{L_i}} [K_c - K] K_c^{-S} \tag{3.7}$$

where we have set K equal to its critical value $K_c = \mu^{-1}$ whenever possible. We just have to convert $[z]$ into length units $[S]$. This is done with the help of the well-known correlation length exponent ν such that

$$z \sim S^\nu \tag{3.8}$$

where z is the typical size of the network, or of any fraction of it. On the other hand the distance to the critical point K_c governs the actual length of the network in monomeric units, whence

$$S \sim (K_c - K)^{-1}, \tag{3.9}$$

an infinite network corresponding to the critical point K_c. The usual basic equivalence is thus

$$z \sim S^{\nu} \sim (K_c - K)^{-\nu}, \tag{3.10}$$

which implies in (3.7)

$$\mathcal{Z}_{\mathcal{G}}^{\text{poly.}} \sim K_c^{-S} (K_c - K)^{1-\gamma_{\mathcal{G}}^{\text{poly.}}} \tag{3.11a}$$

$$\sim \mu^S \, S^{\gamma_{\mathcal{G}}^{\text{poly.}}-1} \tag{3.11b}$$

with

$$\gamma_{\mathcal{G}}^{\text{poly.}} \equiv \nu \left(2(\mathcal{V}-1) - \sum_{i=1}^{\mathcal{V}} x_{L_i} \right) \tag{3.12}$$

Recall that in (3.11b) S is the total length of the polydisperse network with fluctuating individual lengths of the $\mathcal{N}$ branches. The monodisperse case (3.2) is obtained from relation (3.1) yielding

$$\gamma_{\mathcal{G}} - 1 = \gamma_{\mathcal{G}}^{\text{poly.}} - \mathcal{N} \tag{3.13}$$

It is also convenient to use the numbers n_L of $L-$leg vertices in a given network $\mathcal{G}$, and the topological relations $\sum_{L\geq 1} n_L = \mathcal{V}$, $\sum_{L\geq 1} n_L \; L/2 = \mathcal{N}$, to write finally

$$\gamma_{\mathcal{G}} - 1 = -2\nu + \sum_{L\geq 1} n_L \left\{ \nu (2 - x_L) - L/2 \right\} \tag{3.14}$$

which illustrates the basic principle of the factorization[8] of ("infrared") divergences of the partition function (3.2) of a given graph $\mathcal{G}$ over the vertices of $\mathcal{G}$.

It is important to mention several points. All the above analysis is fairly general and applies to *any* $O(n)$ model, where the problem is generalized to the configuration number of a self-avoiding graph in presence of vacuum loops. In this case the correlation length exponent ν in (3.14) is replaced by the exponent ν_2

$$\nu_2^{-1} \equiv 2 - x_2 \tag{3.15}$$

associated with the fractal dimension D_F of the self-avoiding lines in the $O(n)$ model

$$D_F = \nu_2^{-1} = 2 - x_2 = 1 + 1/2g \tag{3.16}$$

where $n = -2 \cos \pi g$, $g \in [1, 2]$ (dilute), $g \in [0, 1]$ (dense) (Eq.(2.5)). The exponent ν_2 differs from the standard thermal exponent ν associated with the energy operator, except for the polymer case $n = 0$. Notice that this choice (3.15) gives a curly bracket contribution for $L = 2$ in (3.14), $\nu_2 (2 - x_2) - 1 \equiv 0$, as it must since the number n_2 of two-leg insertions in a graph is arbitrary and corresponds to any occupied bond in the high-temperature expansion of the $O(n)$ model.

For standard dilute SAW, one plugs the values (2.10) of the x_L exponents into (3.14) using also (see (3.15)) the Nienhuis value[5]

$$\nu = 3/4 \tag{3.17}$$

to get

$$\gamma_{\mathcal{G}} = -\frac{1}{2} + \frac{1}{64}\sum_{L\geq 1} n_L\,(2-L)\,(9L+50) \tag{3.18}$$

This formula is very well checked from numerical simulation results. For instance for network having the topology of a star, this gives $\gamma_L = \frac{68+9L(3-L)}{64}$, hence $\gamma_1 = \gamma_2 \equiv \gamma = \frac{43}{32}$ (usual susceptibility exponent of a linear chain[5]), $\gamma_3 = \frac{17}{16} = 1.0625$, $\gamma_4 = \frac{1}{2}$, $\gamma_5 = -\frac{11}{32} = -0.34374$ and $\gamma_6 = -\frac{47}{32} = -1.46875$. The numerical results are[44] $\gamma_3 = 1.07 \pm 0.02$, $\gamma_4 = 0.52 \pm 0.04$, $\gamma_5 = -0.29 \pm 0.04$ and $\gamma_6 = -1.33 \pm 0.05$. The γ_H exponent of a H–comb is $\gamma_H = \frac{25}{32} = 0.78125$, and numerically[45] $\gamma_H = 0.79 \pm 0.02$.

Of course, the vertex decomposition formula generalizes[6,46] to any space dimension. A general proof in the realm of standard perturbative renormalization theory is still lacking however. It would require a careful selection of the irreducible vertex operator associated with the branching of L lines in the $O(n)$ model, among all operators mixing with φ^L in a φ^4 theory. Let us finally mention that we shall encounter in the case of the $O(n)$ model embedded in a fluctuating surface, a decomposition formula entirely similar to (3.14), which is established there by a direct solution.

3.2 Pinching Points in Percolation

As a second application of the watermelon formalism described in part II, let us return to the percolation problem (i.e. the low-temperature phase of the $O(1)$ model, or the $Q = 1$ Potts model) and to some specific topological questions in it[8]. One can ask: what is the typical length of a hull perimeter near the critical threshold p_c? Or, what is the probability that a point belongs to the hull of the infinite incipient cluster? Or that a point $\vec{X}$ is a *pinching point* of order $L = 2k$, where k clusters come close together (Fig.1b)? Let us recall the values (2.12) of the percolation geometrical exponents associated with k clusters $x_L \equiv x'_k = (L^2-1)/12 = (4k^2-1)/12$. By standard scaling analysis[31], one first shows that the hull perimeter length diverges as

$$\langle \ell(\mathcal{P})\rangle \sim |p-p_c|^{-\gamma_1}, \quad \gamma_1 = (2-2x'_1)\,\nu = 2,$$

where ν is the percolation thermal exponent $\nu = 4/3$[47], and x'_1 the one-cluster watermelon exponent. Accordingly the hull fractal dimension is $D_H = 2 - x'_1 = 7/4$, as mentioned above, and the probability that a point belongs to the hull of the infinite cluster grows like $P_1 \sim (p-p_c)^{\beta_1}$, $\beta_1 = \nu x'_1 = \frac{1}{3}$. One can go to higher topologies and consider the *pinching problem* (Fig.1b). The singular part of the mean number of clusters, the external perimeter of which has the special topology of k bands pinched at their extremities (Fig.6) is

$$\langle n_k\rangle \sim |p-p_c|^{-\gamma_k}, \quad \gamma_k = (2-2x'_k)\,\nu = \frac{2}{9}\left(13-4k^2\right)$$

One can also consider the probability P_k that a point belongs to a region of the perimeter of the infinite cluster, where the latter has the special topology of k bands ("peninsulas") coming close together (Fig.1b). It grows as $P_k \sim (p-p_c)^{\beta_k}$, where $\beta_k = \nu - \frac{1}{2}\gamma_k \equiv \nu x'_k = \frac{1}{9}\left(4k^2-1\right)$ (Eq.(1.4)). For $k = 2$, it is interesting to note that two touching peninsulas are equivalent to a *cutting bond.* We find $x'_2 = \frac{5}{4}$; hence we obtain a fractal dimension $D_{\text{red}} = 2 - \beta_2/\nu = \frac{3}{4} = 1/\nu$, thus giving another determination of a well-known result[9].

IV. INTERSECTIONS OF RANDOM WALKS

In probability theory, and also in the representation of field theory by intersecting random walks, a simple but non trivial problem plays an important role. Consider two random walks (R.W.) in $\mathbf{Z}^d$, w_1, w_2, starting at the origin. What is the probability $P_2(t)$

$$P_2(t) \equiv P(w_1(0,t] \cap w_2(0,t] = \emptyset) \tag{4.1}$$

that after a given number of steps t their *paths have no mutual intersections?* (Fig.10).

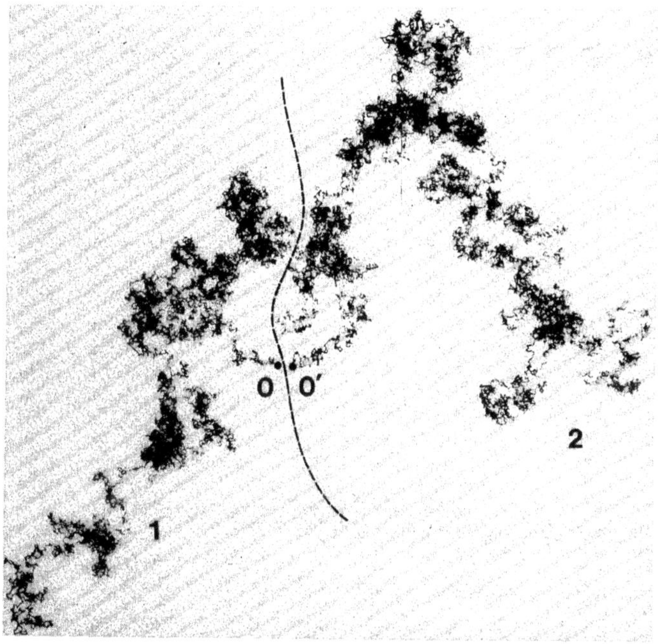

Fig.10. Two random walks, or Brownian paths starting at close points 0 and 0′, and nonintersecting.

The notation $w(0,t]$ represents the set of points

$$w(0,t] = \{w(t'),\ 0 < t' \leq t\}, \tag{4.2}$$

the origin being excluded. For large time t one expects $P_2(t)$ to decay algebraically as

$$\underset{t \longrightarrow \infty}{P_2(t)} \sim t^{-\zeta_2} \tag{4.3}$$

where ζ_2 is a universal critical exponent associated with *mutually-avoiding* walks. That ζ_2 is universal means that it depends only on the space dimension d and not on the lattice representation, and keeps its well-defined value in the continuum limit of Brownian motions. In this latter case however, it is possible that there are infinitely many intersections at short distance with probability one in *two-dimensions*, if the two paths start at the same point. So the equivalent problem to mutually-avoiding walks in the continuum Brownian case, is to consider Brownian paths starting at very close but different points. The non intersecting random walks constitute a critical system in a *new* universality class. The upper critical dimension is the same $d = 4$, since two Brownian paths having a fractal Hausdorff dimension $D_H = 2$, their intersection set is non empty only if $d \leq 2D_H = 4$. Hence $P_2(t) \equiv 1$ for $d > 4$ and $\zeta_2 = 0$ for $d > 4$. Several years ago, Lawler[48] proved that in four dimensions, the decay of $P_2(t)$ is logarithmic

$$P_2(t) \sim (\ell n\ t)^{-1/2} \tag{4.4}$$

This was generalized to the non-intersection probability of L walks in $d = 4$[49]

$$P_L(t) \sim (\ell n\ t)^{-L(L-1)/4} \tag{4.5}$$

For L walks, one expects in the same way for $d < 4$ a non trivial exponent ζ_L generalizing ζ_2 in (4.3)

$$\underset{t \longrightarrow \infty}{P_L(t)} \sim t^{-\zeta_L} \tag{4.6}$$

By using a direct renormalization method, the asymptotic expansion of ζ_L was obtained near four dimensions[49], $d = 4 - \varepsilon$

$$\zeta_L = \frac{L}{2}(L-1)\frac{\varepsilon}{4} + \frac{1}{2}L(L-1)(5-2L)\left(\frac{\varepsilon}{4}\right)^2 + O\left(\varepsilon^3\right) \qquad \varepsilon \equiv 4 - d > 0 \tag{4.7}$$

For $L = 2$, this gives in particular the $\varepsilon-$expansion $\zeta_2 = \frac{\varepsilon}{4} + \left(\frac{\varepsilon}{4}\right)^2 + O\left(\varepsilon^3\right)$.

In *two-dimensions* progresses have been made recently. On the mathematical side[50] it was proved that 1) $\lim_{t \longrightarrow \infty} \ell n\ P_2(t) / \ell n\ t$ exists i.e. the exponent ζ_2 exists, (and the ζ_L), 2) rigorous bounds can be given to ζ_2 :

$$\frac{1}{2} < \zeta_2 \leq \frac{3}{4} \tag{4.8}$$

On the theoretical physics side, the idea appeared[51] to use conformal invariance methods to try and determine the basic probabilistic exponents ζ_L in two-dimensions.

The essential idea is that there should be a special conformal operator ϕ'_L associated with the source of L mutually-avoiding walks (MAW) originating at a given point. This assumption is quite similar to that above concerning the existence of operators ϕ_L (2.4) in the case of the $O(n)-$model. The $n = 0$ limit gave us source operators for L *self- and mutually* avoiding lines. From the scaling dimensions x'_L of the watermelon correlator in the case of MAW, one can deduce by scaling and renormalization group arguments the probability exponents ζ_L [51] :

$$\zeta_L = \nu\, x'_L = \frac{1}{2} x'_L$$

where $\nu = 1/2$ is the trivial correlation length exponent of simple Brownian paths. As a result, one conjectures that the exponents ζ_L (which "acts" in time t, see (4.6), while the scaling dimensions x'_L "act" in space, see (2.4)) are themselves elements of a conformal Kac table. The central charge of the underlying conformal theory is easily seen to be identically zero: $c = 0$. Indeed, e.g. two mutually-avoiding walks can be represented by an interacting field theory with Lagrangian $\sum_{\alpha,\beta} (\varphi_\alpha)^2 (\psi_\beta)^2$, for two fields φ, ψ with components $\alpha, \beta = 1, ..., n$, and in the limit $n = 0$. Hence the field partition function will be trivially $Z(\varphi, \psi) \equiv 1$, and thus $c = 0$ since c can be seen as a universal finite-size scaling correction amplitude of the free energy $\ell n\ Z \equiv 0$ (see [22] and references therein). One cannot use standard transfer matrix techniques to study the MAW spectrum x'_L, since each random walk on a strip requires multiple bond occupancy, nor Coulomb gas techniques since each random walk makes infinitely many closed loops, forbidding a simple mapping onto an SOS model and then a Coulomb gas. So we resorted to Monte-Carlo simulations to study directly in 2D the probabilistic exponents ζ_L. The outcome was the conformal conjecture for the spectrum ζ_L :

$$\zeta_L = h_{0,L}^{(c=0)} = \left(4L^2 - 1\right)/24 \qquad (L \geq 2) \tag{4.9}$$

where $h_{p,q}$ is the standard Kac formula (2.8) taken for $c = 0$ and integer parameter $m = 2$. Again we are in the same conformal table $c = 0$, $m = 2$ as for polymers and percolation, which extends the Friedan, Qiu and Shenker classification for unitary minimal models $c < 1$, $m \geq 3$ to non unitary geometric critical phenomena. This shows that the RW intersections in two dimensions are actually deeply related to conformal invariance, which can be used to obtain new and exact results in probability theory. Furthermore, this provides perhaps the most simple model of a conformally invariant theory. If it were solved rigorously in the future, it would be a good test for conformal invariance methods.

Two remarks: we conjecture for two walks $\zeta_2 = 5/8$, which fits into the bounds (4.8), being even equal to their arithmetic mean. Second, the series (4.9) gives a non trivial value $\zeta_1 = 1/8$. This exponent cannot correspond to an intersection property of several walk and should be associated with a single walk property. It is possible[52] that it governs the probability $P_1(t) \sim t^{-1/8}$ that a Brownian path or random walk *does not encircle* its origin, i.e. that the origin of the path is accessible from infinity without crossing the Brownian path (Fig.11).

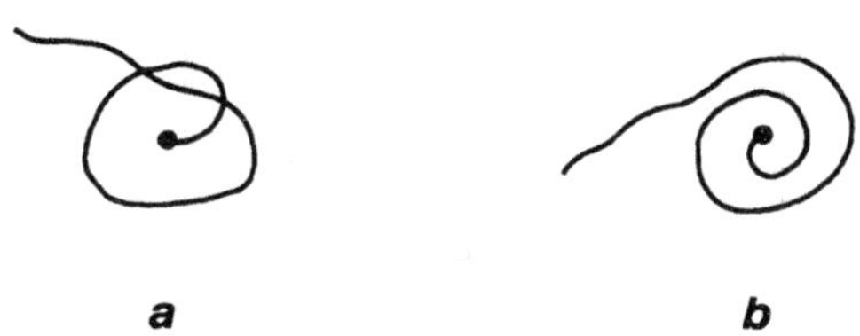

Fig.11. The random walk a) encircle, or b) winds about its origin. In case a) the origin cannot be reached from infinity without crossing the path.

Recently Burdzy and Lawler have also reconsidered the problem of the fractal dimension of the hull of a 2D (closed) Brownian motion[50]. This hull is the closed Jordan curve which is the borderline of the infinite open set exterior to the planar Brownian motion. Mandelbrot[4] called this *Brownian perimeter* the "self-avoiding Brownian motion", since the computer simulations indicated that its Hausdorff dimension $D_{BP} \approx 4/3$, which is that of actual 2D SAW. Burdzy and Lawler[50] used $D_{BP} \leq 2 - \zeta_2$, which can be shown by a conformal mapping, and where ζ_2 is the nonintersection exponent of two walks, together with their lower bound $\zeta_2 \geq 1/2 + 1/\left(4\pi^2\right)$, to get $D_{BP} \leq 3/2 - 1/\left(4\pi^2\right)$. Using our conjecture $\zeta_2 = 5/8$, we get instead the presumably exact bound

$$D_{\text{Brown.Peri.}} \leq 11/8 = 1.375$$

This value is quite close to the numerical estimate $D_{BP} \approx 1.33$, and could be the exact one.

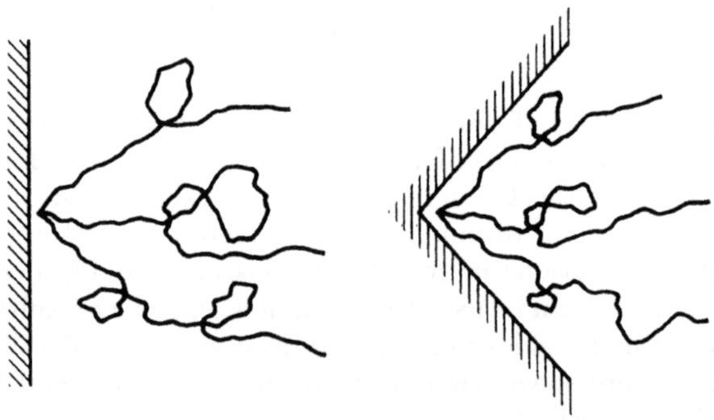

Fig.12 . Mutually-avoiding walks starting at a Dirichlet boundary line, or in the apex of a wedge α, after a conformal mapping $w(z) = z^{\alpha/\pi}$. The associated exponents are ζ_L^S (4.10) and $\zeta_L(\alpha)$ (4.11).

Many other probabilistic exponents are obtained by this approach. One can take L walks all starting at a same point near the boundary line of a half-plane. In this case one obtain surface critical exponents and the probability of no intersection scales as (Fig.12)

$$\begin{aligned} P_L^S(t) &\sim t^{-\zeta_L^S} \\ \zeta_L^S &= \frac{1}{2}\left(h_{1,2L+2}^{(c=0)} - L\right) = \frac{1}{3}L(L-1) \end{aligned} \tag{4.10}$$

If the walks all start in the apex of a wedge angle α (Fig.12), the probability of no further encounter scales as $P_L^W(t,\alpha) \sim t^{-\zeta_L(\alpha)}$, with

$$\zeta_L(\alpha) = \frac{\pi}{\alpha}\frac{1}{3}L(L-1) \tag{4.11}$$

a formula which can be obtained from (4.10) by the conformal mapping $z \longrightarrow z^{\alpha/\pi}$. It is interesting to remark that the case $\alpha = 2\pi$ corresponds to L mutually-avoiding walks in presence of a forbidden half-line. In the many walks limit $L \longrightarrow \infty$ one expects the exclusion of the half-line to be irrelevant when compared to the mutual avoidance effect for $L \longrightarrow \infty$. In this case (4.11) gives a dominant contribution

$$\zeta_L(2\pi) \sim \frac{1}{6}L^2 \quad , \quad L \longrightarrow \infty \tag{4.12}$$

which is the same as the dominant contribution in the bulk exponent ζ_L (4.9) for $L \longrightarrow \infty$, as expected.

As in the case of SAW, one can consider networks of mutually-avoiding walks[49]. If one takes for instance $\mathcal{N}$ independent Brownian motions and ask about the probability that their paths at time t form a certain network $\mathcal{G}$, characterized by the set of numbers $\{n_L\}$ of $L-$walk vertices. In absence of mutual-avoidance, the probability scales as in (3.3)

$$P_{\mathcal{G}}^{RW}(t) \sim t^{-\frac{1}{2}d\mathcal{L}} \tag{4.13}$$

where $\mathcal{L}$ is the number of independent loops in $\mathcal{G}$

$$\mathcal{L} = \frac{1}{2}\sum_{L\geq 1} n_L(L-2) + 1$$

Now, one can implement mutual-avoidance between all the $\mathcal{N}$ walks building up $\mathcal{G}$. Then the probability will scale as[49]

$$P_{\mathcal{G}}(t) \sim t^{-\frac{1}{2}d\mathcal{L} - \sum_{L\geq 2} n_L\zeta_L} \tag{4.14}$$

where ζ_L are the MAW exponents defined above for L walks starting at a same point. This formula describes the factorization over the vertices and is entirely similar to (3.14) for SAW. The relative probability that, knowing that the $\mathcal{N}$ RW form a given graph $\mathcal{G}$, they further have no mutual intersection, is simply the ratio of (4.13) and (4.14)

$$\begin{aligned} P'_{\mathcal{G}} = P_{\mathcal{G}}/P_{\mathcal{G}}^{RW} &\sim t^{-\sum_{L\geq 2} n_L\zeta_L} \\ &= t^{-\sum_{L\geq 2} n_L\frac{4L^2-1}{24}} \end{aligned} \tag{4.15}$$

Notice that if one further introduces the constraint that the free extremities of the walks (corresponding to $L=1$) are *not encircled*, this gives $n_{L=1}$ new constraints which are simply taken into account by a supplementary factor $t^{-n_1\zeta_1} = t^{-n_1/8}$ in (4.14) or (4.15), completing the summation over L down to $L=1$.

As an application, we can, for instance, calculate the probability $P_{\mathcal{W}_L}$ that L independent random walks starting together meet again anywhere at time t without having any mutual crossing point in between (watermelon $\mathcal{W}_L$). It scales like $P_{\mathcal{W}_L}(t) \sim t^{\gamma_{\mathcal{W}_L}-1}$, where the scaling theory of (4.14) gives

$$\begin{aligned} \gamma_{\mathcal{W}_L} - 1 &= -(L-1) - 2\zeta_L \\ &= -\frac{1}{12}\left(4L^2 + 12L - 13\right). \end{aligned} \tag{4.16}$$

It follows from (4.6) and (4.16) that the (conditional) probability that L mutually-avoiding RW starting at the same point enjoy a reunion at time t at any point scales like

$$P_{\mathcal{W}_L}/P_L \sim t^{\gamma_{\mathcal{W}_L}-1+\zeta_L} \sim t^{-(4L^2+24L-25)/24}. \tag{4.17}$$

Directed. Note that the solution for (symmetric) *directed* walks[53] gives different exponents for probabilities (4.6), (4.16), and (4.17), $\tilde{\zeta}_L = \frac{1}{4}L(L-1)$, $\tilde{\gamma}_{\mathcal{W}_L} - 1 = -\frac{1}{2}(L^2-1)$, $\tilde{\gamma}_{\mathcal{W}_L} - 1 + \tilde{\zeta}_L = -\frac{1}{4}(L-1)(L+2)$, which are also quadratic in L, but of course differ from ours. These directed MAW's are extremely sensitive to non-symmetric diffusion constants, which lead to nonuniversal and continuously varying exponents[54]. There the space anisotropy forbids conformal invariance, in contrast to our work.

V. STATISTICAL MECHANICS ON A FLUCTUATING LATTICE

5.1 Brief History

The consideration of statistical mechanics on a random lattice originated from studies of such two-dimensional lattices as models of random surfaces. The first example of critical phenomena on a surface with fluctuating geometry ($2d$ quantum gravity) is given by the bosonic string in the Polyakov's formulation[55]. The matter field is represented by d free bosons (Gaussian fields) living on the surface, where d is the dimension of the equivalent embedding space. The discretization of the model is obtained by replacing the integration over the metrics representing the quantum gravitational field, by a sum over arbitrary (planar) discrete graphs[56−58]. Notice that one has to fix the topology of the world-surface in order to prevent divergences in the sum over topologies, otherwise unavoidable; and the planar (spherical) topology is the simplest one. It became also clear that the graphs generated by any set of local rules (like φ^3, φ^4 etc... vertices) would have the same critical behaviour[56,59,60].

Pure gravity (an abstract random surface with a fluctuating intrinsic metric and not embedded, i.e. in zero dimension) is thus described by the ensemble of abstract planar graphs. Exact results were obtained in $d=0$ or $d=-2$ dimensions for the string susceptibility exponent γ_{string} of the free energy near criticality[57,61,62]. Then the idea of putting more general statistical models on a random surface occured in the first example of the Ising model treated by V.A. Kazakov[63], who obtained critical exponents different from those of Onsager in two-dimensions. Some exact results were also obtained for the Q−state Potts model[64].

Recently, another continuum approach to 2D-critical phenomena in presence of gravity has been developped by Polyakov[65], and Knizhnik, Polyakov and Zamolodchikov[10] (KPZ). It is the generalization of the standard conformal invariance in the plane associated with the Virasoro algebra, to conformal invariance in presence of an (annealed) fluctuating metric. A spectacular prediction by KPZ is that the conformal dimensions of the usual Kac spectrum (2.8)

$$h_{p,q} \equiv \Delta^{(0)}_{p,q} = \frac{(\kappa p - q)^2 - (\kappa - 1)^2}{4\kappa} \tag{5.1}$$

which are associated with a central charge $c \leq 1$

$$c = 1 - 6\frac{(\kappa-1)^2}{\kappa}, \quad \kappa \geq 1 \tag{5.2}$$

are *linearized in presence of (critical) quantum gravity* into the new ones

$$\Delta_{p,q} = \frac{1}{2}\left(|\kappa p - q| - (\kappa - 1)\right), \tag{5.3}$$

satisfying the KPZ quadratic relation

$$\Delta - \Delta^{(0)} = \Delta\left(1 - \Delta\right)/\kappa \tag{5.4}$$

We have distinguished here the dimensions $\Delta^{(0)}$ in the plane from those Δ dressed by gravity. Also, we use the notation

$$\kappa \equiv \frac{m+1}{m} \geq 1 \tag{5.5}$$

in place of the usual conformal parameter m in (2.8). The quite striking idea that critical phenomena in the 2D plane and on a critical random surface are acutally organically related led then immediately to a burst of exact solutions for other statistical models on a random lattice: self-avoiding walks[11], $O(n)$ model[66,67], $Q = 1$ Potts model and bond percolation[68].

All these solvable models, including the former Ising case[63], produced conformal dimensions in presence of gravity which fully satisfy KPZ relation (5.4). Of particular interest is the polymer, or more generally the $O(n)$ model case, where the complete spectrum of the watermelon dimensions Δ_L can be obtained, and compared then to the dimension $\Delta_L^{(0)} = \frac{1}{2}x_L$ in the regular plane (2.7) (2.8) obtained by Coulomb gas techniques. We shall describe here more precisely how the geometrical $O(n)$ loop model or SAW model can be resolved in a fluctuating 2D-lattice, and the watermelon exponents determined. Actually, all sorts of *geometrical* questions, like the embedding of a topological network $\mathcal{G}$ in a random surface, are very well suited to the method[67]. We shall in particular describe the analog on a fluctuating surface of the scaling properties of polymer networks described in section III as well as those of percolation clusters on a random surface. One can there prove basic relationships like (3.12).

5.2 Geometrical Model on a Random Lattice

As an illustration, and to parallel the study of section II in the regular plane, we shall start from the $O(n)$ model on a fluctuating lattice. Instead of considering the partition function (2.1) in the infinite regular lattice, one first has to define it on an arbitrary 3-coordinate planar graph G (i.e. with the topology of the sphere)

$$Z_{O(n)}(G) = \int \prod_{i \in G} \mathrm{d}\vec{S}_i \prod_{\langle j,k \rangle} \left(1 + K\, \vec{S}_j \cdot \vec{S}_k\right) \tag{5.6}$$

where i, j, k are arbitrary sites of lattice G and $\langle j, k\rangle$ denotes nearest neighbours as before. Now we have to take into account the fluctuations of the lattice by summing over all planar graphs G made of e.g. φ^3-type vertices, possibly with a symmetry factor $1/S(G)$. The total *annealed* partition function is therefore.

$$Z_{O(n)}(\beta, K) = \sum_G \frac{1}{S(G)} \mathrm{e}^{-\beta|G|} Z_{O(n)}(G) \tag{5.7}$$

where β is the "cosmological constant" which is conjugated to the "area" or "volume" or "mass" $|G|$ of the fluctuating lattice

$$|G| = \#\text{ vertices of } G. \tag{5.8}$$

The system is thus defined in terms of two fugacities: K (the inverse temperature of the $O(n)$ model) and $e^{-\beta}$ (that of the lattice). The $K-$expansion of the $O(n)$ model is of course still given by a self-avoiding loop representation on each graph G

$$Z_{O(n)}(G) = \sum_{\substack{\text{nonintersecting} \\ \text{loops on } G}} n^{\mathcal{N}_L} K^{\mathcal{N}_B}, \tag{5.9}$$

exactly as in Eq.(2.2) (Fig.13). Notice that we consider a φ^3-lattice for definiteness, but it can be shown be explicit calculations (like on a φ^n-lattice) that the critical behaviour described below is universal. Notice also that here the only difference from the standard honeycomb case (Fig.3) is that the local constraints of closing little hexagons after six e.g. right turning bonds are relaxed on the fluctuating lattice (Fig.13). This suppression of constraints makes the problem solvable.

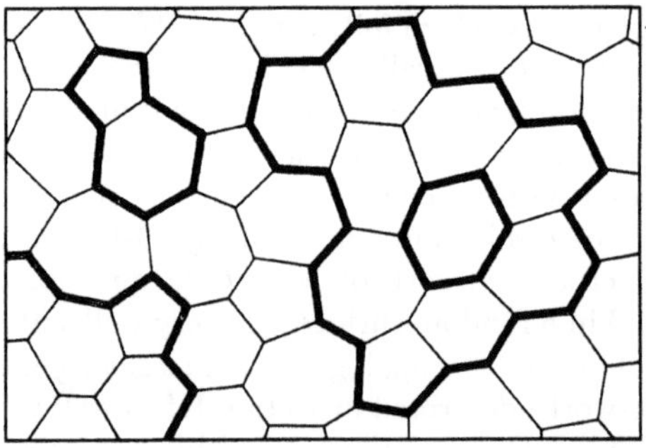

Fig.13. Loop expansion (5.9) of the $O(n)$ model on the random φ^3-lattice.

When one considers only the empty loop configuration ($K = 0$), one gets the partition function of the random surface only

$$Z(\beta) = \sum_G \frac{1}{S(G)} e^{-\beta|G|} \tag{5.10}$$

It exists a critical potential β_c such that the characteristic fluctuations of $|G|$ diverge, and where the partition function Z (5.10) develops a non analyticity

$$Z(\beta) \sim (\beta - \beta_c)^{2-\gamma_{\rm str}} \quad , \beta > \beta_c, \tag{5.11}$$

$\gamma_{\rm str}$ being the string susceptibility exponent, and the random surface model being defined only for $\beta \geq \beta_c$.

For the $O(n)$ model, the loop and graph expansion (5.7) (5.9) reads explicitly

$$Z_{O(n)}(\beta, K) = \sum_G \sum_{\text{loops on } G} n^{\mathcal{N}_L} \left(e^{-\beta}\right)^{\mathcal{N}_E} \left(e^{-\beta}K\right)^{\mathcal{N}_B} \tag{5.12}$$

where $\mathcal{N}_L$ is the number of loops, $\mathcal{N}_B$ that of the occupied bonds on G, $\mathcal{N}_E$ that of the empty vertices of G. The two fugacities $g \equiv e^{-\beta}$, $z \equiv e^{-\beta}K$ thus control the complete phase behaviour of the system.

If, for a fixed and low enough value of z, g increases, one will enconter a critical point $g_c(z,n)$ where the fluctuations of the random surface diverge. This is the usual infinite random surface point, with the same universality class, and only the nonuniversal position of the critical point $g_c(z,n)$ depends on the presence of the $O(n)$ model at temperature K^{-1}. If one fixes on the contrary g (and small enough) then one shall meet by increasing K or z another critical phase $z_c(g)$ where the mean length of the $O(n)$ loops diverges but not the nonfilled part of the random lattice, still governed by a non critical g. This naturally corresponds to the dense phase of the $O(n)$ model (see part II) where the self-avoiding loops fill the (here fluctuating) lattice with a non vanishing density. Finally only when one approaches the intersection point of the two critical lines $g_c(z^*) = g^*$, $z_c(g^*) = z^*$, is a simultaneous double critical behaviour possible, when the lattice and loop volumes diverge independently. This will correspond to the standard dilute critical point of the $O(n)$ model, here on an infinite surface. The shape of the lines $g_c(z,n)$, $z_c(g,n)$ is in general complicated for arbitrary n. Notice that one expects a second order phase transition in the $O(n)$ model only for $-2 \leq n \leq 2$, even on the random surface[66]. We shall later concentrate on the polymer i.e. $n = 0$ model, in which case the phase diagram is simpler[67]. Indeed since for $n = 0$, there are no vacuum loops in the partition function (5.12) the critical surface line $g_c(z, n=0)$ is a constant $g_c(z,n=0) = g_c$ $(= \left(12\sqrt{3}\right)^{-1/2}$ in the case of a φ^3 lattice[59]), corresponding to the empty lattice critical point. The polymer critical line $z_c(g, n=0)$ is determined below from an explicit solution.

5.3 Random Matrices

Most statistical models on a fluctuating lattice can be represented in terms of models of random $N \times N$ matrices in the large N limit[59–64,66,68,69], the action of the matrix model depending on the statistical model considered, and on the type of connectivity of the lattice. We shall not develop this aspect here, which will not be used explicitly in the specific case of self-avoiding walks. For completeness in the general introduction of the $O(n)$ model (5.6) (5.7) (5.12), let us simply add that after a representation in terms of a large N matrix integral, evaluated at its saddle point, the partition function reads explicitly[66]

$$\begin{aligned} Z_{O(n)}(\beta, K) &= \int_a^b \mathrm{d}\lambda\, \rho(\lambda) \left(-\frac{1}{2}\lambda^2 + \frac{g}{3}\lambda^3\right) \\ &+ \int_a^b \mathrm{d}\lambda\, \rho(\lambda) \int_a^b \mathrm{d}\mu\, \rho(\mu) \left(\ell\mathrm{n}\,|\lambda-\mu| - \frac{n}{2}\ell\mathrm{n}\left(\frac{1}{z} - \lambda - \mu\right)\right) \end{aligned} \tag{5.13}$$

where $\rho(\lambda)$ is the normalized eigenvalue density of the random matrix at the saddle point

$$\begin{gathered} \lambda - g\,\lambda^2 = 2\int_a^b \mathrm{d}\mu\, \rho(\mu) \left(\frac{P}{\lambda-\mu} + \frac{n}{2}\frac{1}{\frac{1}{z} - \lambda - \mu}\right) \\ \int_a^b \rho(\lambda)\, \mathrm{d}\lambda = 1 \end{gathered} \tag{5.14}$$

(P means principal value). Notice that solving ρ in Eq.(5.14) requires also the determination of the support $[a,b]$ outside of which ρ vanishes. The solution of (5.14) for general n is not an easy task[69] and is known only along the critical line $\frac{1}{z} = 2b$.

From (5.13) (5.14) it is indeed possible to see the expected characteristics: the critical surface line $g_c(z,n)$ corresponds to the singularity of the end point b in terms of g : $\left.\frac{\partial g}{\partial b}\right|_z = 0$. This end-point b plays an important role since for $\lambda = \mu = b$ the nearest singularity of the integrand in (5.13) (5.14) is at $\frac{1}{z} = 2b(g,z)$, yielding $z_c(g,n)$. From (5.13) (5.14) one can show also that the equations make sense only for $n \in [-2,2]$ as expected[66,69].

5.4 Self-Avoiding Walks on a 2D-Random Lattice

a) *Watermelon partition function.* We now consider specifically the $n=0$ case and calculate the scaling dimensions Δ_L of the operator source if L self-avoiding lines on the random lattice. However the method we follow[11] can be generalized identically to the $O(n)$ model[66,67]. For this, we consider as usual the watermelon network, but this time on the fluctuating lattice (Fig.14).

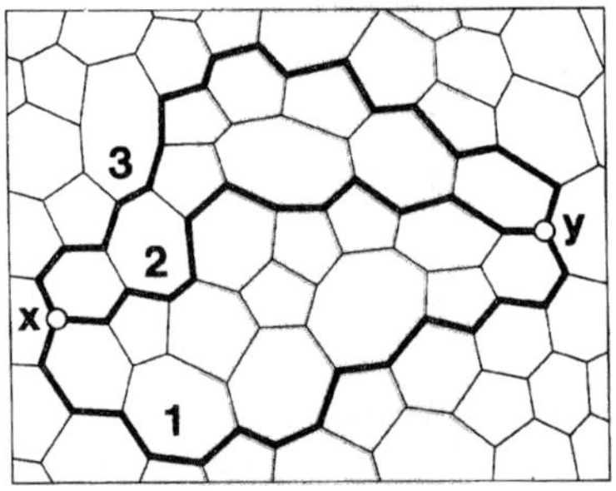

Fig.14. Watermelon network on the random φ^3-lattice.

The total partition function of the lattice and of the L SAW is defined as

$$Z_L(\beta,K) = \sum_G \frac{1}{S(G)} e^{-\beta|G|} \sum_{i,j} \sum_{\substack{\Gamma_{ij}^{(\ell)} \\ \ell=1,\dots,L}} K^{|\Gamma|} \tag{5.15}$$

where the sum extends on all graphs G with the topology of the sphere, made of φ^3 vertices, and over all polymer sets of lines $\Gamma_{ij}^{(\ell)}$, $\ell = 1,\dots,L$, joining any two points i,j on G. In the absence of SAW ($K=0$) the random surface itself has a critical point β_c where the typical size $|G|$ diverges, with a partition function (5.10) behaving as in (5.11), where the string susceptibility exponent γ_{st} has been calculated exactly[56,57] for embedding space dimensions $d=-2$, $\gamma_{st}=-1$, and $d=0$, $\gamma_{st}=-1/2$. Note that here the embedding space dimension is formally $d=0$, but will be replaced by the central charges $c=-2$ or $c=0$.

The key point is that the partition function Z_L can be calculated exactly. For this, one fixes first the SAW lengths and sums over the L lattice connected pieces between successive polymer lines ℓ and $\ell+1$ (Fig.15).

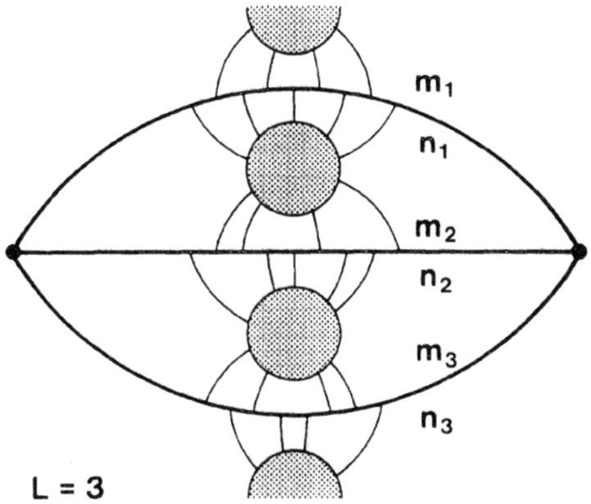

Fig.15. Illustration of the convolutive sum (5.17) on the spherical lattice. Each bubble $\ell = 1, 2, 3$ corresponds to a connected piece of lattice with a Green function $G_{n_\ell + m_{\ell+1}}$ (5.16). The bold lines are the SAW.

Each of these planar pieces contributes a factor $G_{n_\ell + m_{\ell+1}}$ to the partition function, where G_n is the Green function of random graphs with n external legs

$$G_n(\beta) = \sum_{n-\text{leg planar } G} e^{-\beta|G|} \tag{5.16}$$

and where n_ℓ and $m_{\ell+1}$ are the number of legs attached to the ℓ and $\ell + 1$ SAW respectively. As a result, Z_L is the convolutive sum

$$Z_L(\beta, K) = \sum_{m_\ell, n_\ell} (e^{-\beta} K)^{\sum_\ell m_\ell + n_\ell} \prod_{\ell=1}^{L} \binom{m_\ell + n_\ell}{m_\ell} G_{n_\ell + m_{\ell+1}}(\beta) \tag{5.17}$$

with the cyclic convention $L + 1 \equiv 1$. (The combinatorial factors are the numbers of relative positions of m_ℓ and n_ℓ lattice legs branched on each side of the ℓth SAW). Now the second key point is that the planar random lattice Green function, G_n, can be calculated from the thermodynamic limit of matrix integrals. It is simply the nth moment of the eigenvalue density (5.14)[59]

$$G_n = \int_a^b d\lambda\, \lambda^n \rho(\lambda) \tag{5.18}$$

Notice that all the calculations so far are valid for any loop model when the connected pieces of lattice between the lines of the watermelon bear vacuum loops. The density ρ in (5.18) is then simply the solution of (5.14). Now a very simple algebra allows to resum (5.17) once (5.18) is inserted. One gets the integral representation of Z_L

$$Z_L(\beta, K) = \int_a^b \dots \int_a^b \prod_{\ell=1}^{L} \rho(\lambda_\ell)\, d\lambda_\ell \prod_{\ell=1}^{L} \left[1 - z(\lambda_\ell + \lambda_{\ell+1})\right]^{-1} \tag{5.19}$$

where $z \equiv e^{-\beta} K$ is the effective polymer fugacity. The integrals are defined for $z < (2b)^{-1}$, $z_c(\beta) \equiv e^{-\beta} K_c(\beta) = [2b(\beta)]^{-1}$ giving the critical point where the SAW lengths diverge. Hence only the vicinity of the upper boundary $\lambda = b$ will matter for the critical behaviour of (5.19). In the case of polymers ($n = 0$) the solution of (5.14) has been calculated ten years ago for counting planar diagrams[59]

$$\rho(\lambda) = \frac{1}{2\pi}\left[1 - e^{-\beta}\left(\frac{a+b}{2} + \lambda\right)\right]\sqrt{(\lambda - a)(b - \lambda)} \tag{5.20}$$

and the endpoints a, b of the support of ρ are functions of β through

$$\begin{aligned} 2\, e^{-2\beta} &= \sigma(1-\sigma)(1-2\sigma) \\ a + b &= 2\sigma\, e^{\beta} \\ b - a &= 4(1-2\sigma)^{-1/2} \end{aligned} \tag{5.20a}$$

The critical point of the empty surface corresponds to the first singularity of the parametric representation where $\frac{\partial g}{\partial b} = 0$, which is found to be $e^{-\beta_c} = \left(12\sqrt{3}\right)^{-1/2}$. So from (5.19) one already observes the two kinds of possible critical behaviours: one (that of the surface) is hidden in the singularities of $\rho(\lambda)$ (5.20) near β_c; the second one, associated with the SAW, occurs when z approaches its critical upper value $z_c(\beta) = 1/2b(\beta)$, the dominant contribution to the multiple λ–integral in (5.19) coming from all $\lambda_\ell \longrightarrow b^-$, $\ell = 1, ..., L$. Hence the only features we will need are the two distinct critical behaviors of ρ near the upper end b of interval $[a, b]$ for $\beta > \beta_c$ or $\beta = \beta_c$

$$\rho(\lambda) \sim (\beta - \beta_c)^{1/2}(b - \lambda)^{1/2} + \text{const.}\,(b - \lambda)^{3/2} \tag{5.21}$$

Notice the difference in the two critical exponents 1/2 or 3/2.

b) *Critical behaviours.* We shall not give here all details of the analysis[11] of (5.19) (5.21), but it is easy to understand that there will be two different critical behaviours corresponding to (5.21). First, if $\beta > \beta_c$ the part of the surface unoccupied by the SAW remains finite, while one can reach the critical point $K_c(\beta)$ where the SAW become *infinite*. This corresponds to a *dense* polymer phase. Second, if one puts $\beta = \beta_c$ and $K = K_c(\beta_c)$, both the surface not occupied by the polymers and the SAW are infinite. Using the edge behaviour (5.21) in (5.19) and a standard power counting argument one finds the critical behaviour

$$Z_L(\beta, K) \sim \left[(K_c - K)^{1/2}(\beta - \beta_c)^{1/2} + \text{const}\,(K_c - K)^{3/2}\right]^L \tag{5.22}$$

For $\beta > \beta_c$ the first term dominates the *dense* SAW phase. Hence

$$Z_L(\beta, K) \sim (K_c - K)^{L/2}, \quad K \longrightarrow K_c(\beta) \tag{5.23}$$

When the surface is first infinite, $\beta = \beta_c$ and in this dilute polymer phase

$$Z_L(\beta_c, K) \sim |K_c - K|^{3L/2}, \quad K \longrightarrow K_c(\beta_c) \tag{5.24}$$

Note that the two different exponents 1/2, 3/2 in (5.23) and (5.24) correspond directly to those governing the eigenvalue density $\rho(\lambda)$ in Eq.(5.21). Another way to reach the dilute polymer phase is to let the non-filled surface and polymers become infinite simultaneously in the *finite size scaling regime* $\beta - \beta_c \sim (K_c - K)^2$, such that both terms of (5.22) are equivalent. Then the characteristic surface and SAW sizes $|G| \sim (\beta - \beta_c)^{-1}$ and $|\Gamma| \sim |K_c - K|^{-1}$ respectively, are related by

$$\beta - \beta_c \sim |K_c - K|^{\nu D}, \qquad \nu D = 2 \tag{5.25}$$

where ν is the polymer size exponent and D the fractal dimension of the surface. This shows that the respective surface size $|G|$ and polymer size $|\Gamma|$ scale like $|\Gamma| \sim |G|^{1/2}$, thus leading to a dilute polymer phase with vanishing density $|\Gamma| / |G| \sim |G|^{-1/2} \longrightarrow 0$. Notice that for the other dense phase one has $|G| \sim |\Gamma|$, hence

$$\nu D = 1 \tag{5.26}$$

5.5 Conformal Invariance on a Random Surface

It remains to identify the conformal dimensions underlying the two exact behaviours (5.23) (5.24) of Z_L in the dense and dilute critical phases. The watermelon partition function Z_L can be viewed as that of two conformal operators $\phi_L(i)$, $\phi_L(j)$ associated with the $L-$leg polymer vertex, as in the plane, integrated over the points i and j of the random lattice. Hence one expects it to scale with the cosmological constant β like

$$Z_L(\beta, K) \sim (\beta - \beta_c)^{2\Delta_L - \gamma_{st}} \tag{5.27}$$

where Δ_L is the conformal weight of ϕ_L on the random surface, the insertion of the two points on the random surface giving a further factor $Z''(\beta) \sim (\beta - \beta_c)^{-\gamma_{st}}$ in (5.27). Eq.(5.27) holds in the FSS regimes (5.25) or (5.26). Hence one can also rewrite it as

$$Z_L \sim |K_c - K|^{\nu D(2\Delta_L - \gamma_{st})} \tag{5.28}$$

where $\nu D = 1\,(\beta > \beta_c)$ or $\nu D = 2\,(\beta = \beta_c)$. To identifying the values of Δ_L requires the further information[11] $\nu D = (1 - \Delta_2)^{-1}$ which is nothing but hyperscaling. One thus finds for the dimensions and string susceptibilities

$$\begin{aligned} \Delta_L^D &= (L-2)/4, \quad \gamma_{st} = -1, \quad\ \ c = -2 \text{(dense phase)} \\ \Delta_L &= (3L-2)/8, \quad \gamma_{st} = -1/2, \quad c = 0 \ \ \text{(dilute)} \end{aligned} \tag{5.29}$$

Notice that γ_{st} itself is deterined here from the exact solution. We have recalled the associated central charges and the values of γ_{st} are also those of free random surfaces embedded in $d = -2$ or $d = 0$ dimensions since the latter have the same central charge $c = d = \#$ components of a Gaussian field.

Let us now compare these results to Knizhnik, Polyakov and Zamolodchikov's relationship (5.4) between a critical system in the plane and its counterpart on a random $2D$ lattice (i.e dressed by quantum gravity). The conformal dimensions $\Delta^{(0)}$ in the plane and Δ on the random surface of a conformal operator satisfy the simple quadratic relation (5.4) $\Delta - \Delta^{(0)} = \Delta(1 - \Delta)/\kappa$, where κ parametrizes the central charge (5.2) $c = 13 - 6\kappa - 6/\kappa$. Note that $\Delta^{(0)}$ here is KPZ notation for the Kac spectrum $h = x/2$ as in (2.8). Let us collect the conformal dimensions found for an $L-$leg vertex in the *plane* from Coulomb gas technique (Eq.(2.10)) $\Delta_L^{(0)D} = x_L^D/2 = (L^2 - 4)/32$ (dense), and $\Delta_L^{(0)} = x_L/2 = (9L^2 - 4)/96$ (dilute). It is easy to see that in the dense phase, for all L, $\Delta_L^{(0)D}$ and Δ_L^D satisfy KPZ relation for $c=-2$, $\kappa=2$, while in the dilute phase $\Delta_L^{(0)}$ and Δ_L satisfy it for $c=0$, $\kappa=3/2$. In terms of the *linear* KPZ conformal dimensions (5.3), one finds explicitly for (5.29)

$$\begin{aligned}\Delta_L^D &\equiv \Delta_{0,\frac{L}{2}}(\kappa=2)\\ \Delta_L &\equiv \Delta_{\frac{L}{2},0}(\kappa=\frac{3}{2})\end{aligned}\tag{5.30}$$

i.e. the same indices as in the plane (Eqs.(2.8) (2.10)), QED.

Notice that this provides a full series ($L \geq 1$) of cross checks of the validity of Coulomb gas methods in the plane, of KPZ conformal theory on fluctuating continuum surfaces, and also of the equivalence of critical random lattices to the continuum Polyakov's summation over metrics in 2D quantum gravity. Note also that relation (5.4) can be derived in the conformal gauge of the Liouville theory of random surfaces[70,71].

5.6 $O(n)$ Model Watermelon Exponents

For the $O(n)$ model in the Euclidean plane, we know the values of the watermelon scaling dimensions (2.8)

$$x_L = g\ L^2/8 - (1-g)^2/2g$$

$$n = -2\cos \pi g$$

$$\begin{aligned}x_L &= 2\Delta_{L/2,0}^{(0)} \equiv 2h_{L/2,0}, \quad g=\frac{m+1}{m}, \quad g\in[1,2] \ \text{(dilute)}\\ &= 2\Delta_{0,L/2}^{(0)} \equiv 2h_{0,L/2}, \quad g=\frac{m}{m+1}, \quad g\in[0,1] \ \text{(dense)}\end{aligned}$$

Comparing this to Eq.(5.5), we find that in the dilute and dense phases respectively

$$\begin{aligned}\kappa &= g \quad &&\text{for} \quad g\in[1,2]\\ \kappa &= 1/g \quad &&\text{for} \quad g\in[0,1]\end{aligned}$$

and we expect the conformal dimensions (5.3) dressed by gravity predicted by KPZ theory

$$\begin{aligned}\Delta_L \equiv \Delta_{L/2,0} &= g\ L/4 - (g-1)/2\\ \Delta_L^D \equiv \Delta_{0,L/2} &= \frac{L}{4} - \left(\frac{1}{g}-1\right)\frac{1}{2}\end{aligned}\tag{5.31}$$

These values can be obtained directly from the solution of the $O(n)$ model (5.12) (5.13) on the random 2D-lattice[66], by a technique entirely similar to that presented in section (V.4) for polymers, providing a check of both KPZ and Coulomb gas approaches in the case of all $O(n)$ models for $n\in[-2,2]$.

As an application, we can calculate the fractal dimension D_F of the loops in the high-temperature expansion of the $O(n)$ model. The critical exponent $\nu_2 D$ (where, as above, D is the fractal dimension of the random surface and where $\nu_2 = 1/D_F'$ is the inverse fractal dimension of the loops) is given by the two-leg conformal operator[11,67]

$$\nu_2 D = \frac{1}{1-\Delta_2}\tag{5.32}$$

From Eq.(5.31) we find in the dilute and dense phase respectively

$$\begin{aligned} &\nu_2 D = 2 \qquad (\text{dilute } O(n)) \\ &\nu_2 D = 2g \qquad (\text{dense } O(n)) \qquad g \in \left[\frac{1}{2}, 1\right], \qquad n \geq 0 \end{aligned} \tag{5.33}$$

in agreement with the values found for the polymer phases (5.25) (5.26). Hence we find for the fractal dimension $D'_F = 1/\nu_2$ in presence of a fluctuating metric

$$\frac{D'_F}{D} = \frac{1}{2} \quad (\text{dilute}) \ , \quad \frac{D'_F}{D} = 1/2g \quad (\text{dense}) \tag{5.34}$$

This is to be contrasted to the results (3.16) in the Euclidean plane ($D = 2$) $\frac{1}{2} D_F = \frac{1}{2} + \frac{1}{4g}$, valid in both phases.

In particular let us reconsider the percolation model described in sections (II.4) and (III.2). We have indicated that the geometrical properties of the hulls of percolation clusters were described equivalently by a $Q = 1$ Potts model or an $O(n = 1)$ model in the low-temperature phase. The Coulomb gas coupling constant is then $g = \frac{2}{3}$ and (5.34) yields the *hull fractal dimension on a fluctuating surface*

$$D'_H / D = 3/4 \tag{5.35}$$

to be compared to $D_H/2 = 7/8$ for the standard hull of $2D$ percolation. *The hull thus fills more space in the plane than on the fluctuating critical surface.*

It is also interesting to compute the gravitational exponents Δ'_L for the nonintersection probabilities of L random walks or Brownian motions (see section IV). We had Eq.(4.9)

$$\zeta_L = h_{0,L}^{c=0} \equiv \Delta_{0,L}^{(0)}$$

with $m = 2$. Hence the parameter κ (5.5) is $\kappa = \frac{3}{2}$ here as for dilute SAW, and the gravitational dimensions (5.3) are

$$\zeta'_L = \Delta_{0,L} = \frac{1}{4}(2L - 1) \tag{5.36}$$

It would be very interesting to calculate these values directly, since it would provide an indirect derivation of the conjectured exact values (4.9). However, for describing random walks on a lattice, one has to admit loops and multiple occupancy of the random lattice bonds by the walks, which gives a statistical problem rather more complicated that the self-avoiding case.

5.7 Higher Topologies

a) *Polymer networks.* We consider a general polymer network $\mathcal{G}$ of arbitrary but fixed topology, embedded in the random surface (of e.g. genus zero) (Fig.16).

In section III, we have shown how general SAW networks can be handled in the plane, and in particular their configuration exponents $\gamma_{\mathcal{G}}$ calculated as functions of the set of scaling dimensions $\{x_L\}$ (Eqs.(3.12) (3.14)). On a random critical surface, a similar decomposition in terms of vertices exists. It can be shown by an exact solution[67] that on a random surface

$$\mathcal{Z}_{\mathcal{G}}^{\text{poly}} \sim |K_c - K|^{-\gamma_{\mathcal{G}} - \nu D} \tag{5.37}$$

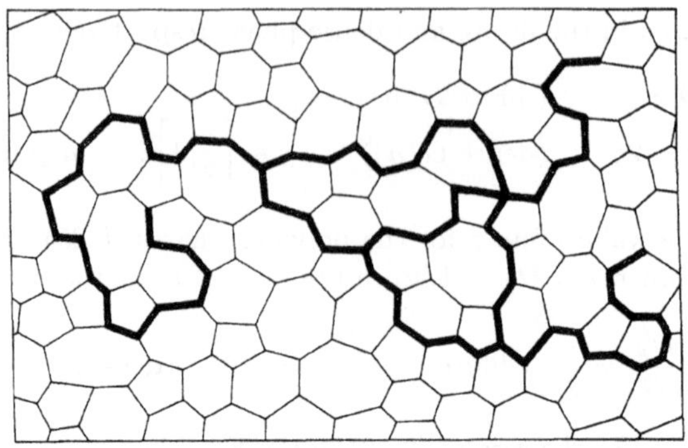

Fig.16. A polymer network embedded in the planar random φ^3–lattice.

with a critical exponent

$$\gamma_{\mathcal{G}}^{\text{random}} = \nu D \left[\mathcal{V} - 1 - (2 - \gamma_{\text{st}}) - \sum_{L \geq 1} n_L \Delta_L \right] \tag{5.38}$$

where, as in part III, $\mathcal{V}$ is the total number of vertices of $\mathcal{G}$, and n_L that of type L. Formula (5.38) for a network on a random surface is then very similar to that obtained in the Euclidean plane. Eqs.(5.38) and (3.12) are indeed identical, provided one replaces $2\nu\,(\equiv d\nu)$ by νD, $x_L \equiv 2\Delta_L^{(0)}$ by $D\,\Delta_L$, and adds a contribution $2 - \gamma_{\text{st}}$ coming from the free energy of the random surface itself (Eqs.(5.11)). This is of particular interest since the exact solution on a random surface provides an (indirect) check of the scaling theory (3.14) in the plane.

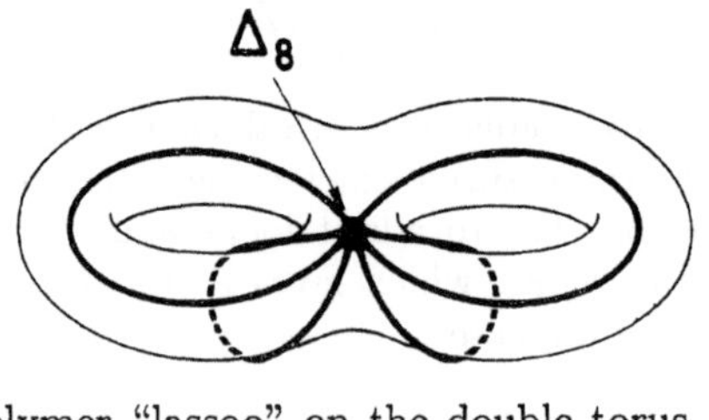

Fig.17. A minimal polymer "lassoo" on the double torus. The extraction of the conformal dimension Δ_8 yields the value of γ_{st} for the double torus.

b) *Higher surface genus.* Formula (5.38) is also valid for any topology $\mathcal{T}$ of the fluctuating membrane itself. $\gamma_{\mathcal{G}}^{\text{random}}$ depends on $\mathcal{T}$ only through γ_{st}, since the conformal dimensions Δ_L are local and independent of the global topology. Eq.(5.38) is then interesting since it allows the determination of $\gamma_{\text{st}}(\mathcal{T})$, by a direct calculation of $\gamma_{\mathcal{G}}$ and then identification with (5.38). For example, if one considers a double torus

(Fig.17), one can draw a "lasso" polymer network on it, whose only vertex conformal operator is ϕ_8 with known dimension Δ_8. The exponent γ_G can be computed by the generalization of technique (5.19). One finds then for any topological genus of Euler characteristics $\chi = 2(1-H)$ (H handle number or genus) the string susceptibility exponent

$$2-\gamma_{st} = \frac{3}{2}\chi, \qquad d=c=-2$$

$$2-\gamma_{st} = \frac{5}{4}\chi, \qquad d=c=0$$

in agreement with a former exact solution for $d=0,-2$[62]. All of this can be generalized to e.g. the $O(n)$ model with central charge $c = 1-6(1-g)^2/g = 13-6\kappa-6/\kappa$ and one finds[67]

$$2-\gamma_{st} = \frac{1}{2}\chi(\kappa+1) \tag{5.39}$$

where $\kappa = 1/g$, $g \in [0,1]$ in the dense phase, and $\kappa = g$, $g \in [1,2]$ at the critical point. Eq.(5.39) can be rewritten as

$$2-\gamma_{st} = \chi\frac{1}{24}\left[25-c+\sqrt{(1-c)(25-c)}\right] \tag{5.40}$$

For the sphere topology ($\chi=2$) one recovers the result conjectured by KPZ[10]

$$\gamma_{st}(\text{sphere}) = \frac{1}{12}\left[c-1-\sqrt{(1-c)(25-c)}\right]$$

while the general result (5.40) for arbitrary genus was obtained in the conformal gauge in the continuum Liouville theory of random surfaces[70] (see also Ref.[71]). Notice that the geometrical methods presented here allow for a direct calculation of (5.38) (5.39) for any genus[67].

ACKNOWLEDGEMENTS

It is a pleasure to thank F. David, I. Kostov, K.H. Kwon and H. Saleur with whom different aspects presented here were developed. I also benefited from stimulating discussions with B. Mandelbrot and B. Sapoval at the Erice meeting, and an interesting correspondance with K. Burdzy.

REFERENCES

[1] P. Lévy, "Processus Stochastiques et Mouvement Brownien", Gauthier-Villars (Paris, 1965).
[2] A.M. Polyakov, J.E.T.P. Lett. 12, 381 (1970).
[3] A.A. Belavin, A.M. Polyakov and A.B. Zamolodchikov, Nucl. Phys. B241, 333 (1984).
[4] B.B. Mandelbrot, "The Fractal Geometry of Nature", W.H. Freeman and Co. (New York, 1983).
[5] B. Nienhuis, Phys. Rev. Lett. 49, 1062 (1982); J. Stat. Phys. 34, 731 (1984).
[6] B. Duplantier, Phys. Rev. Lett. 57, 541 (1986).

[7] A. Ludwig, Saclay preprint SPhT/89-041
B. Duplantier and A. Ludwig (in preparation).
[8] H. Saleur and B. Duplantier, Phys. Rev. Lett. 58, 2325 (1987).
[9] A. Coniglio, J. Phys. A15, 3829 (1982).
[10] V.G. Knizhnik, A.M. Polyakov and A.B. Zamolodchikov, Mod. Phys. Lett. A3, 819 (1988).
[11] B. Duplantier and I. Kostov, Phys. Rev. Lett. 61, 1433 (1988).
[12] E. Domany, D. Mukamel, B. Nienhuis and A. Schwimmer, Nucl. Phys. B190 [FS3], 279 (1981).
[13] B. Nienhuis, in "Phase Transitions and Critical Phenomena", edited by C. Domb and J.L. Lebowitz (Academic, London, 1987) Vol.11.
[14] H. Saleur, J. Phys. A20, 455 (1987); A19, L807 (1986).
[15] B. Duplantier, J. Stat. Phys. 49, 411 (1987).
[16] B. Duplantier and H. Saleur, Nucl. Phys. B290 [FS20], 291 (1987).
[17] B. Duplantier and F. David, J. Stat. Phys. 51, 327 (1988).
[18] M.T. Batchelor and H.W.J. Blöte, Phys. Rev. Lett. 61, 138 (1988).
[19] Vl.S. Dotsenko and V.A. Fateev, Nucl. Phys. B240 [FS12], 312 (1984).
[20] V.G. Kac, Lecture Notes in Physics 94, 441 (1979) (Springer Verlag, Berlin, Heidelberg).
[21] D. Friedan, Z. Qiu and S. Shenker, Phys. Rev. Lett. 52, 1575 (1984).
[22] See J.L. Cardy, in "Phase Transitions and Critical Phenomena", edited by C. Domb and J.L. Lebowitz (Academic London, 1987) Vol.11.
[23] D.A. Huse, Phys. Rev. B30, 3908 (1984).
[24] J. Cardy and H.W. Hamber, Phys. Rev. Lett. 45, 499 (1980).
[25] B. Duplantier and H. Saleur, Phys. Rev. Lett. 60, 2343 (1988).
[26] M.E. Fisher, V. Privman, S. Redner, J. Phys. A17, L569 (1984).
[27] F. Spitzer, Trans. Am. Math. Soc. 87, 187 (1958).
[28] C. Bélisle, University of Michigan, preprint (1988).
[29] J.W. Pitman and M. Yor, Ann. Probab. 14, 733 (1986).
[30] B. Duplantier and H. Saleur, Phys. Rev. Lett. 59, 539 (1987).
See also A. Coniglio, N. Jan, I. Majid and H.E. Stanley, Phys. Rev. B35, 3617 (1987).
[31] R.M. Ziff, Phys. Rev. Lett. 56, 545 (1986).
[32] B. Sapoval, M. Rosso and J.F. Gouyet, J. Phys. Lett. (France) 46, L149 (1985).
[33] J.L. Cardy, Nucl. Phys. B240, 514 (1984).
[34] B. Duplantier and H. Saleur, Phys. Rev. Lett. 57, 3179 (1986).
[35] I. Guim and T.W. Burkhardt, Temple University preprint (1988).
[36] B. Duplantier and H. Saleur, in preparation.
[37] F.Y. Wu, Rev. Mod. Phys. 54, 235 (1982).
[38] M. den Nijs, Phys. Rev. B27, 1674 (1983); J. Phys. A12, 1857 (1979)..
[39] P.W. Kasteleyn and C.M. Fortuin, J. Phys. Soc. Jpn 26 (Suppl.), 11 (1969).
[40] B. Nienhuis, J. Phys. A15, 199 (1982).
[41] B. Duplantier; B. Nienhuis (unpublished).
[42] B. Duplantier and H. Saleur (to be published).
[43] A.L. Stella, C. Vanderzande, Phys. Rev. Lett. 62, 1067 (1989).
[44] M.K. Wilkinson, D.S. Gaunt, J.E.G. Lipson and S.G. Whittington, J. Phys. A19, 789 (1986).
[45] D.S. Gaunt, J.E.G. Lipson, S.G. Whittington and M.K. Wilkinson, J. Phys. A19, L811 (1986).

[46] B. Duplantier, J. Stat. Phys. 54, 581 (1989).
[47] M. den Nijs, J. Phys. A12, 1857 (1979).
[48] G.F. Lawler, Comm. Math. Phys. 86, 539 (1982).
[49] B. Duplantier, Comm. Math. Phys. 117, 279 (1988).
[50] K. Burdzy, G.F. Lawler and T. Polaski, preprint (1988); K. Burdzy and G.F. Lawler, preprint (1989).
[51] B. Duplantier and K.H. Kwon, Phys. Rev. Lett. 61, 2514 (1988).
[52] B.Duplantier and K. Kwon, (unpublished).
[53] D.A. Huse and M.E. Fisher, Phys. Rev. B29, 239 (1984). M.E. Fisher, J. Stat. Phys. 34, 667 (1984).
[54] M.E. Fisher and M.P. Gelfand, J. Stat. Phys. 53, 175 (1988).
[55] A.M. Polyakov, Phys. Lett. 103B, 207 (1981).
[56] F. David, Nucl. Phys. B257, 45 (1985); ibidem 543.
[57] V.A. Kazakov, I.K. Kostov and A.A. Migdal, Phys. Lett. 157B, 295 (1985); D. Boulatov, V. Kazakov, I. Kostov and A. Migdal, Nucl. Phys. B275, 641 (1986); Phys. Lett. B174, 87 (1986).
[58] J. Fröhlich, in Lecture Notes in Physics, Vol.216, L. Garrido Ed. (Springer, Berlin, 1985); J. Ambjorn, B. Durhuus and J. Fröhlich, Nucl. Phys. B257, 433 (1985).
[59] E. Brézin, C. Itzykson, G. Parisi, J.B. Zuber, Comm. Math. Phys. 59, 35 (1978).
[60] I. Kostov, Nucl. Phys. B (Proc. Suppl.) 4, 98 (1988).
[61] F. David, Phys. Lett. B159, 303 (1985).
[62] I. Kostov and M. Mehta, Phys. Lett. 189B, 118 (1987).
[63] V.A. Kazakov, Phys. Lett. 119A, 140 (1986); D.V. Boulatov and V.A. Kazakov, Phys. Lett. 186B, 379 (1987).
[64] V.A. Kazakov, Nucl. Phys. B (Proc. Suppl.) 4, 93 (1988).
[65] A.M. Polyakov, Mod. Phys. Lett. A2, 899 (1987).
[66] I. Kostov, Modern Phys. Lett. A4, 217 (1989).
[67] B. Duplantier and I. Kostov, in preparation.
[68] V.A. Kazakov, Niels Bohr Institute preprint (1988).
[69] M. Gaudin and I. Kostov, Saclay preprint SPhT 88/234
[70] F. David, C.R. Acad. Sci. (Paris) 307 (1988) 1051, Saclay preprint SPhT 88/132.
[71] J. Distler and H. Kawai, Cornell preprint CNLS 88/853.

FRACTAL STRUCTURE OF ISING AND POTTS CLUSTERS: STATIC AND DYNAMIC APPROACH

Antonio Coniglio

Dipartimento di Scienze Fisiche, Università di Napoli
and Gruppo Nazionale di Struttura della Materia (CNR)
Mostra D'Oltremare Pad. 19, 80125 Napoli, Italy

I. INTRODUCTION

How to characterize geometrically a fluctuation near a critical point is a longstanding problem[1-8] that recently has received renewed attention,due to a novel experiment in which direct visual observation of critical fluctuations was possible[9]. Here I want to describe a static and dynamic approach to this problem. The static approach is based on a particular site bond correlated percolation model which was previously introduced as a model for sol gel transition[10]. For a particular value of the bond probability[4], this approach can be related to a formalism developped by Kasteleyn and Fortuin[3,11] and gives the correct definition of the Ising and Potts clusters for a geometrical description of the phase transition. I will first review the main results and show how the formalism can be extended to the case of non zero magnetic field. In Sect. III-V I will present exact results[12] on the fractal structure of the Ising and Potts clusters based on a mapping[13] from the Potts model to the Coulomb gas. In Sec. VI it will be shown that a model originally introduced by Mandelbrot and Given[14] for percolation clusters is found extremely good to describe the fractal structure of the Potts clusters. Finally Sec. VII is devoted to a dynamical approach which has been recently[15] introduced and is based on the propagation of "damage" in a spin system.

II. THE CORRECT CLUSTERS

It is now well established that in an Ising model the naive definition of clusters made of nearest neighbor parallel spins is not satisfactory[2]. These clusters are in fact too large, representing both correlations and pure geometrical effects.As an example at $T = \infty$ in a typical configuration clusters of parallel spins are present although there is total absence of correlations. To eliminate the pure geometrical effect a different definition of cluster was proposed[4] for the Ising model and generalised to the q-state

Fractals' Physical Origin and Properties
Edited by L. Pietronero
Plenum Press, New York

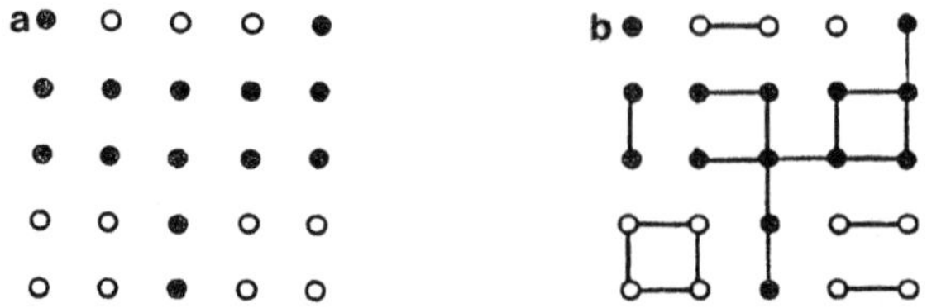

Figure 1. a) Ising configuration: "up" spins and "down" spins are represented respectively by filled and empty circles. b) Correct clusters obtained from the configuration given in a) by putting bonds between sites in the same state with probability $p = 1 - e^{-K}$.

Potts model[5] whose hamiltonian is given by

$$-\mathcal{H}/kT = K \sum_{<ij>} \delta_{\sigma_i \sigma_j} + H \sum_i \delta_{\sigma_i 1}, \tag{1}$$

where $\sigma_i = 1, 2 \ldots q$ are discrete variables assuming q possible states. For $H = 0$ these new clusters are defined as nearest neighbour sites in the same state connected by bonds, each bond beeing present with probability p Fig(1). By chosing

$$p = 1 - e^{-K}, \tag{2}$$

the clusters behave correctly at the critical point T_c, namely their radious and the density of sites in the infinite cluster behave critically as function of $|T - T_c|$ respectively with the correlation length exponent $\nu(q)$ and the order parameter exponent $\beta(q)$ of the q-state Potts model. In particular they coincide with the clusters of the tree percolation problem for $q = 0$ of the random percolation problem for $q = 1$ and of the Ising model for q=2[3]. The interest in the geometrical description of the fluctuations has gone much beyond the original motivation. Recently Swendsen and Wang[16] introduced a new dynamics which instead of fliping one spin at a time, flips altoghether the spins in same cluster. The resulting algoritm has proved to be extremly fast compared with the Glauber dynamics, with a drastic reduction of the critical slowing down. Using geometrical concept, a scaling ansatz was proposed relating the exponents of the two dynamics.

It has been shown[4,5] that the statistics of the Potts clusters can be obtained from the following hmiltonian

$$-\mathcal{H}/kT = J \sum_{<ij>} (\delta_{\tau_i \tau_j} - 1)\delta_{\sigma_i \sigma_j} + K \sum_{<ij>} \delta_{\sigma_i \sigma_j}, \tag{3}$$

where the second term, which controls the distribution of the spin variables, is the q-state Potts hamiltonian, whereas the first term contains auxiliary Potts variables $\tau_i = 1, 2 \ldots s$ and controls the bonds distribution. More specifically it can be shown[4,5] that by taking the derivative of the free energy of the hamiltonian model (3) with respect to s and taking the limit $s = 1$, one obtains the distribution of the clusters defined as sites in the same state connected by bonds present with probability $p = 1 - e^{-J}$. By taking $J = K$ the bond probability assumes the particular value (2) for which the clusters correctly describe the fluctuations. Note that for this value of J, hamiltonian (3) assumes a simplified form which in part explains why the bond probability given by (2) is so special.

So far we have defined the clusters in absence of an external magnetic field H. If for $H \neq 0$ one defines the clusters in the same way one finds a critical line above T_c in the $H - T$ plane[6] where the cluster size diverges without a corresponding divergence of the correlation length. If the percolation properties of the correct clusters must reflect the thermodynamic properties everywhere in the $H - T$ plane, one needs to extend correctly the definition of the clusters in the presence of a magnetic field. Following Fortuin and Kastelyn we define a ghost site in state 1 which has probability

$$p_G = 1 - e^{-H} \tag{4}$$

of being connected to a site in state 1 and $1 - p_G$ of being disconnected. The ghost site is always disconnected from all the other sites which are in a state different from 1. Note that a site connected to the ghost site belongs to the infinite cluster. Therefore the correct finite clusters are defined now as a finite set of n.n. sites in the same state connected by bonds present with probability given by (2) and disconnected by the ghost site with probability $1 - p_G$. With this definition, the only place where the percolation transition occurr is at the Potts critical temperature $T = T_c$. In the following we will consider Potts clusters at $T = T_c$ and $H = 0$.

III. CLUSTER STRUCTURE

It has been shown[4,5] that at the critical point the Potts clusters are fractals with fractal dimension[17] $D(q) = d - \beta(q)/\nu(q)$ where $\beta(q)$ and$\nu(q)$are the order parameter and the correlation length exponents of the q-state Potts model and d is the euclidean dimension. This follows from the fact that the number of sites in the infinite cluster scales as the total magnetization M which scales at T_c as $L^{d-\beta(q)/\nu(q)}$ where L is the sistem size. Note also that $D(q)$ coincides with the magnetic scaling exponent $y_H(q)$. This reduces to the well known result for percolation that is obtained by putting $q = 1$.

It is interesting to note that $D(q)$ does not vary substantially with q, as shown in table 1 for $d = 2$[18]. This observation can be understood by noting that using this geometrical approach, the driving mechanism of the critical behavior can be viewed as coalescence of clusters just like in a percolation transition. Then one would expect for any q that the fractal dimension should be close to the fractal dimension of the critical clusters in the percolation problem. This also explains the observation, known as strong universality[19] made by Suzuky that over a large class of models the ratio γ/ν or β/ν do not vary appreciably. Since these ratios of critical exponents for fixed d depend only on the magnetic scaling exponent which is identical to the fractal dimension, the strong universality is consequence of the quasi universal feature of the fractal dimension as discussed above[20,21].

We will see now that there are other geometrical properties which change substantially when q goes from zero to the the critical value q_c above which the transition is of first order. At T_c the clusters of the q-state Potts model are found[20] to have a structure made of links and blobs just like in percolation. To be more precise in a given box of linear dimension L one has to distinguish the spanning configurations which cross the system in a given direction and the non spanning configurations which are all the others. The spanning configurations are characterized by the dangling bonds and a backbone. The backbone is made of links which are singly connected bonds, commonly called "red" bonds[22,23]. and the blobs which are made of multiply connected bonds.. The fractal dimension of the red bonds D_R coincide with the scaling exponent $y_B(q)$ associated to the bond probability considered as an indipendent variable.

$$D_R(q) = y_B(q) \tag{5}$$

To be more precise $y_B(q) = \nu_B^{-1}(q)$ where $\nu_B(q)$ is the critical exponent associated to the divergence of the radious of the clusters in which the temperature is fixed at its critical value K_c and the bond probability p as an indipendent variable approaches from below $p_c = 1 - e^{-K_c}$ i.e.$\xi \sim (p_c - p)^{-\nu_B(q)}$. Note that $\nu_B(q)$ must not be identified with the correlation length exponent $\nu(q)$. The latter describes the divergence of the correlation length associated to the spin-spin pair correlation function, or in view of the properties of the clusters $\nu(q)$ is also associated to the divergence of the cluster radious ξ when $p = 1 - e^{-K}$ and K is used as a variable i.e.$\xi \sim |K - K_c|^{-\nu}$. Only for $q = 1$ $\nu_B(1) = \nu(1)$.[5] The result of eq.(5) is based on the following relation

$$p\frac{dp_{ij}}{dp} =< \lambda_{ij} > \tag{6}$$

where $p_{ij} =< \gamma_{ij} >$ is the probability that i and j are connected and γ_{ij} is 1 if i and j are in the same Potts cluster 0 otherwise, λ_{ij} is the number of red bonds between i and j. The brakets denote the average over all Potts variables and bond configurations namely

$$< ... >= \frac{1}{Z}\sum_{\sigma_i} e^{-\beta\mathcal{H}} \sum_{G} ...p^B(1-p)^D \tag{7}$$

where $Z = \sum_{\sigma_i} e^{-\beta\mathcal{H}}$, the first sum is over all Potts variables, the second sum is over all graph G contained in the graph $E\{\sigma_i\}$ made of all bonds connecting n.n. sites in the same state, for a fixed configuration $\{\sigma_i\}$ B is the number of bonds in the graph G and D the number of empty bonds. In eq.(6) the derivative is made with respect to the bond probability, considered as an indipendent variable and then p is put equal to $1 - e^{-K}$. Relation (6) follows from a general result valid for random bond percolation for any graph which relate the pair connectedness to the average number of red bonds like in (6). Therefore by writing such a relation for any graph $E\{\sigma_i\}$ and averaging over all configurations $\{\sigma_i\}$ we obtain a relation (6) valid for Potts clusters. From (6) using the same procedure as for random percolation[23] it follows eq.(5).

IV. HULL AND BRIDGE BONDS

The typical non spanning configurations are characterized by almost spanning clusters. For each cluster the hull or external perimeter is made of all the absent bonds surrounding the cluster. The absent bonds are of two types, those between sites in the same state and those between sites in different states. The "bridges"[24] instead are absent bonds such that if one was present two clusters would merge in one single spanning cluster. The absent bonds that we consider here are only those between two sites in the same state. It is possible to show that the fractal dimension of the red bonds and of the bridge bonds is identical $D_B(q) = D_R(q)$. This is a generalization of a result valid in percolation[24] ($q = 1$) and follows from a relation similar to (2)

$$(1-p)\frac{dp_{ij}}{dp} =< \mu_{ij} > \tag{8}$$

where μ_{ij} is the number of brige bonds between the clusters to which i and j belong, such that if one was present the two sites would be connected. Since relation (4) has been proved for random percolation defined on any graph, using the same reasoning as for the red bonds, relation (4) can be extended to the Potts clusters and therefore as for random percolation[24] it follows $D_B(q) = D_R(q)$. For $d = 2$ and $q = 1$ (percolation) we know the exact value of $D_R(1) = 3/4$ and the exact[13] value of the fractal dimension of the hull $D_H(1) = 7/4$ as was conjectured in ref.(25). The next question is to found the values of $D_R(q)$ and $D_H(q)$ for all values of q.

It is possible to identify $D_R(q)$ and $D_H(q)$ with some of the exponents obtained by Saleur and Duplantier[19] by mapping the Potts model on the Coulomb gas. The result is the following

$$D_H(q) = (g+2)/g, \tag{9}$$

$$D_R(q) = (8g - 3g^2 + 16)/8g, \tag{10}$$

with $q = 2 + 2cos(\pi g/2)$ and $g \in [2,4]$. $D_H(q)$ and $D_R(q)$ as function of q are plotted in fig(2) and their values for discrete $q = 0, 1, 2, 3, 4$ are given in table I. For $q = 1$ eqs.(9) and (10) give the well known results for random bond percolation[13]. So far no results are known for the other exponents except for the fractal dimension of the red bonds of the correct Ising clusters. This has been calculated by de Arcangelis[26], who found,using Montecarlo methods, $D_R(2) = 0.52 + 0.03$ in good agreement with the exact result 0.5417.

From fig(2) and table 1 it appears that, unlikely the fractal dimension of the whole cluster $D_R(q)$ and $D_H(q)$ do change substantially and characterize the different models as function of q. Particularly sensitive to q is the fractal dimension of the red bonds, which has its largest value at $q = 0$ (tree percolation), where the backbone is made only of links. As q approaches q_c the cluster becomes less ramified untill the red bonds

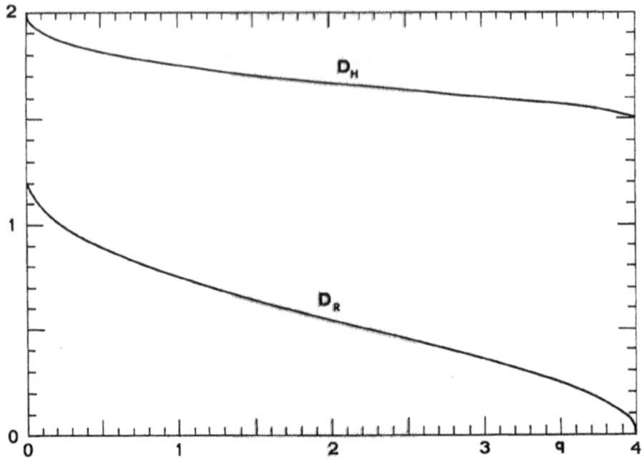

Figure 2. Fractal dimensions of the singly connected bonds (red bonds) $D_R(q)$ and the hull $D_H(q)$ for the Potts clusters.

vanish ($D_R(4) = 0$). This result in a drasting structural change from a links and blobs picture to only blobs, anticipating a first order transition[5].

V. ACCESSIBLE PERIMETER

Another quantity of interest is the accessible perimeter[27,28], which corresponds to that part of the hull that can be reached by any incoming particle from infinity following all possible trajectories, in which the unit step connects two nearest neighbor sites. An argument[13,27] predicts for the fractal dimension of the accessible perimeter $D_{AP}(1) = 4/3$ for percolation in $2d$ in agreement with numerical results[27,28]. Here I want to give a simple estimate, although not exact, for the the fractal dimension of the accessible perimeter $D_{AP}(q)$ for any q. In the non spanning configurations the intersection of the accessible perimeter of two critical clusters coincides with the set of bridges bond. Applying the rule that the sum of the codimension of two fractals equals the codimension of the intersection, one easily find $D_{AP}(q) = (D_R(q)+d)/2$. For $d = 2$ $D_{AP} = 13/8, 11/8, 61/48, 47/40, 1$. Clearly this is only an aprroximation since the above rule applies only when the two fractals are not correlated with each other, however for $2d$ percolation this approximation gives $D_{AP}(1) = 11/8$ in good agreement with the numerical result.

Table I

q	D	D_H	D_R
0	2	2	5/4
1	91/48	7/4	3/4
2	15/8	5/3	13/24
3	28/15	8/5	7/20
4	15/8	3/2	0

Fractal dimensions of the whole cluster (D) of the Hull (D_H) and of the red bonds (D_R) for the Potts clusters.

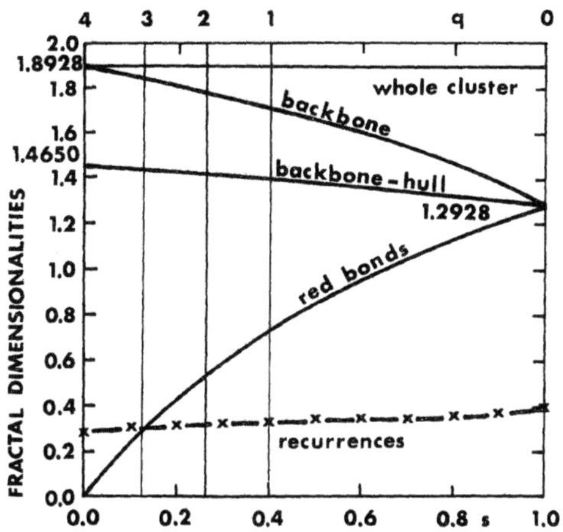

Figure 3. Adapted from fig.(3) of ref.(14). Fractal dimensionalities of different quantities as function of the parameter s in the Mandelbrot Given model. The vertical line correspond to the values of s which maps on $q = 0, 1, 2, 3, 4$, as eplained in the text.

VI. FRACTAL MODEL

Is there a satisfactory model for the Potts clusters? Mandelbrot and Given[14] (MG) proposed a fractal model for percolation clusters in $2d$. However this model as, we will see, it turns out to be much reacher than expected and can describe Potts clusters besides percolation clusters. The MG model is constructed from a Sierpinsky gasket of base $b = 3$ with fractal dimension $log_3 8 = 1.8928$. This carpet has no dangling bonds and is infinitely ramified. The idea was to reduce ramification by successive random deletion of bonds, without changing the fractal dimension. The deletion is controlled by a parameter s, in a range of values between 0 and 1. For more details see the original papers[14]. Mandelbrot and Given calculated the fractal dimension of various quantities as function of s on this model such as red bonds, backbone and backbone hull. Using s as adjustable parameter they chose $s = 0.4$ for which they obtained results which better fitted the available data for percolation.

I want to show here that by changing s from 0 to 1 the MG model can well describe the fractal structure of the clusters of the Potts model for the values of q between 4 and 1. First note that changing s in the MG model the fractal dimension does not change. Similarly in the Potts model the clusters have a fractal dimension about 1.9 for all values of q.

We can map $s = 1$ to $q = 0$ since both values correspond to a tree structure. The mapping between the other values of s and q can be done via the implicit equation $D_R^{MG}(s) = D_R(q)$ where $D_R^{MG}(s)$ is the fractal dimension of the red bonds as function of s in the MG model and $D_R(q)$ is the exact value of the fractal dimension of the red bonds in the q-state Potts model (fig.3).

We can compare now the properties of the MG model with those of the corresponding Potts model. The MG model for $s = 1$ gives the fractal dimension of the red bonds about 1.293 which well compare with the exact value $D_R(0) = 1.25$ for the corresponding $q = 0$ state Potts model. In the MG model for $s = 0$ the backbone and the whole cluster coincide, with a fractal dimension of the hull of 1.465 which compare extremely well with the exact value $D_H(4) = 1.5$ for the corresponding $q = 4$ state Potts model.

From the MG model one can calculate other properties which might be difficult to calculate in the q state Potts model. For example the MG model predicts for $s = 1$ absence of dangling bonds, one would expect that this would be the case also in the $q = 4$ state Potts model. Moreover the MG model exhibits a nice example of fractals with the same fractal dimension but with different structures, quantified by different fractal dimensions of subsets of the whole cluster. The study of this model can give a way for a better understanding of the origin of the strong and weak universality.

VII. DYNAMIC APPROACH: DAMAGE SPREADING

Here I want to discuss a dynamic approach which has been introduced recently to describe in terms of geometrical concept how a perturbation propagates in a spin system. Dynamics of statistical systems (e.g.Glauber Metropolis,etc.) define trajectories in phase space and a classical way to study such dynamical systems and to distinguish chaotic behavior is to see if two initially closed configurations move on trajectories in phase space that are always close or not. This kind of analysis has become known under the name of "damage spreading". The concept of "damage spreading" in the Ising model has been introduced[29,30] in analogy to the use of this concept in cellular automata[31]. Let $\sigma_i = +1$ be the variable on site i, one considers two different configurations $\{\sigma^A\}$ and $\{\sigma^B\}$ on a lattice of N sites and define a distance or damage between these two configurations as

$$D = \frac{1}{4N} \sum (\sigma_i^A - \sigma_i^B)^2. \tag{11}$$

The two configurations evolve in time according to some dynamics submitting them to exactly the same noise. In this ay one can study the time evolution of the relative distance $D(t)$ between the two configurations in phase space. Different results are obtained depending on which dynamics is used. In most cases the damage seems to have some critical behaviour at or near the Ising critical point. The concept of damage has been applied also to spin glasses where it seems very promising[30,32].

More recently exact results[15] were found relating the damage to thermodynamical properties in an Ising model. More precisely at $t = 0$ let $\{\sigma^A\}$ be one configuration and $\{\sigma^B\}$ the second one identical to $\{\sigma^A\}$ except at the origin, for which we shall fix $\sigma_o^B = -1$. This value at the origin in configuration B will be kept fixed during all times. If we let the two configurations evolve toward equilibrium according to the heath bath dynamics using the same random number, the following relation holds:

$$D_{oi} = \frac{C_{oi}}{2(1-m)}, \tag{12}$$

where D_{oi} is the probability that site i is damaged under the condition that the spin at the origin is fixed to be down in one of the two parallel configurations, $m = \langle \sigma_o \rangle$

is the average magnetization at the origin and $C_{oi} =< \sigma_o \sigma_i > - < \sigma_o >< \sigma_i >$ is the pair correlation function. By taking at each time step the damaged sites The physical picture which arise is the following. At each time step a cloud of damage evolves in time. The source of the damage is at the origin where one spin is kept fixed in one of the two configurations. Above T_c the damage grows and shrinks around some tipical size. At T_c this tipical size diverges and a power law distribution sets in. The set of the damaged sites define a new type of fractal with fractal dimension given by $D = d - \beta/\nu$ with a distrtibution of size given by

The cloud of damaged sites can be identified as the set of sites that are correlated to the fixed spin at a given time. An intuitive explanation why this is so is the following. The fixed spin at the origin in the B configuration tend to aligne the spin around. However not all down spins are correlated to the central spin. Those down spins which are down not because of correlation effect are down also in configuration A. Therefore the damage sites which are those down spins in configuration A, which are up in configuration B represent the correlated spins.

A second result relates the damage to the spontaneous magnetization . If in an Ising model we fix the bounadry condition $\{\sigma_i^A\} = +1$ and $\{\sigma_i^B\} = -1$, after reaching equilibrium the damage is identical to the magnetization calculated in a system with $+1$ boundary condition.

In conclusion I have presented a static and dynamic approach to characterize geometrically a fluctuation near a critical point. In the first approach I have shown that the fractal sructure of the Potts clusters is made of links and blobs like in percolation. The fractal dimension of the clusters coincide with the magnetic scaling field $y_H(q)$, whereas the fractal dimension of the red bonds coincides with the bond probability scaling exponent $y_J(q)$. This exponent is distinct from the thermal scaling exponent $y_K(q)$ except for $q = 1$. What is the geometrical quantity related to the thermal scaling exponent for $q \neq 1$ is still an open problem. Note that the fractal dimension of the red bonds goes to zero at q_c, showing a drastic change in the fractal structure due to the appearence of the first order transition, whereas $y_H(q)$ is roughly constant and $y_K(q)$ is an increasing function of q, without showing any pecularity at q_c.

In the second approach the clusters still have a fractal dimension given by the magnetic scaling exponent, however their structure is rather differentfrom the previous one. What is then the structure that one might observe in a real experiment? This is still an open question, however I believe that also in a real experiment what one observes depends on the operative definition of the experimental cluster.

ACKNOWLEDGEMENTS

I would like to thank B. Duplantier for interesting discussions,and my collaborators in this field L. de Arcangelis, R. Figari, H.Herrmann, N. Jan, F.di Liberto, G.Monroi, W. Klein , J.Kertesz, F. Peruggi, H.E. Stanley and D. Stauffer. This work was supported in part by a CNR/NSF grant.

References

1. M.E.Fisher, Physics (N.Y.) **3**,225 (1967).
2. K.Binder, Am.Phys. (N.Y.) bf 98, 390 (1976) and ref. therein.
3. C.M.Fortuin and P.W.Kasteleyn, Physica (Utrecht) **57**, 536 (1972).
4. A.Coniglio and W.Klein, J.Phys. A **12**, 2775 (1980).
5. A.Coniglio and F.Peruggi, J.Phys A **15**, 1873 (1982).
6. J.Kertesz, D.Stauffer and A.Coniglio, Ann. Isr. Phys. Soc. **5**, 121 (1983).
7. C.H.Ku, Phys. Rev. B **29**, 5103 (1984).
8. Z.Alexandrowicz, Phys.Rev.Lett. **60**, 669 (1988).
9. P.Guenon, F.Perrot and D.Beysens.Preprint (1988).
10. A.Coniglio, H.E.Stanley and W.Klein, Phys. Rev. Lett.**42**, 518 (1979).
11. S.Alexander, J. Phys. A **11**,1803 (1978).
12. A.Coniglio, Phys. Rev. Lett. **62**, 3054 (1989); A.Coniglio, F. di Liberto, G.Monroy and F. Peruggi, J. Phys.A **22**, L837, (1989).
13. H.Saleur and B.Duplantier, Phys. Rev. Lett. **58**, 2325 (1987).
14. B.B. Mandelbrot and J.Given, Phys. Rev. Lett **52**, 1853 (1954); see also B.B. Mandelbrot, J.Stat.Phys. **34**, 895 (1984).
15. A.Coniglio, L. de Arcangelis, H.J. Herrmann and N.Jan, Europhysics Letters **8**, 315 (1989).
16. R.H.Swendsen and J.S.Wang, Phys.Rev.Lett **58**, 86 (1987).
17. B.B.Mandelbrot, The fractal geometry of nature, (Freeman, San Francisco,1982).
18. M.den Nijs, Phys. Rev. B **27**, 1674 (1983).
19. M.Suzuki, Progr. Theor. Physics (Kioto)**51**, 1992 (1974).
20. A.Coniglio and R.Figari, J.Phys. Lett. A **16**, L535 (1983).
21. F.Family, J.Stat.Phys. **36**, 881 (1984).
22. H.E.Stanley, J.Phys. A **10**, l211 (1977).
23. A.Coniglio, Phys. Rev. Lett. **46**, 250 (1981) and J.Phys A **15**, 3829 (1982).
24. A.Coniglio, Springer Verlag, 1985 Proceedings Les Houches Conference, N. Boccara and M.Daoud, eds.

25. B.Sapoval, M.Rosso and J.F.Gouyet, J. Phys. Lett. (Paris) **46**, L149 (1985).

26. L.de Arcangelis, unpublished.

27. T.Grossmann and H.Aharony, J.Phys.A **19**, L745 (1986).

28. P.Meakin and F.Family, Phys. Rev. A **34**, 2558 (1986).

29. H.E.Stanley, D.Stauffer, J.Kertesz and H.J. Herrmann, Phys. Rev. Lett.**59**, 2326 (1987).

30. B.Derrida and G.Weisbuch, Europhys. Lett.**4**, 657 (1988).

31. B.Derrida and D.Stauffer, Europhys. Lett.**2**, 739 (1986). L. de Arcangelis, J. Phys. A **20**, L369,(1987).

32. L. de Arcangelis, A. Coniglio, H. Herrmann, Europhys. Lett. **9**, 794 (1989).

Part 3

Fractal Growth Models: General Features

DIFFUSION-LIMITED AGGREGATION: RECENT DEVELOPMENTS

Paul Meakin and Susan Tolman

E. I. du Pont de Nemours and Company
Wilmington, DE 19880-0356

INTRODUCTION

The development of the diffusion-limited aggregation (DLA) model by Witten and Sander[1] has stimulated interest in a broad range of non-equilibrium growth and aggregation processes (see references 2-12 for recent books, reviews and conference proceedings). Since that time a wide range of physical realizations of the DLA model has been found including fluid-fluid displacement[13] in Hele-Shaw cells[14] and porous media[15], dielectric breakdown[16], electrodeposition[17,18] and the dissolution of porous materials[19]. Brief surveys of these and other applications can be found in references 9 and 20. A variety of theoretical approaches including mean field theories[21-24] and position space renormalization models[25,26] have been applied to the DLA process. Recently, a variety of promising new ideas have been applied to DLA[26-31] and closely related models.[32] Despite these advances, we still do not have a widely accepted general theory for DLA though a quite successful theory for noise reduced DLA has been developed.[32]

During the past few years increasingly efficient models for DLA have been developed[33-36] and the size of square lattice DLA clusters that can be generated has increased from only a few thousand sites in 1981 to more than 10^7 sites. Figure 1 shows a cluster containing 1.27×10^7 sites grown[37] using the algorithm of Ball and Brady.[35] Despite this advance in our ability to generate very large DLA clusters, we still do not have an unambiguous picture for the structure of either square lattice or off-lattice two dimensional DLA clusters.

Apart from some relatively small scale simulations ($\leq 10^4$ sites or particles) of DLA in spaces and/or lattices with Euclidean dimensionalities in the range $3 \leq d \leq 6$[33] and the generation of about 100 5×10^4 site cubic lattice DLA clusters,[38] almost all DLA simulations have been restricted to two dimensional models. Recently, we have developed improved algorithms for both off-lattice and hypercubic lattice DLA in dimensions 3-8[36]. With these algorithms quite large numbers of clusters have been generated with about 10^5 particles or sites for d = 3-8 and much larger clusters have been grown for d = 3 and 4. Figure 2 shows a projection of and a cross-section through a 3×10^6 site cluster grown on a cubic lattice and Figure 3 shows a cross-section and a projection for a 10^6 site four dimensional DLA cluster grown on a hypercubic lattice.

Despite the quite large number of investigations which have been carried out to measure the scaling properties and other characteristics of both

Fractals' Physical Origin and Properties
Edited by L. Pietronero
Plenum Press, New York

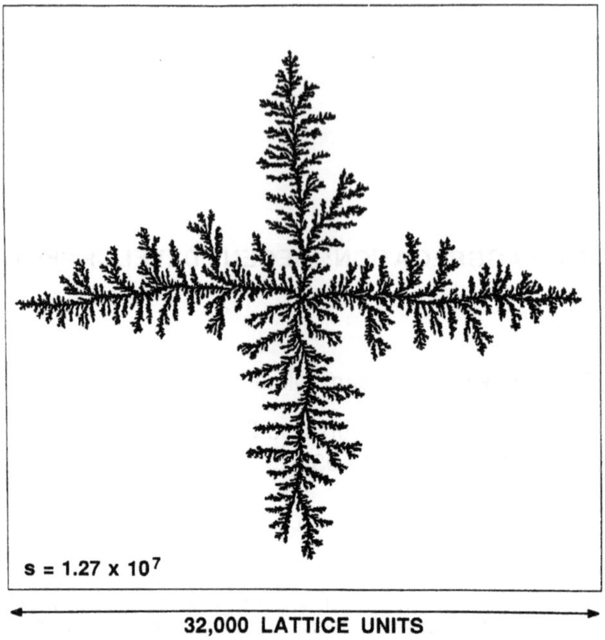

Figure I. A square lattice DLA cluster containing 1.27×10^7 sites. This figure was generated using the algorithm of Ball and Brady.[35]

off-lattice and square lattice DLA, considerable uncertainties remain. For example, it is not clear if one or more than one exponent is needed to describe the geometric scaling properties (fractal geometry)[39]. Here we discuss some of these investigations and describe the results obtained from simulations that have been carried out in an attempt to obtain a better description of the asymptotic structure of two dimensional DLA. Some of the results obtained recently from large scale DLA simulations using spaces and lattices with a Euclidean dimensionality (d) ≥ 3 are also presented. In addition, some recent results obtained from noise reduced DLA models and DLA models in which the growth probability is proportional to ϕ_i^{η} where ϕ_i is the value of a scalar Laplacian field (or field gradient) associated with the ith unoccupied perimeter site are presented.

THE STRUCTURE OF TWO DIMENSIONAL DLA CLUSTERS

In the diffusion-limited aggregation (DLA), model particles are added, one at a time, to a growing cluster or aggregate of particles via random walk trajectories originating from outside of the region occupied by the cluster. Since the introduction of this model by Witten and Sander[1] in 1981, a quite large number of attempts have been made to develop a simple picture for the fractal[39] structure of the clusters generated by these models. Using six square lattice clusters containing 2079-3609 particles, Witten and Sander[1] obtained an effective fractal dimensionality (D_α) of 1.657 ± 0.004 from the two point density-density correlation function (C(r)), which was found to have a power law form

$$C(r) \sim r^{-\alpha} \qquad (1)$$

for intermediate lengths (r) larger than a few lattice units and smaller than the overall size of the clusters. The corresponding fractal dimensionality, D_α,

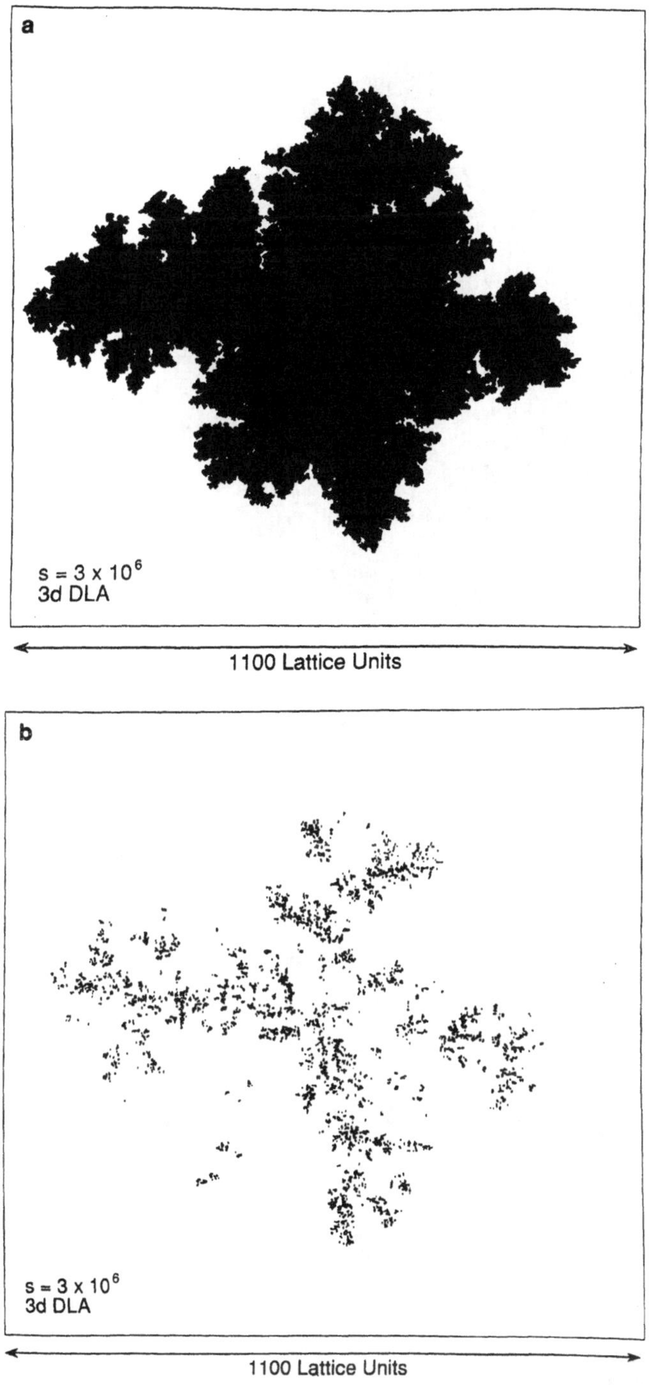

Figure 2 A projection and a cross section of a 3×10^6 site cubic lattice DLA cluster. The cross section passes through the origin of the cluster along one of the natural (001) planes of the cubic lattice. The projection is onto the same plane.

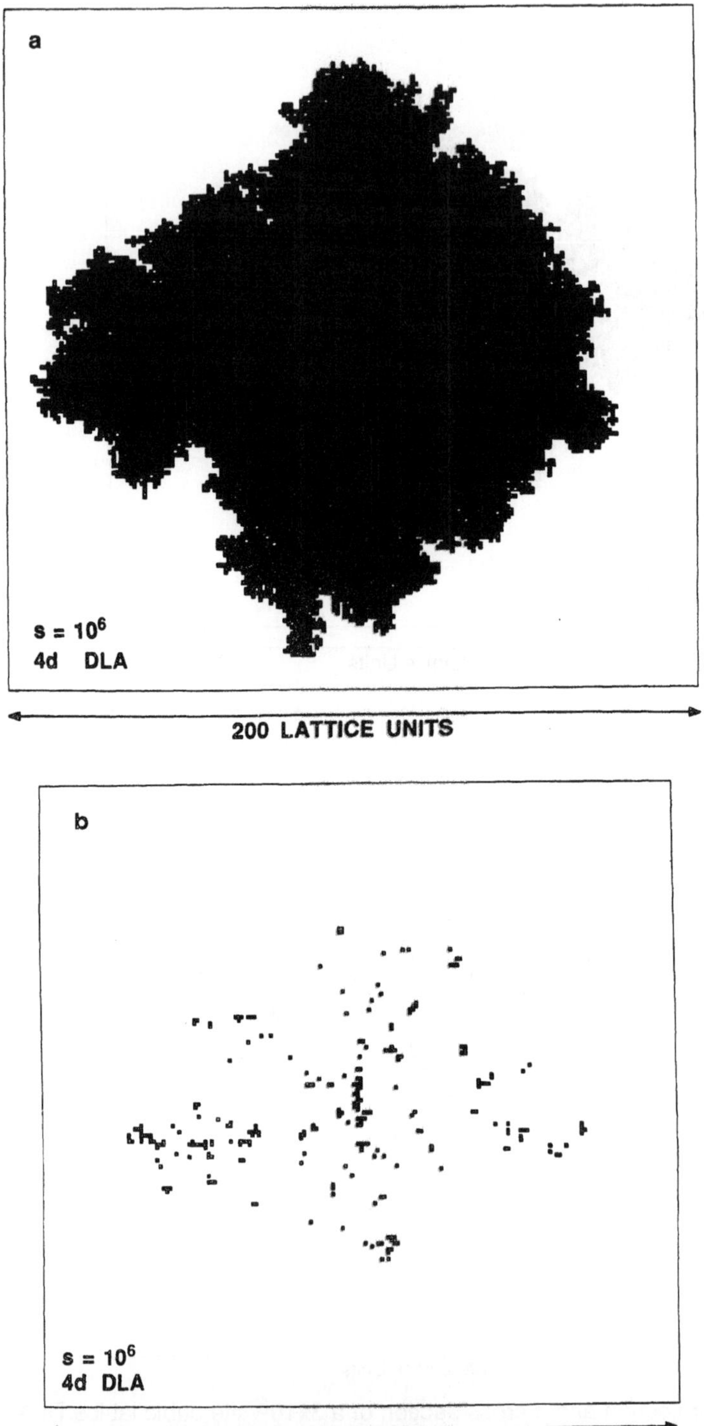

Figure 3. A projection and a cross-section obtained from a 10^6 site four dimensional hypercubic lattice DLA cluster.

is given by $D_\alpha = d - \alpha$ where d is the dimensionality of the Euclidean embedding space or lattice. Witten and Sander also measured the dependence of the cluster radii of gyration (R_g) on their sizes or number of particles (s) and found that

$$R_g \sim s^\beta \quad (2)$$

The power law relationship between R_g and s can be used to obtain a second estimate of the fractal dimensionality (D_β) from the relationship $D_\beta = 1/\beta$. In this fashion a fractal dimensionality of 1.70l±0.02 was obtained.[1,40]

Using slightly larger clusters (about l0,000 particles or sites), Meakin[33] obtained a value of about 1.71 for D_β from both square lattice and off-lattice simulations. Values of 1.68±0.05 and 1.68±0.03 were obtained for D_α from the square lattice and off-lattice simulations respectively. Meakin and Wasserman[41] also measured the fractal dimensionalities D_0, D_2, D_3 for ten square lattice DLA clusters with an average size of 9580 occupied sites. Here the dimensionalities D_q[42] are determined from the definition

$$D_q = \{d\ln[C_q(\lambda)]/d\ln(\lambda)\}/(q-1) \quad (3)$$

by covering the fractal with a grid whose elements have sides of length λ and measuring the qth moments $C_q(\lambda)$ of the masses contained in the grid elements

$$C_q(\lambda) = \sum_i [N_i(\lambda)]^q \quad (4)$$

Here $N_i(\lambda)$ is the number of occupied sites in the ith grid element with sides of length λ and the sum is over all occupied elements. In this fashion, values of 1.6l±0.02, 1.65±0.0l and 1.65±0.0l were obtained for D_0, D_2 and D_3. The quantity D_2 is closely related to D_α. Despite the fact that D_β was consistently found to be larger than D_α and D_q ($q = 0\text{-}3$), these results were interpreted in terms of a homogeneous[43] self-similar fractal geometry with a single fractal dimensionality ($D_\alpha = D_\beta = D_q \simeq 5/3$). A fractal dimensionality of 5/3 was consistent with the, then extant[21,22] mean field theories which predicted a fractal dimensionality given by $D = (d^2+1)/(d+1)$ where d is the dimensionality of the embedding space or lattice.

As more efficient algorithms for DLA were developed[34,35], it became possible to generate much larger numbers of larger clusters and reduce the uncertainties due to both statistical and finite size effects. Using four thousand, 2500 site square lattice DLA clusters, Plischke and Racz[44] measured the growth of both the radius (r_a) and width (ξ_a) of the "active zone" (region where growth is occurring) with increasing mass for square lattice DLA. The radius $r_a(s)$ is the mean deposition radius of the sth particle and $\xi_a(s)$ is the variance in $r_a(s)$. Plischke and Racz found that both $\xi_a(s)$ and $r_a(s)$ exhibited an algebraic dependence on s

$$r_a(s) \sim s^\upsilon \quad (5a)$$

$$\xi_a(s) \sim s^{\bar{\upsilon}} \quad (5b)$$

They found that the exponent υ had a value of 0.584±0.02 corresponding to a fractal dimensionality of 1.7l±0.06 (essentially the same values were obtained for β). However, the exponent $\bar{\upsilon}$ was found to have a value of 0.48±0.01. As a result of these simulations, Plischke and Racz suggested that two diverging lengths or two distinct exponents are needed to describe the active zone of DLA clusters.

Meakin and Sander[45] used one thousand 50,000 particle off-lattice DLA clusters (to avoid potential complications arising from the effects of lattice anisotropy[34,35]) to measure the exponents β, υ and $\bar{\upsilon}$. Values of 0.584±0.002 ($D = 1.712\pm0.006$) were obtained for the exponents β and υ for all clusters containing more than about 1000 particles. More recent simulations have confirmed these results for clusters containing up to 10^6 particles[36] (a value of 1.715±0.004 was obtained for D_β from 377 clusters in the size range $10^5 \leq s \leq 10^6$ particles). The exponent $\bar{\upsilon}$, on the other hand, was found to have an effective value of about 0.48 for small clusters, but had a value of about 0.54 for clusters in the size range $25{,}000 \leq s \leq 50{,}000$. These results are consistent with the idea that $\beta = \upsilon = \bar{\upsilon} \simeq 1.71$ in the limit $s \to \infty$.

Meakin and Vicsek[46] measured the density correlations inside off-lattice DLA clusters in the tangential (angular) direction. They found that the density correlation function $C(\Theta)$ can be expressed as

$$C(\Theta) \sim \Theta^{-\alpha'} \quad (6)$$

for $\Theta \ll 1$. However, the exponent α' has a value (0.41±0.04) which is significantly different from the exponent α obtained from the density-density correlation functions averaged over all angles. A similar result ($\alpha'-\alpha$ = 0.16±0.05) was obtained by Kolb.[47]

The effects of lattice anisotropy have a strong effect on the asymptotic shape of DLA clusters[27,28,35,48]. In the asymptotic limit ($s \to \infty$), the cluster grows into a star or cross-like pattern with n distinct arms, where n is the number of growth directions on the lattice[48,49]. Large scale simulations indicate that the length (ℓ) and width (w) of the cluster arms may grow with different exponents

$$\ell \sim s^{\upsilon_{\|}} \quad (7a)$$

$$w \sim s^{\upsilon_{\perp}} \quad (7b)$$

with $\upsilon_{\|} > \upsilon_{\perp}$. However, simulations carried out with noise reduction[50,51] indicate that in the limit $s \to \infty$, the exponents $\upsilon_{\|}$ and $\upsilon_{\perp}$ may be equal.[52-54]

Though lattice anisotropy has a dramatic effect on the asymptotic shape of DLA clusters and seems to change the value of the radius of gyration fractal dimensionality (D_β) from 1.71 to a value only slightly larger than 1.5, this is a weak effect and it seems that small square lattice DLA clusters have a structure that is quite similar to that of off-lattice DLA clusters. In addition, it seems quite probable that the internal structure of square lattice DLA clusters is very similar to that found for off-lattice clusters on all but quite long length scales.

There is a variety of other evidence that DLA clusters may have a more complex structure than that normally associated with random self-similar fractals such as infinite percolation clusters at the percolation threshold. For example, Meakin and Havlin[55] have measured the distribution of mass, $N_s(r)$, contained within a distance r from a particle or occupied site for a variety of random aggregates. Here $N_s(r)$ is the number of circles of radius r containing s particles. For a self similar fractal $N_s(r)$ can be described by the scaling form

$$N_s(r) \sim s^{-1} f(s/r^D) \quad (8)$$

For screened growth model clusters[56,57] grown on a square lattice and clusters generated using a two dimensional off-lattice[58] hierarchical[59] model for diffusion-limited cluster-cluster aggregation[60,61] a quite good data collapse was obtained by using the scaling form given in equation (8). In this work, the distributions $N_s(r)$ were obtained for a number of radii (r) and these distributions were scaled onto the scaling function f(x) using equation (8). For off-lattice DLA clusters, a good scaling collapse could not be obtained. The best results were obtained with the scaling form

$$N_s(r) \sim s^{-\gamma} f(s/r^{\delta}) \quad (9)$$

with $\gamma \simeq 0.9$ and $\delta \simeq 1.60$.

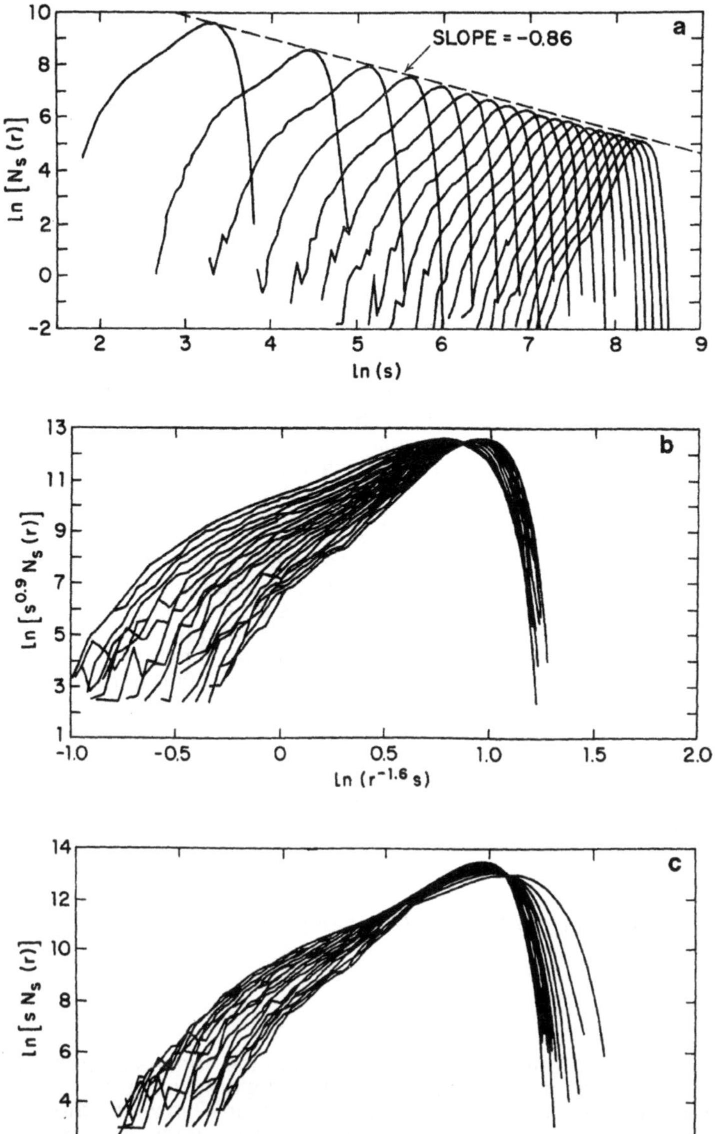

Figure 4. Figure 4a shows the mass distributions $N_S(r)$ obtained from two dimensional off-lattice DLA clusters. The distances r were measured from the centers of particles added when the clusters were 10% to 40% complete. Distributions are shown for lengths (r) of $5d_0$, $10d_0 \ldots 100d_0$. Figures 4b and 4c show the results of attempts to scale these curves using the scaling form given in equation (9) with the scaling exponent $\gamma = 0.9$, $\delta = 1.6$, and $\gamma = 1.0$, $\delta = 1.70$ respectively. These results were obtained using 50 100,000 particle clusters.

Similarly, if a self-similar fractal is covered by a grid with elements of (linear) size λ and the distribution of mass ($N_s(\lambda)$) is measured, we expect that the mass distribution ($N_s(\lambda)$) should be described by the scaling form

$$N_s(\lambda) \sim s^{-2} g(s/\lambda^D) \tag{10}$$

Again, the scaling form given in equation (10) does not work well for off-lattice DLA clusters.

The results discussed above do not by any means represent an exhaustive survey of all the attempts which have been made to characterize DLA clusters. However, they are sufficient to illustrate the fact that no simple, self-consistent picture for the structure of DLA has yet emerged which is consistent with all (or most) of the simulation results.

Recently, attention has been drawn to the inconsistencies in our description of DLA by Argoul et al.[62] and by Ramanlal and Sander[63]. Using relatively small (12,500 site) square lattice DLA clusters, Argoul et al. measured the effective fractal dimensionality D_β from the dependence of the radius of gyration on cluster size and obtained a value of 1.70±0.04 in good agreement with earlier work. They also measured the fractal dimensionalities D_q (equation (3)) for q in the range $-15 \leq q \leq 15$ and obtained a q independent value of 1.60±0.01. However, the data presented by Argoul et al. do indicate that the effective values for the D_qs do increase as the length scale (λ) over which they are measured increases. Because of this and the small cluster sizes used in this work (to avoid the effects of lattice anisotropy), the results obtained by Argoul et al. are not inconsistent with a limiting ($s \to \infty$, $\lambda \to \infty$) value of about 1.71 for two dimensional (off-lattice) DLA. Similarly, Hinrichsen et al.[64] have examined the structure of ten 250,000 particle two dimensional off-lattice DLA clusters. From the dependence of the radius of gyration on cluster size a fractal dimensionality (D_β) of 1.71±0.005 was found, but a simple "box counting" procedure gave the result D_o (D_q, $q = 0$) = 1.59±0.05. A fractal dimensionality D_b was determined from the branching ratio (r_N) and length ratio r_L for branches of different order.[65] The value for this dimensionality is given by

$$D_b = -\log(r_N)/\log(r_L) \tag{11}$$

and in this way the result $D_b = 1.55 \pm 0.10$ was obtained.

MASS DISTRIBUTION

Because of the apparent inconsistency between the various attempts to characterize the structure of two dimensional DLA clusters, we were motivated to repeat the simulations of Meakin and Havlin[55] in which the mass distributions $N_s(r)$ and $N_s(\lambda)$ were determined. The simulations were repeated on a slightly larger scale (using 100,000 instead of 50,000 particle off-lattice clusters) and the range of length scales over which $N_s(r)$ was determined was extended from $2d_o$-$20d_o$ to $5d_o$-$100d_o$ where d_o is the particle diameter. As in the earlier work, 5,000 particles were selected randomly (from those added when the cluster growth process was 10%-40% complete so as to avoid particles near to the possibly anomalous[66] center and also the outer region of the clusters which are far from complete) and the distribution $N_s(r)$ was obtained from the number of particles contained within circles of radius r measured from these randomly selected particles. Figure 4a shows the distributions $N_s(r)$ obtained in this way and Figures 4b and 4c show the results of two attempts to scale these curves using the scaling form given in equation (9). The data collapses shown in Figures 4b and 4c are both quite poor and no better results could be obtained with any other combination of the exponents γ and δ.

Figure 5 shows the results obtained from a similar simulation in which the particles about which the distributions ($N_S(r)$) were measured were selected randomly from all of the particles in the clusters. In these simulations 11 clusters were used. Figure 5b shows that now a quite good data collapse can be obtained using the scaling forms given in equations (8) and (9) (i.e., $\gamma = 1$ and $\delta = D = 1.71$). Taken together Figures 4 and 5 show that the distributions $N_S(r)$ scale in the way expected for a self-similar fractal if they are averaged over the entire cluster, but that the interior of the cluster does not have a simple self-similar structure.

Figure 6 shows the distributions $N_S(\lambda)$ obtained by covering the clusters used to obtain the results shown in Figure 4 using grids with scales of length λ. Results are shown for 13 different values of λ in the range $4d_0 \leq \lambda \leq 200d_0$. Figures 6b and 6c show the results of attempts to scale these curves using the scaling form

$$N_S(\lambda) \sim s^{-\gamma'} h(s/\lambda^{\delta'}) \qquad (12)$$

for 7 values of λ in the range $4d_0\lambda \leq 40d_0$. Neither data collapse is particularly good. But Figure 6c does indicate that for larger clusters and larger values of λ it might be possible to obtain a good data collapse using the scaling form given in equation (10).

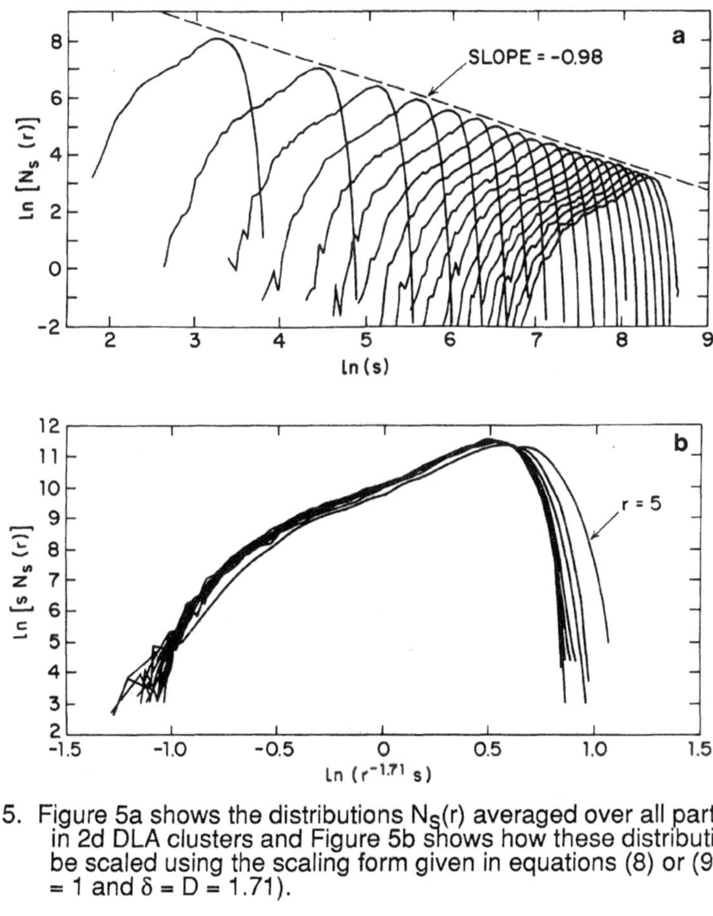

Figure 5. Figure 5a shows the distributions $N_S(r)$ averaged over all particles in 2d DLA clusters and Figure 5b shows how these distributions can be scaled using the scaling form given in equations (8) or (9) (with $\gamma = 1$ and $\delta = D = 1.71$).

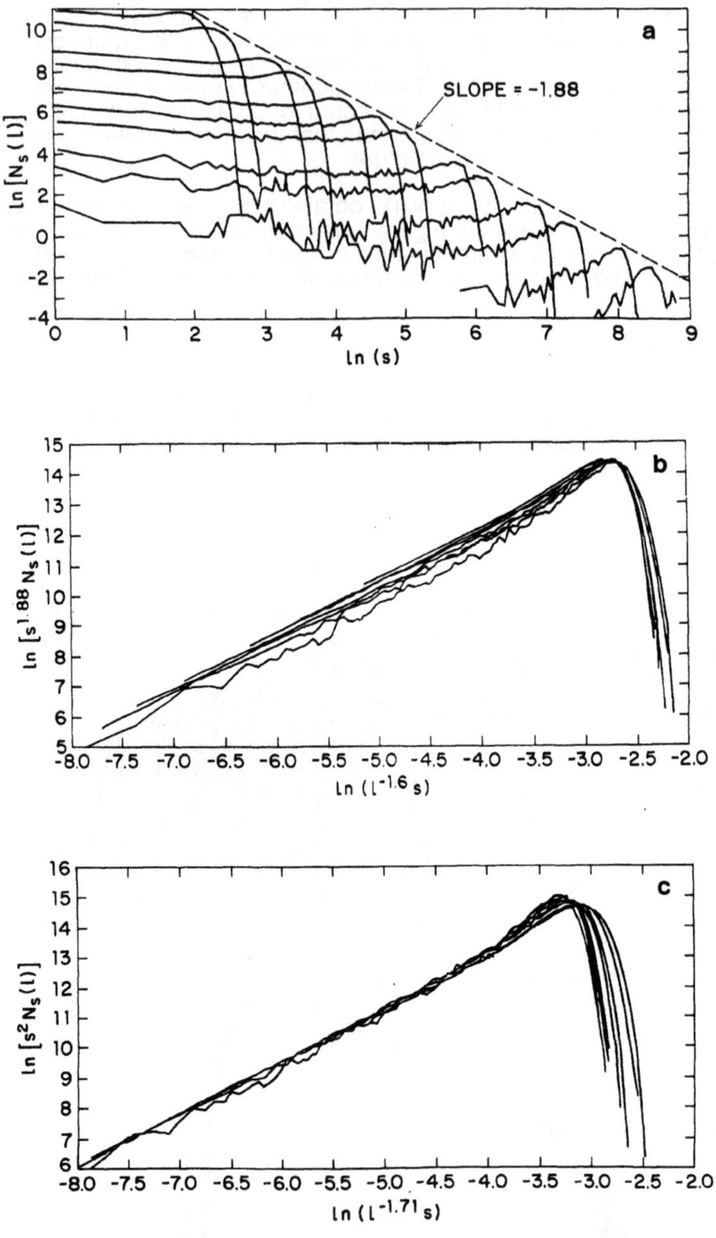

Figure 6. This figure shows the distributions $N_S(\lambda)$ (Figure 6a) and the results of two attempts to scale them onto a common curve using the scaling form given in equation (11) (Figures 6b and 6c). These results were obtained from the simulations used to generate the results displayed in Figure 4. Here ℓ is λ.

THE DIMENSIONALITIES D_q

With G. Li and L. M. Sander we have measured the generalized dimensionalities[42] (D_q) defined by equations (3) and (4). Figure 7 shows some of the results obtained from this work. The quantities d_q ($q = 0$-8) were obtained by covering each cluster with grids with sides of length λ ($\lambda =$ 1,2,3...lattice units or diameters) and measuring the mass within each grid element. For the off-lattice DLA clusters the number of particles whose centers fell within a particular grid element was taken as the mass. For each cluster the procedure was repeated 5 times with randomly placed grids.

The quantities D_q were obtained from the qth moments of the masses $C_q(\lambda)$ within the grid elements by least squares fitting the dependence of these moments on λ over the range $L_1 \leq \lambda \leq (L_2 = 1.5\, L_1)$ (see equations (3) and (4)). Figure 7 shows the results obtained by using 140 12,500 particle clusters, 80 25,000 particle clusters, 21 50,000 particle clusters and 26 100,000 particle clusters. Results are shown for $q = 0$, 2 and 8. In all of these cases D_q increases as λ increases and the values obtained for the larger values of λ are consistent with the idea that all of the generalized dimensionalities might have an asymptotic value equal to D_β (i.e., about 1.71) in the limit $s \to \alpha$, $\lambda \to \infty$. Very similar results were obtained from lattice model simulations with clusters of the same sizes.

DLA IN DIMENSIONALITIES 2-8

We have recently developed improved algorithms for both off-lattice and hypercubic lattice DLA in dimensionalities 2-8. Figure 8 shows a 10^6 particle two dimensional off-lattice DLA cluster. Quite a large number of clusters of this size were generated and used to investigate the size dependence of both the radius of gyration and the width of the active zone[44] (ξ). Here ξ is the variance in the deposition radius. Earlier simulations using clusters containing up to 50,000 particles[45] had indicated that the effective fractal dimensionality (D_β) obtained from the dependence of R_g on s was essentially cluster size independent. The new results indicate that D_β has a value of about 1.71 for clusters in the size range 10^3-10^6 particles and there is no indication that D_β is changing as the cluster size is increased. The exponent υ which describes the dependence of ξ on s

$$\xi \sim s^{\bar{\upsilon}} \tag{13}$$

continues to increase with increasing s and for clusters containing 10^6 particles $\bar{\upsilon}$ has reached a value of about 0.56 and we now believe more strongly that in the limit $s \to \infty$ the exponents β and $\bar{\upsilon}$ will converge to the same value of about 0.585 (1/1.71). For $d = 3$-8 we have been able to generate quite large numbers (typically between 50 and several hundred) of clusters containing about 10^5 particles or sites. Using these clusters effective fractal dimensionalities D_β which describes how the radius of gyration grows with increasing cluster size (s) has been measured. Figures 9 and 10 show typical results obtained from both off-lattice and hypercubic lattice models for $d = 3$ and $d = 5$. To obtain the effective fractal dimensionality D_β the mean radius of gyration was measured at each 5% increment in the cluster mass and the effective fractal dimensionality was obtained by least squares fitting a straight line to the dependence of $\ln(R_g)$ on $\ln(s)$ for clusters in the size range $s_1 \leq s \leq s_2 (s_2 = 1.05^9\, s_1)$ to obtain $D_{eff}(s)$ where $s = (s_1 s_2)^{1/2}$.

The results shown in Figures 9 and 10 indicate that the fractal dimensionalities obtained from the off-lattice models are in good agreement with the values predicted by mean field theories[21,22,24] which lead to the prediction

$$D = (d^2+1)/(d+1) \tag{14}$$

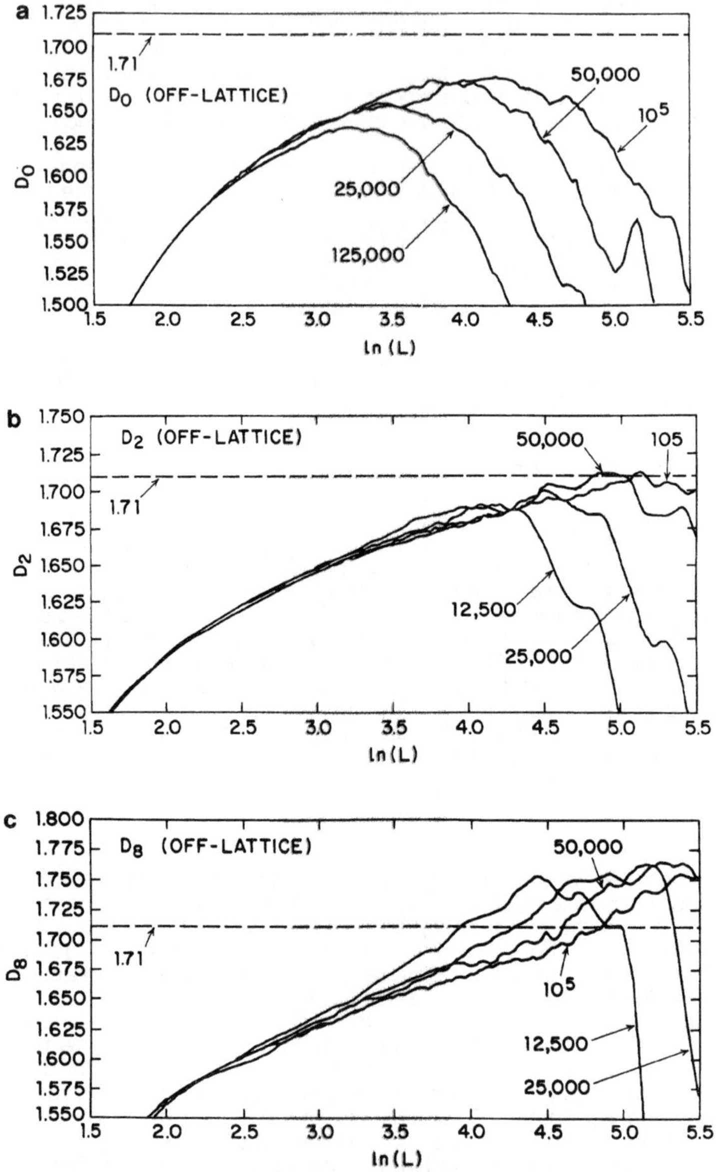

Figure 7. Dependence of the effective values of the fractal dimensionalities D_q (q = 0 Fig.7a, q = 2 Fig 7b and q = 8 Fig 7c) on the grid length scale ($L = \lambda$) obtained for off-lattice DLA clusters containing 12,500, 25,000 50,000 and 100,000 particles.

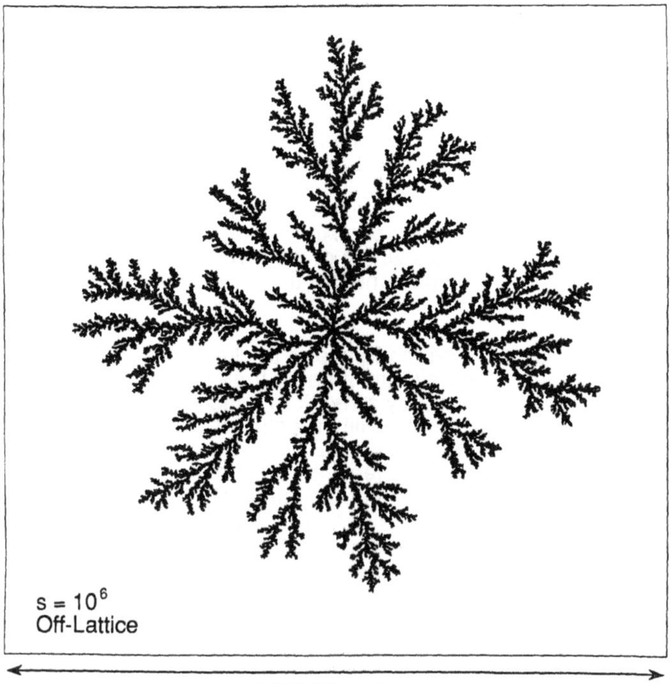

Figure 8. A 10^6 particle off-lattice two dimensional DLA cluster.

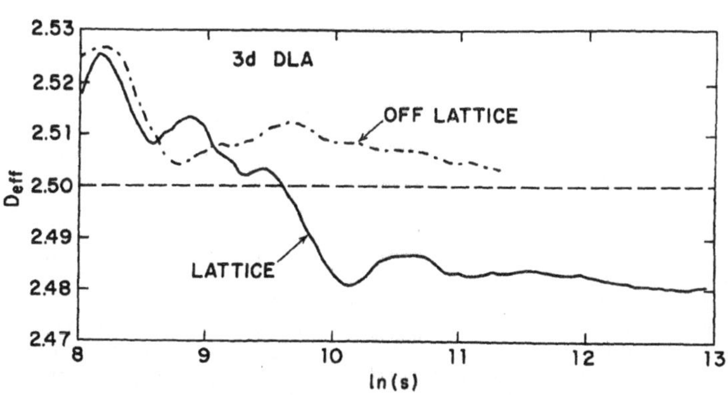

Figure 9. Dependence of the effective fractal dimensionality (D_β) on the cluster size s obtained from 169 100,000 particle off-lattice three dimensional clusters and 98 1.25×10^6 site cubic lattice model clusters.

For d = 2 the simulation result D = 1.715±0.004 seems to be significantly larger than the mean field value. For d = 2, 3, 4 and 5 the effective fractal dimensionality (D_β) at first increases quite rapidly with increasing cluster size. As the cluster size continues to increase, the increase in D_β slows down and finally D_β decreases slowly to an apparently asymptotic value in good agreement with the mean field theory predictions. For d≥6 only the first part of the curve is seen and the effective value for D_β at the largest practical cluster size is substantially in excess of the mean field theory predictions. However, we believe that our results are consistent with an asymptotic value for D_β in substantial agreement with the mean field values For d>6, it was not practical to generate large numbers of clusters containing 10^5 particles or sites. Consequently, somewhat smaller clusters were used. The comparison with the results of mean field theories (equation (14)) is not meant to be an endorsement of this theoretical approach. At this stage equation (14) should be regarded as an empirical formula which gives a value for D that is in good agreement with the simulation results and the theoretical asymptotic limit (D $\rightarrow$ d - 1 as d $\rightarrow \infty$).

For d≤5 the hypercubic lattice models lead to clusters with effective fractal dimensionalities which are slightly smaller than those obtained from the off-lattice models. This is probably a result of lattice anisotropy effects. For d = 3 the effective fractal dimensionality for clusters containing 1.25×10^6 sites is about 2.48 (vs a mean field value of 2.50). It is clear that enormous clusters would be required to see an effective fractal dimensionality close to the values obtained from noise reduced cubic lattice DLA simulations (see below). Turkevich and Scher[67] have extended their theory[27] for two dimensional lattice model DLA to lattices with dimensionalities (d) greater than 2. For the three dimensional cubic lattice, they find that D = 2.4630986---. This is certainly consistent with the results shown in Figure 9, but it is evident that this value will not be seen in simulations carried out on a practical scale. The results shown in Figure 9 do not provide an adequate test of this theory. However, it appears (see Figure (2)) that the cubic lattice DLA clusters eventually evolve into a structure with six distinct arms. This is not the asymptoic shape used by Turkevich and Scher to obtain their theoretical result for D.

On the basis of much smaller scale simulations, Meakin[33] suggested that the fractal dimensionality of DLA clusters might be given by D = 5d/6. For d = 2 and d = 3 this equation gives the same values as the mean field theory and for d = 4 a value of 3.333, instead of 3.40 is obtained. However, our 4d simulation results give much better agreement with the mean field value. For d = 5 5d/6 is 4.166... which is substantially smaller than the mean field value of 26/6 or 4.333... and our simulation results are in much better agreement with the mean field theory prediction. A fractal dimension of 5d/6 would also be in serious disagreement with the theoretical result of Ball and Witten[68,69] (D $\rightarrow$ d-1 as d $\rightarrow \infty$) which seems to be the only quantitatively reliable theoretical result for DLA. Using mean field arguments, Hentschel[23] has predicted that D = $(8+5d^2)/(6+5d)$ for d<5.1 and D = $(8-4d+d^2)/(d-2)$ for d>5.1. This leads to the predicted values of 1.75 for d = 2, 2.524 for d = 3, D = 3.385 for d = 4 and D = 4.290 for d = 5. For d = 2 our results are in about equally poor agreement with this mean field theory and with equation (14). For d = 3 our simulation results are in better agreement with equation (14) than with Hentschel's prediction. For d = 4 Hentschel's mean field theory and equation (14) give predicted values which are numerically very close to each other. For d = 6 Hentschel predicts a fractal dimensionality of 5.0. Our simulation results are in much better agreement with the value of 5.286 obtained from equation (14), but we do not believe that they accurately represent the asymptotic value for D_β. The prediction D = $(8-4d+d^2)/(d-2)$ gives an asymptotic (d $\rightarrow \infty$) value of d-2 for D.

OTHER LAPLACIAN GROWTH MODELS

The DLA model does not represent diffusion-limited growth from a finite concentration field. Instead, it describes a random growth process in which

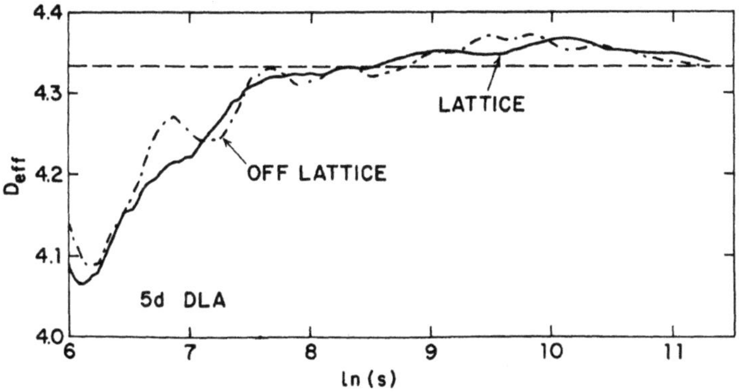

Figure 10. The dependence of the effective fractal dimensionality on the cluster size obtained from 100,000 particle 5d off-lattice DLA clusters and 100,000 site 5d hypercubic lattice DLA clusters.

the growth probabilities P_i for the unoccupied perimeter sites are controlled by a scalar field ϕ which obeys the Laplace equation $\nabla^2\phi = 0$ with absorbing boundary conditions on the growing structure and a fixed value for ϕ ($\phi = 1$ for example) at infinity. In the ordinary DLA model the random walkers are used to simulate a field obeying the Laplace equation and the corresponding growth probabilities are proportional to ϕ_i (within a factor of order unity which depends on the local boundary conditions). In the dielectric breakdown model[16] a discretized version of the Laplace equation is solved numerically on a lattice with a fixed value for the scalar field (potential) on a distant surface which encloses the cluster. Unoccupied perimeter sites are then selected at random with appropriate probabilities (P_i) to represent the growth process. Here

$$P_i \propto n\phi_i \tag{15}$$

where n is the number of occupied nearest neighbors for the conventional dielectric breakdown model.[16] A more general growth model can be obtained by replacing equation (15) by[16,70]

$$P_i \propto n(\phi_i)^\eta \tag{16}$$

Unfortunately, the numerical solution of the Laplace equation presents considerable difficulties. Accurate relaxation of the Laplacian field requires large amounts of computer time and this problem is exacerbated if the outer (fixed potential) boundary is placed far from the cluster. In terms of the DLA model, this boundary corresponds to the "killing circle" which can be placed very far from the cluster without substantially increasing the computer time requirements for random walk DLA simulations. In our experience the conjugate gradient method[71] is substantially superior to standard relaxation algorithms.[72]

Matsushita et al.[73,74] have developed a closely related model using random walkers that can be used for small integer values of η. In this model particles (random walkers) are added, one at a time, to a growing cluster using standard DLA algorithms. However, after an unoccupied perimeter site has been reached η-1 random walks are started from the contacted site and only if all of these walks reach the outer boundary at a distance of k R_{max} from the center of the cluster (without contacting the cluster) is that site filled. Using this approach, Hayakawa et al.[74] obtained an effective fractal dimensionality of 1.47$\pm$0.03 for η = 2 using an off-lattice model.

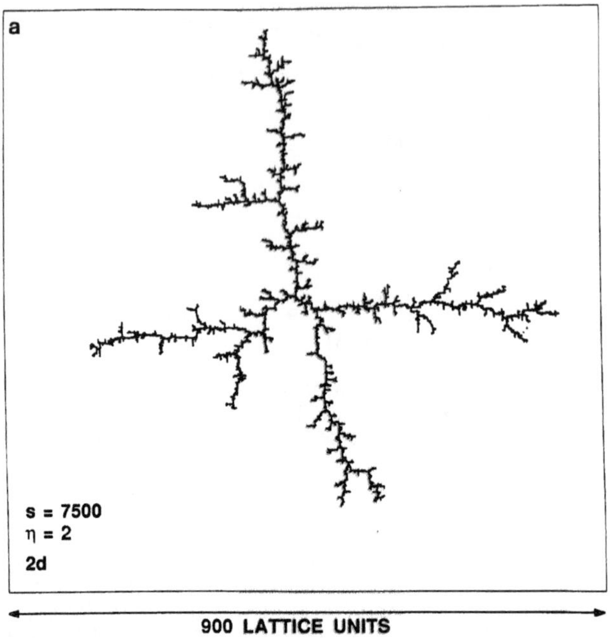

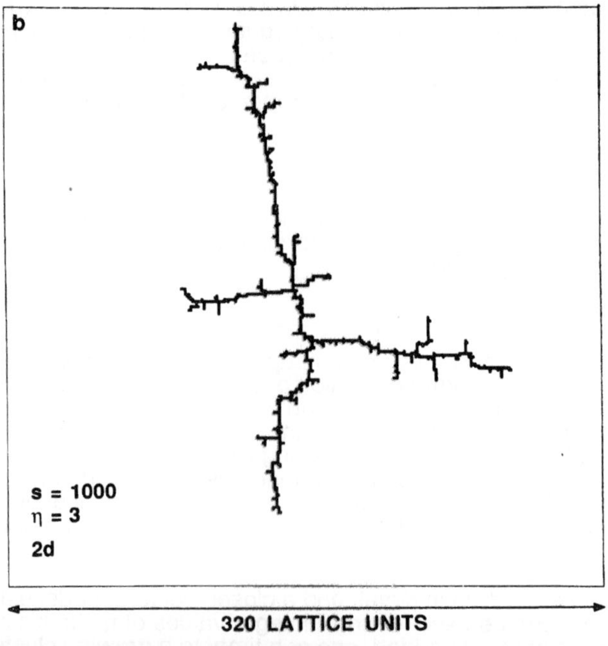

Figure 11. Clusters grown on a square lattice with growth probability exponents (η) of 2 (Figure 11a) and 3 (Figure 11b) using random walkers (Matsushita et al.[73]) instead of numerical relaxation of a harmonic field. The cluster shown in Figure 11a contains 7500 sites and that contained in Figure 11b contains l000 sites.

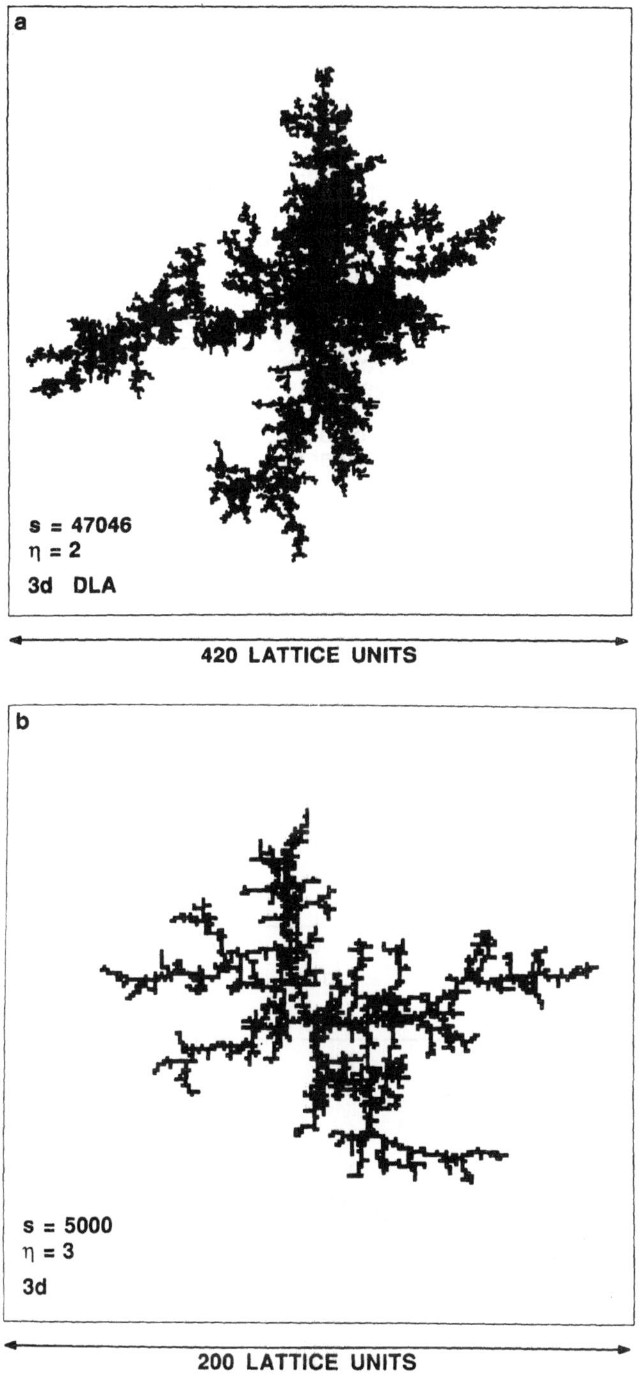

Figure 12. Clusters grown on a cubic lattice with growth probability exponents (η) of 2 (Figure 12a) and 3 (Figure 12b). The cluster shown in Figure 12a contains 47046 sites and that shown in Figure 12b contains 5000 sites.

Figure 11 shows clusters grown on a square lattice with $\eta = 2$ and 3 and Figure 12 shows clusters grown on a cubic lattice also with $\eta = 2$ and 3. To obtain a more quantitative assessment of the structures generated by these models, 75 clusters were grown to a size of 5000 sites using the square lattice model with $\eta = 2$ and 17 clusters were grown to a size of 750 sites with $\eta = 3$. Similarly, using the cubic lattice models, 31 clusters were grown to a size of 25,000 sites with $\eta = 2$ and 29 clusters were grown to a size of 3500 sites with $\eta = 3$. Figures 13 and 14 show the dependence of the cluster radii of gyration (R_g) on the number of occupied sites (s). In all cases the dependence of $\ln(R_g)$ on $\ln(s)$ seems quite linear for all but the smallest clusters indicating that R_g and s are related by equation (2). The values of the exponent β and the corresponding fractal dimensionality $D_\beta \simeq 1/\beta$) obtained from these simulations were $\beta = 0.727 \pm 0.0003$ ($D_\beta \simeq 1.38$) for $d = 2$ and $\eta = 2$, $\beta = 0.814 \pm 0.002$ ($D_\beta \simeq 1.23$) for $d = 2$ and $\eta = 3$, $\beta = 0.4836 \pm 0.0002$ ($D_\beta \simeq 2.07$) for $d = 3$ and $\eta = 2$ and $\beta = 0.549 \pm 0.0004$ ($D_\beta \simeq 1.82$) for $d = 3$ and $\eta = 3$. For the case $\eta = 2$ on a square lattice the effective fractal dimensionality of about 1.38 is significantly smaller than the value of 1.47 ± 0.03 obtained by Hayakawa et al.[71] using an off-lattice model. It is also substantially smaller than the value of about 1.60 obtained for $\eta = 2$ on a square lattice in the pioneering work of Niemeyer, Pietronero and Wiesmann[16,75]. The value of 1.43 obtained

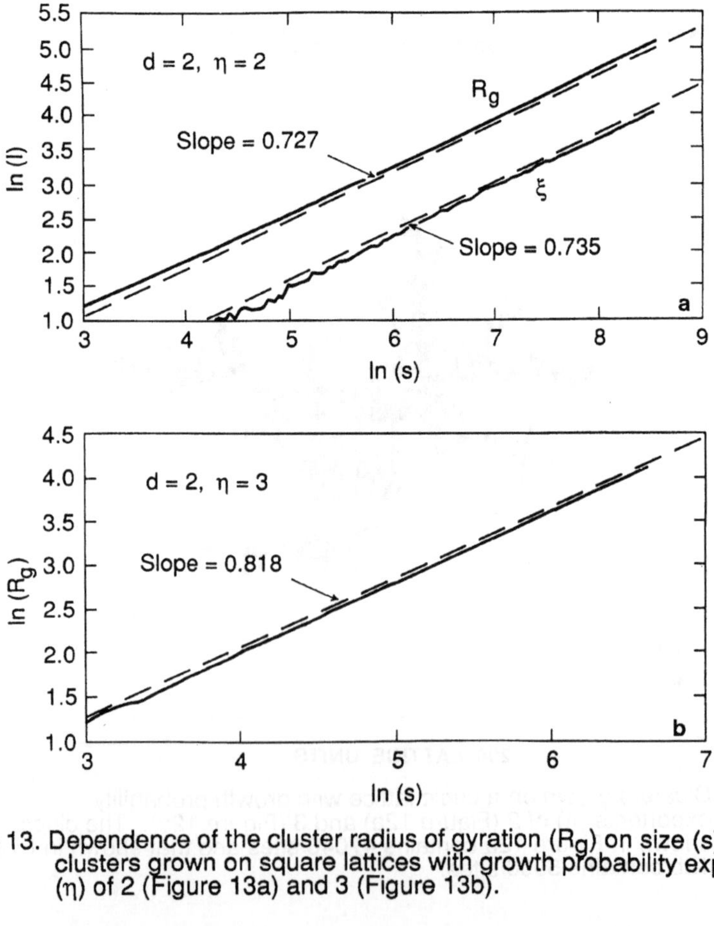

Figure 13. Dependence of the cluster radius of gyration (R_g) on size (s) for clusters grown on square lattices with growth probability exponents (η) of 2 (Figure 13a) and 3 (Figure 13b).

by Wiesmann and Pietronero[76] using the dielectric breakdown model is in much better agreement with the results reported here as is the value of 1.36±0.05 obtained by Meakin[70] using a diffusion limited growth model which is essentially identical to the dielectric breakdown model. Satpathy[77] has measured the fractal dimensionality D_β for clusters generated on a cubic lattice using a dielectric breakdown model similar to that of Niemeyer et al.[16] Effective values of 2.09±0.06, 1.84±0.07 and 1.79±0.08 were obtained for $\eta = 2$, 3 and 4 respectively. Our results are in excellent agreement with those of Satpathy for $\eta = 2$ and 3. For $\eta = 2$ and $\eta = 3$ the method of Matsushita et al.[73,74] appears to be more efficient than standard dielectric breakdown algorithms. For $\eta \geq 4$ the probability that $\eta - 1$ walkers will escape becomes quite small and relaxation of the Laplacian field is a more efficient procedure.

The values obtained for the fractal dimensionality (D_β) from the two dimensional models are in quite good agreement with simulations carried out earlier by Meakin[78] in which the first site to be contacted η times by random walkers was grown (in this model the contact "score" associated with each perimeter site is set to zero after each growth event). For this model values of about 0.73 and about 0.78 were obtained for $\eta = 2$ and $\eta = 3$ respectively. Matsushita et al.[73] have generalized the mean field theory of Honda et al. to obtain the result

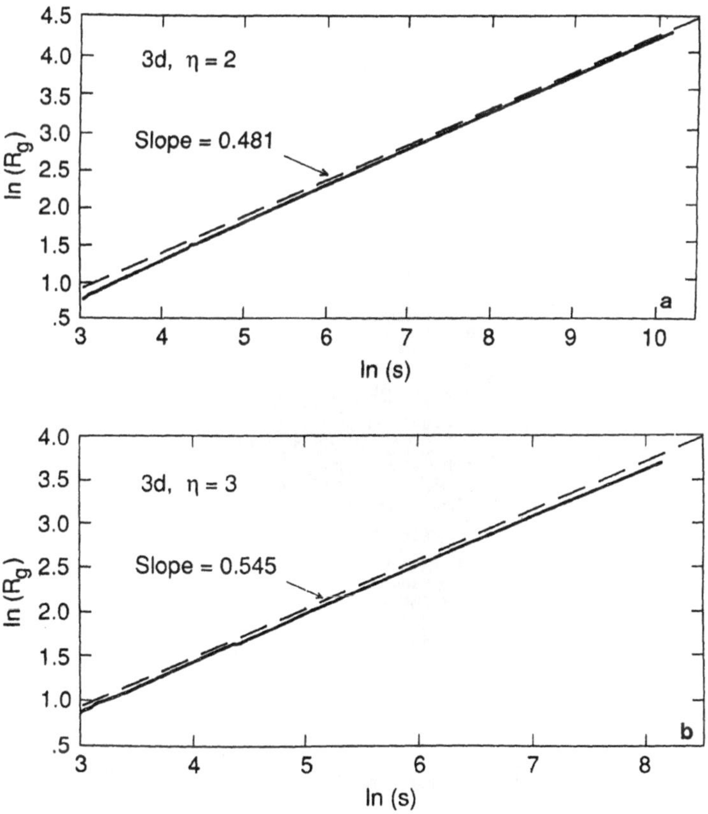

Figure 14. Dependence of the radius of gyration on cluster size for clusters grown on cubic lattices with growth probability exponents (η) of 2 (Figures 14a) and 3 (Figure 14b).

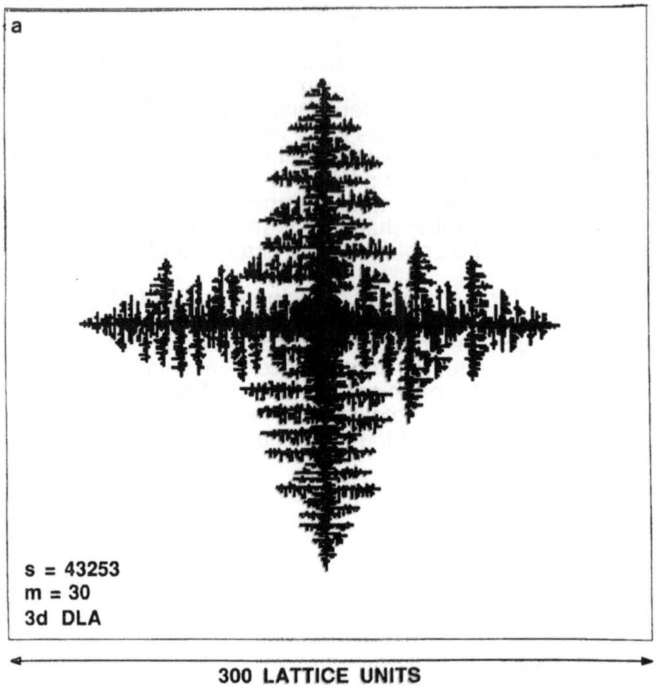
a
s = 43253
m = 30
3d DLA
300 LATTICE UNITS

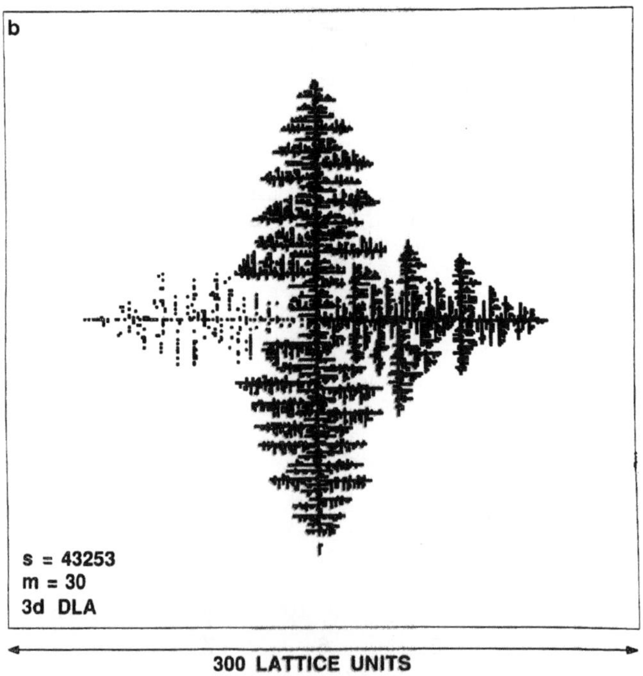
b
s = 43253
m = 30
3d DLA
300 LATTICE UNITS

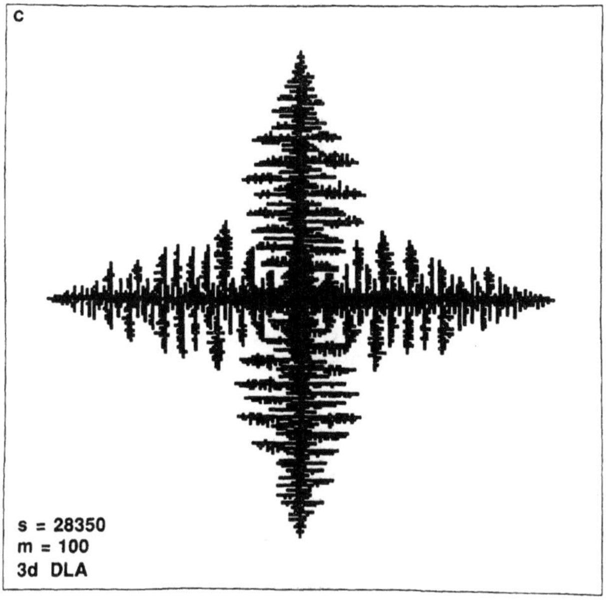

240 LATTICE UNITS

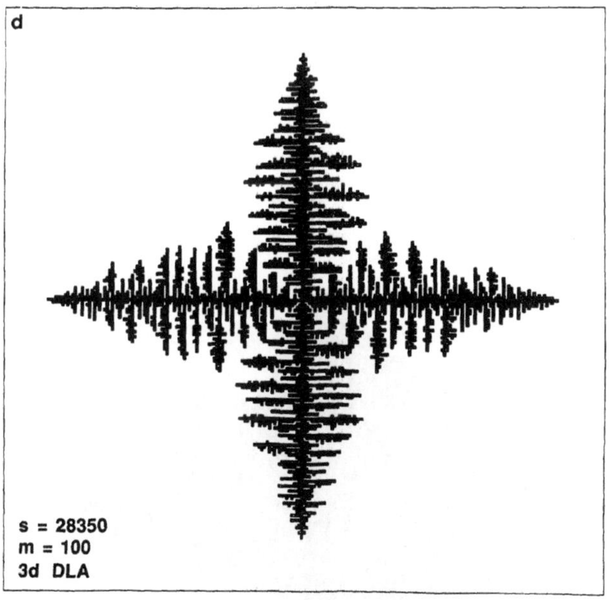

200 LATTICE UNITS

Figure 15. Projections and cross sections for noise reduced cubic lattice DLA clusters. Figures 15a and 15b show results for a 43553 site cluster with a noise reduction parameter of 30 and Figures 15c and 15d show results obtained from a 28350 site cluster grown with a noise reduction parameter of 100. The cross sections are along a plane which intersects the origin. In Figure 15b the core along the center of the cluster arm on the left hand side deviates from this plane.

$$D = [d^2+\eta(Dw-1)]/[d+\eta(Dw-1)] \tag{17}$$

where Dw is the fractal dimensionality of the particle trajectories (2 in our case). This equation leads to the prediction $D = 1.5$ for $d = 2$, $\eta = 2$, $D = 1.40$ for $d = 2$, $\eta = 3$, $D = 2.20$ for $d = 3$, $\eta = 2$ and $D = 2.0$ for $d = 3$, $\eta = 3$. The results from our simulations are all significantly smaller than those predicted by equation (17). This could be a result of lattice anisotropy which is quite evident in Figures 11 and 12.

NOISE REDUCED DLA

In the noise reduced DLA model[50,51] perimeter sites are filled only after they have been contacted m times. A score is kept of how many times each of the unoccupied perimeter sites have been reached by a random walker. After a perimeter site has been reached by a random walker, its score is incremented by 1 and the random walk is terminated. A new random walk is then launched from outside of the region occupied by the cluster. As the cluster grows, the scores associated with each of the perimeter sites continue to accumulate (they are not set to zero after a growth event). The noise reduced DLA model and closely related models[1,32,53] have been quite extensively investigated in two dimensions, but only preliminary results have been reported for d = 3[9]. A quite detailed theoretical understanding of at least one two dimensional noise reduced DLA model has now been obtained.[32]

Figure 15 shows projections and cross-sections through two noise reduced cubic lattice DLA clusters. Figures 15a and 15b show a 43253 site cluster grown with a noise reduction parameter (m) of 30 and Figures 15c and

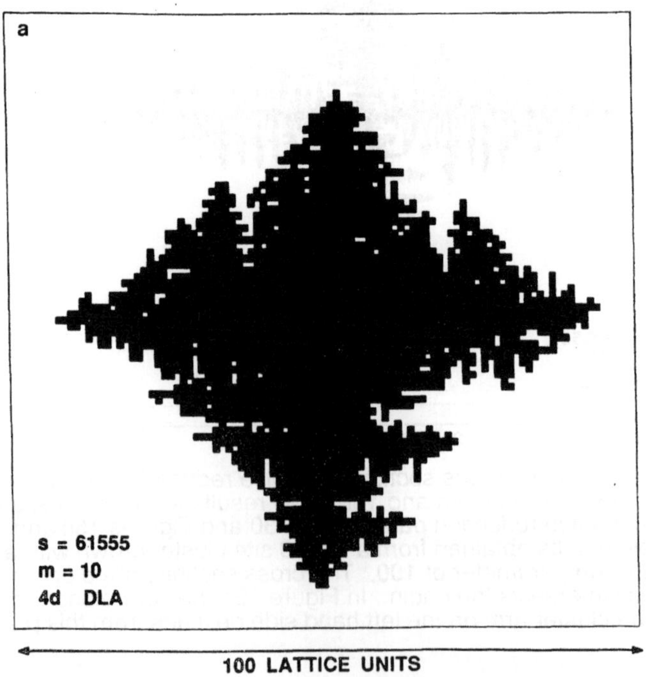

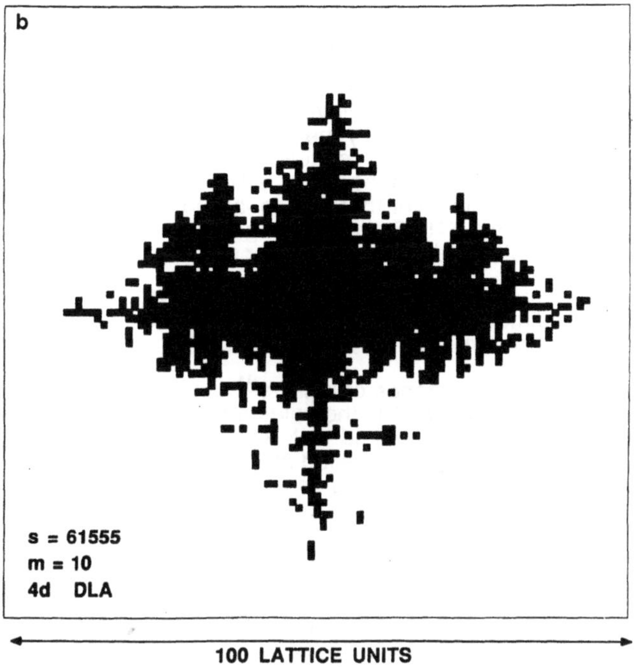

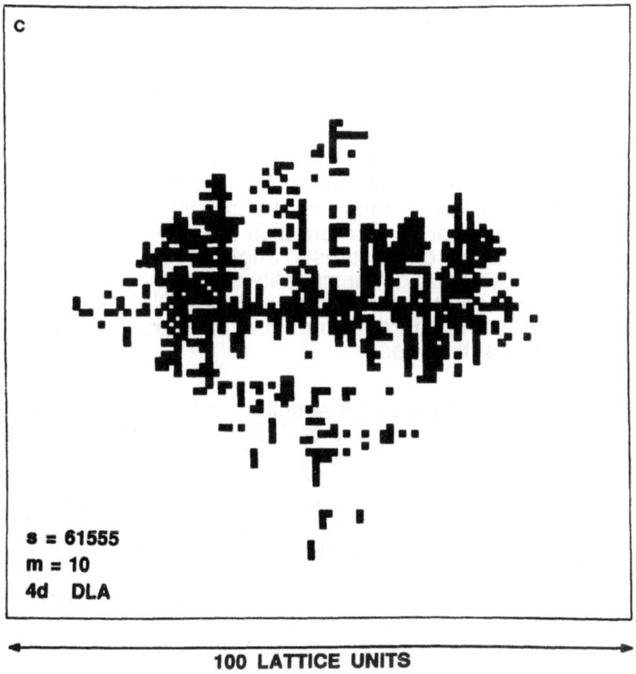

Figure 16. A 61555 site DLA cluster grown on a four dimensional hypercubic lattice with a noise reduction parameter (m) of 10. Figure 16a shows a projection onto a plane, Figure 16b shows a cross section through a projection onto a cubic lattice and Figure 16c shows a cross section through the clusters.

15d show a 28350 site cluster generated with m = 100. It is evident from this figure that noise reduction strongly enhances the effects of lattice anisotropy and for d = 2, at least, small clusters generated with quite modest noise reduction parameters (m = 2 or 3) strongly resemble much larger DLA clusters (m = 1). For this reason it is generally believed that the structure for noise reduced DLA clusters represents faithfully the structure of much larger clusters grown on a lattice without noise reduction. If this is correct, it may be possible to reveal the asymptotic behavior of lattice models for DLA using noise reduced DLA models. However there is, so far, no rigorous proof of this conjecture. Figure 16 shows a 61555 site cluster grown on a four dimensional hypercubic lattice with a noise reduction parameter of 10.

To determine the dependence of the cluster radii of gyration on the cluster size, a number of three dimensional and four dimensional clusters were grown with noise reduction parameters of m = 3, 10 and 30.

Figure 17a shows the dependence of $\ln(R_g/s^{\beta^*})$ on ln(s) obtained from the four dimensional simulations. Here β^* is the value for the radius of gyration exponent corresponding to the "mean field" value for D_{β^*} (equation (14)). For d = 4 β^* has a value of 5/17. The curve labelled m = 1 in Figure 17a was obtained without noise reduction. For large values of s this curve is almost horizontal indicating that the effective value for D_β is quite close to 3.4. Figure 17b shows the dependence of the effective fractal dimensionality (D_β) on ln(s) for noise reduction parameters of 1, 3, 10 and 30. These results were obtained using the same procedures that were used to generate Figures 9 and 10. The results shown in Figure 17b indicate that $D_\beta \simeq 3.4$ for m = 1, $\simeq 3.25$ for m = 3, $\simeq 3.2$ for m = 10 and about 3.0 for m = 30. Unfortunately, the results shown in Figure 17 do not indicate the value of the asymptotic ($s \rightarrow \infty$, $m \rightarrow \infty$) fractal dimensionality. However, they do indicate that D_β may be less than 3.0 for the four dimensional hypercubic lattice for large values of m and s. The observation that the effective value for D_β is almost independent of s (for s larger than a few thousand sites) indicates that clusters of enormous size would be required to attain this asymptotic value for D_β (if indeed the noise reduced DLA model does represent the behavior of very large DLA clusters without noise reduction). The theoretical work of Turkevich and Scher[67] shows that the strength of the singularity in the Laplacian field at the tip of a "needle" with absorbing boundary conditions would lead to a tip growth probability corresponding to a fractal dimensionality of d-1 for $D \geq 3$. This means that d-1 is a theoretical lower limit to the fractal dimensionality. This appears to be a reliable lower limit (in practice the hypercone at the end of the cluster arms should have a characteristic angle greater than 0 leading to a weaker singularity and a fractal dimensionality somewhat larger than d-1). It would be interesting to extend the noise reduced DLA simulations for d = 4 to larger values of m (using a larger number of clusters to reduce statistical uncertainties) to test this idea.

A similar series of noise reduced DLA simulations was carried out using a cubic lattice. Clusters were grown to a size of 50,000 sites with noise reduction parameters in the range $2 \leq m \leq 100$ (52 clusters wih m = 2, 67 clusters with m = 3, 24 clusters with m = 5, 11 clusters with m = 10 and 6 clusters with m = 30). For clusters in the size range $5000 \leq s \leq 50{,}000$, the effective fractal dimensionality (D_β) is approximately 2.43, 2.40, 2.33, 2.26 and 2.22 respectively for m = 2, 3, 5, 10 and 30. It appears that in this case the effective fractal dimensionality is approaching a limiting value (as $m \rightarrow \infty$) which is larger than the theoretical lower limit of 2.0. Again, simulations with larger noise reduction parameters would be desirable.

A noise reduced two dimensional DLA model has been analyzed in detail by Eckmann et al.[32] using conformal mapping. In this model the particles follow off-lattice random walk trajectories, but after a particle in the cluster has been contacted, the contacting particle is rotated about the contacted particle in the cluster until the vector from the contacted particle to the contacting particle points in the nearest of n directions each separated by an angle of

$2\pi/n$ from its nearest neighbors. Each particle in the cluster can be regarded to have n "antennas" associated with the n directions in space. In the noise reduced DLA model the score associated with the appropriate antenna on the contacted particle is incremented after that particle has been contacted. Only when the score associated with a particular antenna on one of the particles in the cluster reaches a value of m is the new particle added to the end of the antenna. The theory of Eckmann et al. indicates that there are two phases of growth. In the first stage the cluster grows as a compact cross and in the second stage branching occurs and a fractal structure is eventually generated. The cluster size s*(m) at which side branching begins to occur is given (according to the theory) by

$$s^*(m) \sim (\log(m))^3 \tag{18}$$

Figure 18 shows a square lattice DLA cluster grown with a noise reduction parameter of 10^4. The compact central core is quite evident for such large values of m. Although equation (18) was not derived for ordinary noise reduced square lattice DLA, it is expected to be appropriate for this model as well. This expectation has been confirmed by computer simulations.[32]

The theory shows that the mass added at a distance x along a branch of length R(s) during the first (compact) stage of growth is given by

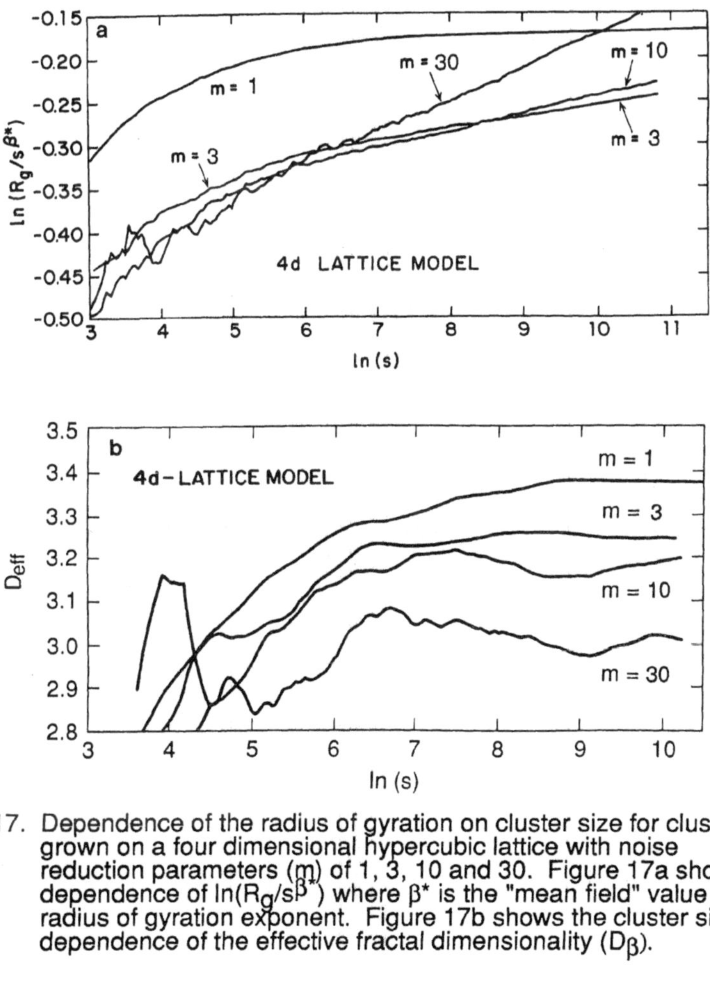

Figure 17. Dependence of the radius of gyration on cluster size for clusters grown on a four dimensional hypercubic lattice with noise reduction parameters (m) of 1, 3, 10 and 30. Figure 17a shows the dependence of $\ln(R_g/s^{\beta^*})$ where β^* is the "mean field" value for the radius of gyration exponent. Figure 17b shows the cluster size dependence of the effective fractal dimensionality (D_β).

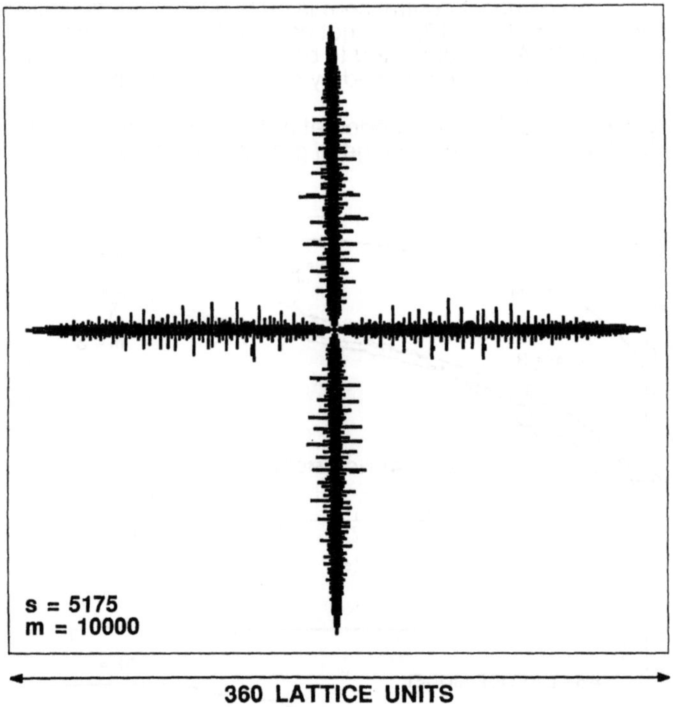

Figure 18. A cluster of 5175 sites grown on a square lattice using a noise reduction parameter (m) of 10,000.

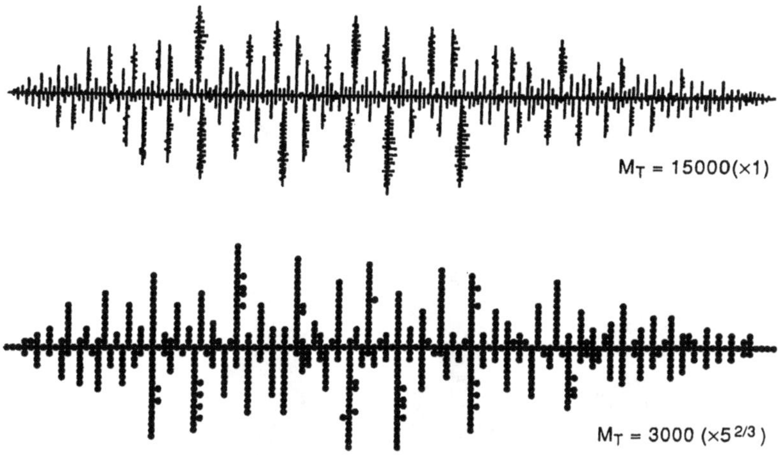

Figure 19. Cluster arms obtained from a DLA model in which particles follow off-lattice trajectories, but growth is restricted to n (n = 4) directions. These cluster arms were generated with a noise reduction parameter of 300 and are displayed on a length scale proportional to $s^{2/3}$ (where s is the cluster size) to illustrate the rescaling of the cluster geometry.

$$M(x, R(s)) = x^{1/2} F(x/R(s)) = (R(s))^{1/2} G(x/R(s)) \tag{19}$$

In the later stages of growth the size (w) of the side branches is given by

$$w(x,R(s)) \sim M^2(x,R(s)) = xF^2(x/R(s)) = R(s)G^2(x/R(s)) \tag{20}$$

This means that the shape of the cluster arms is characterized by the length to width (aspect) ratio which reaches a fixed value as the cluster size increases. The shape of the cluster arms becomes invariant to isotropic rescaling. This is illustrated in Figure 19 which shows two cluster arms generated with a noise reduction parameter of 300 and 4 directions of growth (n = 4). The cluster arms were obtained from clusters grown to a size of 3000 and 15,000 particles that are displayed on a length scale proportional to $s^{2/3}$ (where s is the cluster size).

The end of each arm of a DLA cluster grown using these models with large noise reduction parameters (m) is an "exposed tip" consisting of a linear array of particles with no side branches. Figure 20 shows the 3 tips of a cluster grown with m = 100 and n = 3 (three directions of growth). The theory of Eckmann et al. predicts that the length of this exposed tip should be approximately 6, 4 and 3 (particles) for n = 3, 4 and 5 respectively. This prediction is also in good agreement with simulation results. Providing that m is sufficiently large, the length of the exposed tips is independent of m. The function F in equations (19) and (20) depends on the number of arms (n) in the cluster

$$F(x/R) = \int_{x/R}^{1} \frac{y^{(n/2-5/2)}}{(1-y^n)^{1/2}} dy \tag{21}$$

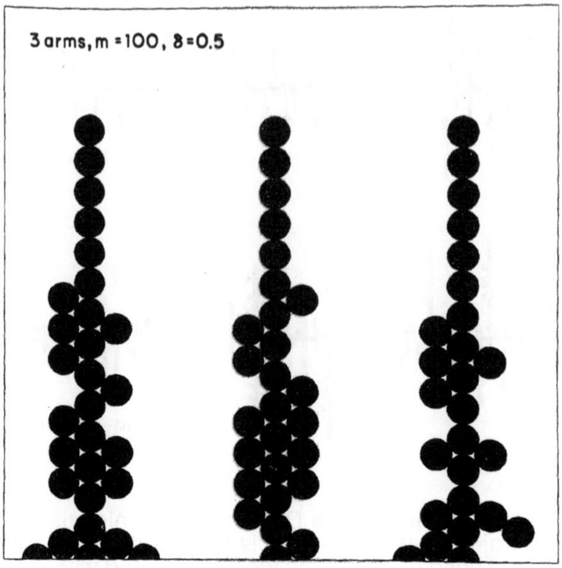

Figure 20. The ends of the three arms of a DLA cluster generated using a DLA model with a noise reduction parameter (m) of 100 in which growth is restricted to 3 directions in the two dimensional embedding space. In this model the "particles" follow off-lattice random walks. The exposed tip containing about 6 particles is shown in this figure.

Fig. 21a

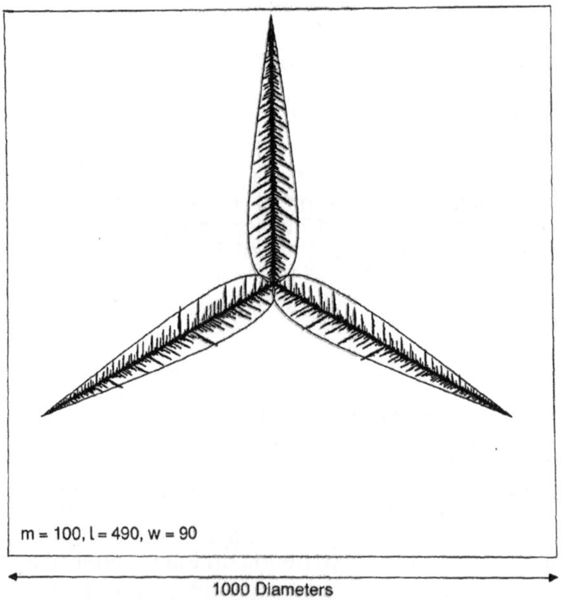

Figure 21. A comparison of the shapes of DLA clusters generated using the "semi-lattice" model (off-lattice walks with growth in n discrete directions) described in the text with a noise reduction parameter (m) of 100. Figures 21a, 21b and 21c show clusters with n = 3, 4 and 5 arms. The cluster envelopes were obtained using equations (21) and (22).

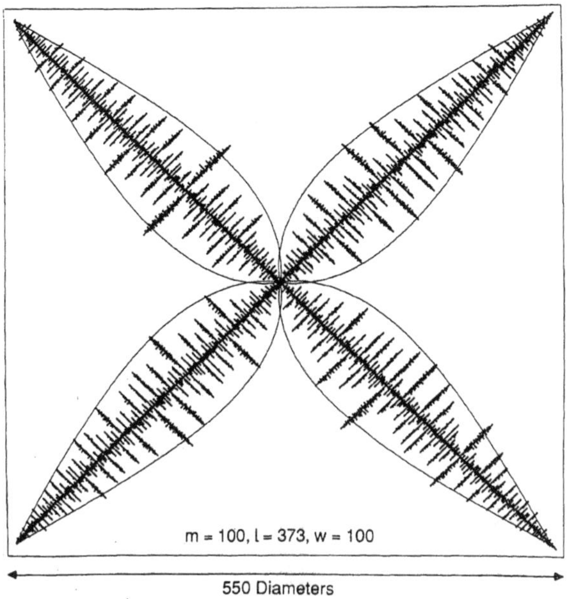

Fig. 21b

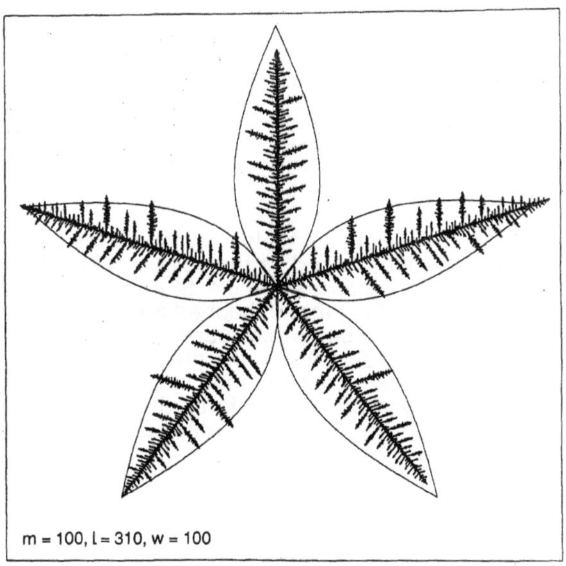

Fig. 21c

The function F(x/R) describes the shape of the cluster arms.

$$w(x,R) = \alpha x F^2 (x/R) \tag{22}$$

Figure 21 compares the shapes of clusters with 3, 4 and 5 arms with the cluster envelopes calculated using equations (21) and (22). The parameter α was adjusted to give approximately the correct ratio between the length and width of the arms. The results shown in Figure 21 show that the theory successfully predicts the overall cluster shapes for n = 3, 4 and 5. It should be emphasized that despite the success of this theory in describing the structure of the highly anisotropic DLA clusters grown with large noise reduction parameters (including some quite detailed features) we still do not have a successful theory for the more isotropic and irregular patterns generated by off-lattice DLA.

SUMMARY

Despite considerable advances in our ability to simulate the growth of DLA clusters, a satisfactory description of their asymptotic scaling properties has not yet emerged. A variety of measurements suggest that more than one exponent is needed to describe the structure of both off-lattice and square lattice two dimensional DLA clusters. However, it appears that in at least some cases this may be an artifact of finite size effects (or measurement over short length scales). At present, there does not seem to be compelling evidence that more than one exponent is needed and the asymptotic structure of both off-lattice and square lattice DLA clusters may be a self-similar fractal. If only one exponent is needed to describe the structure of off-lattice DLA, our simulations indicate that the fractal dimensionality is close to 1.715. For square lattice DLA both computer simulations and theoretical considerations indicate that D has a value much closer to 1.5.

Since most of the theoretical approaches to DLA give numerical values for the fractal dimensionalities D(d) which are in quite good agreement with simulation results, it is difficult to discriminate between them on the basis of a comparison with simulation results. A satisfactory theory for DLA should also be applicable to a variety of other more or less closely related models (such as the noise reduced DLA models and the growth probability exponent (η) model). This provides us with an opportunity to make a more meaningful comparison between simulation results and theoretical predictions. In some cases the differences between the theoretical predictions is larger for models related to DLA than for DLA itself.

We still seem to be quite far from a satisfactory theory for isotropic off-lattice DLA. At present, theories based on the solution of the Laplace equation with simple boundary conditions[27-29,32] seem to be the most successful. The assumptions made in these theories are relatively transparent and they lead to predictions that can be readily tested using computer simulations. Despite simplifying assumptions, the theory of Eckmann et al.[32] provides a particularly successful description of the structure of anisotropic DLA with large noise reduction parameters. Unfortunately, this advance does not seem to bring us closer to understanding off-lattice DLA on lattice models in the noise dominated regime.

ACKNOWLEDGMENT

This work would not have been possible without valuable interactions with a number of colleagues and collaborators. Several of these (J. P. Eckmann, S. Havlin, G. Li, I. Procaccia, L. M. Sander and R. Zeitak) were directly involved in the work described here. We have also benefited considerably from discussions with R. C. Ball concerning the development of efficient DLA algorithms and other aspects of this work.

REFERENCES

1. T. A. Witten and L. M. Sander, Phys. Rev. Lett. 47:1400 (1981).
2. J. Feder, Fractals, Plenum Press, New York (1988).
3. K. Honda, "Fractals in Physics", Osakura Shoten (1987).
4. R. Jullien and R. Botet, "Aggregation and Fractal Aggregates", World Scientific, Singapore (1986).
5. F. Family and D. P. Landau, eds., "Kinetics of Aggregation and Gelation", North Holland, Amsterdam (1984).
6. H. E. Stanley and N. Ostrowsky, eds. "On Growth and Form: Fractal and Non-fractal Patterns in Physics", NATO ASI Series E100, Martinus Nijhoff, Dordrecht (1986).
7. L. Pietronero and E. Tosatti, eds., "Fractals in Physics", Proceedings of Sixth International Symposium on Fractals in Physics, ICTP, Trieste, Italy. North Holland, Amsterdam (1986).
8. H. J. Herrmann, Physics Reports, 136:153 (1986).
9. P. Meakin in "Phase Transitions and Critical Phenomena", C. Domb and J. L. Lebowitz, eds., Vol. 12, p. 335, Academic Press, New York (1988).
10. P. Meakin, Advances in Colloid and Interface Science, 28:249 (l988).
11. R. Pynn and A. T. Skjeltorp, eds., "Scaling Phenomena in Disordered Systems", NATO ASI Series B133, Plenum Press, New York (1986).
12. T. Riste and R. Pynn, eds., "Time Dependent Effects in Disordered Materials", NATO ASI Series B167, Plenum Press, New York (1987).
13. L. Paterson, Phys. Rev Lett. 52:1621 (1984).
14. J. Nittmann, G. Daccord and H. E. Stanley, Nature, 314:141 (1985).
15. K. J. Maloy, J. Feder and T. Jossang, Phys. Rev. Lett. 55:2688 (1985).
16. L. Niemeyer, L. Pietronero and H. J. Wiesmann, Phys. Rev. Lett. 52:1033 (1984).
17. M. Matsushita, M. Sano, Y. Hayakawa, H. Honjo and Y. Sawada, Phys. Rev. Lett. 53:286 (1984).
18. R. M. Brady and R. C. Ball, Nature 309:255 (1984).
19. G. Daccord and R. Lenormand, Nature 325:41 (1987).
20. R. C. Ball in ref. 6, page 69.
21. M. Muthukumar, Phys. Rev. Lett. 50:839 (1983).
22. M. Tokayama and K. Kawasaki, Phys. Lett. 100A:337 (1984).
23. H. G. E. Hentschel, Phys. Rev. Lett. 52:212 (1984).
24. K. Honda, H. Toyoki and M. Matsushita, J. Phys. Soc. Japan, 55:2479 (1986).
25. H. Gould, F. Family and H. E. Stanley, Phys. Rev. Lett. 50:686 (1983).
26. L. Pietronero, A. Erzan and C. Evertsz, Phys. Rev. Lett. 61:861 (1988).
27. L. Turkevich and H. Scher, Phys. Rev. Lett. 55:1026 (1985).
28. R. C. Ball, R. M. Brady, C. Rossi and B. R. Thompson, Phys. Rev. Lett. 55:1406 (1985).
29. T. C. Halsey, P. Meakin and I. Procaccia, Phys. Rev. Lett. 56:854 (1986).
30. I. Procaccia and R. Zeitak, Phys. Rev. Lett. 60:2511 (1988).
31. T. Bohr, P. Cvitanovic and M. H. Jensen, preprint (1988).
32. J. P. Eckmann, P. Meakin, I. Procaccia and R. Zeitak, preprint (l988).
33. P. Meakin, Phys. Rev. A27:604, 1495 (1983).
34. P. Meakin, J. Phys. A18:L661 (1985).
35. R. C. Ball and R. M. Brady, J. Phys. A18: L809 (1985).
36. S. Tolman and P. Meakin, preprint (1988).
37. P. Meakin, unpublished.
38. P. Meakin and L. M. Sander, unpublished.
39. B. B. Mandelbrot "The Fractal Geometry of Nature" W. H. Freeman and Company, New York (1982).
40. T. A. Witten and L. M. Sander, Phys. Rev. B27:5686 (1983).
41. P. Meakin and Z. R. Wasserman, Chemical Physics 91:391 (1984).
42. H. G. E. Hentschel and I. Procaccia, Physica D8:835 (1983).
43. T. A. Witten, J. Poly. Sci., Polymer Symposium 73:7 (1985).
44. M. Plischke and Z. Racz, Phys. Rev. Lett. 53:415, 2053 (1985).
45. P. Meakin and L. M. Sander, Phys. Rev. Lett. 54:2053 (1985).
46. P. Meakin and T. Vicsek, Phys. Rev. A32:685 (1985).
47. M. Kolb, J. Phys. Lett. 46: L631 (1985).

48. P. Meakin, R. C. Ball, P. Ramanlal and L. M. Sander, Phys. Rev. A35:5233 (1987).
49. P. Meakin, Phys. Rev. A33:3371 (1986).
50. C. T. Tang, Phys. Rev. A31:1977 (1985).
51. J. Kertesz and T. Viscek, J. Phys. A19:L257 (1986).
52. B. R. Thompson, unpublished.
53. J. Nittmann and H. E. Stanley, Nature 321:663 (1986).
54. P. Meakin, Phys. Rev. A36:332 (1987).
55. P. Meakin and S. Havlin, Phys. Rev. A36:4428 (1987).
56. P. A. Rickvold, Phys. Rev. B26:674 (1982).
57. P. Meakin, Phys. Rev. B28:6718 (1983).
58. P. Meakin, Phys. Lett. 107A:269 (1985).
59. R. Botet, R. Jullien and M. Kolb, J. Phys. A17:L75 (1984).
60. P. Meakin, Phys. Rev. Lett. 51:1119 (1983).
61. M. Kolb, R. Botet and R. Jullien, Phys. Rev. Lett. 51:1123 (1983).
62. F. Argoul, A. Arneodo, G. Grasseau and H. L. Swinney, Phys. Rev. Lett. 61:2558 (1988).
63. P. Ramanlal and L. M. Sander, J. Phys. A21:L995 (1988).
64. E. L. Hinrichsen, K. J. Maloy, J. Feder and T. Jossang, preprint.
65. R. E. Horton, Geol. Soc. Am. Bull 56:275 (1945).
66. T. C. Halsey and P. Meakin, Phys. Rev. A 32:2546 (1985).
67. L., A. Turkevich and H. Scher, Phys. Rev. A33:786 (1986).
68. R. C. Ball and T. A. Witten, Phys. Rev. A 29:2966 (1984).
69. R. C. Ball and T. A. Witten, J. Stat Phys. 36:873 (1984).
70. P. Meakin, J. Theor. Biol. 118:101 (1986).
71. I. M. Dudkin, I. Rabinovich and I. Vokhutinsky, "Iterative Aggregation Theory", Marcel Dekker, New York (1987).
72. D. M. de G. Allen "Relaxation Methods" McGraw Hill, New York (1954).
73. M. Matsushita, K. Honda, H. Toyoki, Y. Hayakawa and H. Kondo, J. Phys. Soc. Japan 55:2618 (1986).
74. Y. Hayakawa, H. Kondo and M. Matsushita, J. Phys. Soc. Japan 55:2479 (1986).
75. L. Pietronero and H. J. Wiesmann, J. Stat. Phys. 36:909 (1984).
76. H. J. Wiesmann and L. Pietronero in ref. 7, p. 151.
77. S. Satpathy, Phys. Rev. B 33:5093 (1986).
78. P. Meakin, Phys. Rev. A33:4199 (1986).

NEW THEORETICAL METHODS FOR FRACTAL GROWTH

L. Pietronero (a), A. Erzan(b) and C. Evertsz(c)

(a) Dipartimento di Fisica, Universita` di Roma "La Sapienza"
Piazzale A. Moro 2, 00185-Roma, Italy
(b) Solid State Physics Laboratory, University of Groningen
Melkweg 1, 9718 EP Groningen, The Netherlands
(c) Applied Physics, Yale University
Box 2155 Yale Station, New Haven, CT 06520, USA

Abstract

In order to understand the physical origin of fractal structures the first step is to formulate models of fractal growth based on physical mechanisms like the Diffusion Limited Aggregation and the more General Dielectric Breakdown Model. They are based on a simple iterative process governed by the Laplace equation and a stochastic field and they give rise to patterns that spontaneously evolve into random fractal structures of great complexity. In addition one would like to achieve a theoretical understanding of these models similar to that provided by the Renormalization Group for Ising-type models. Recently we have introduced a new theoretical framework for intrinsically critical growth models. This method is based on a Fixed Scale Transformation (with respect to the dynamical evolution) that defines a functional iteration for the distribution of elementary configurations that appear in a coarse graining process. This allows to include screening effects in terms of convergent series and to describe the intrinsic fluctuations of the boundary conditions. This approach clarifies the origin of fractal structures in these models and provides a systematic method for the calculation of the fractal dimension and the multifractal properties. It also makes clear why the usual renormalization schemes are not very suitable for these problems. Here we describe the basic ideas of this new approach and report about recent developments including the application to the fractal dimension of the percolating cluster interpreted as a problem of fractal growth.

Fractals' Physical Origin and Properties
Edited by L. Pietronero
Plenum Press, New York

1. Introduction

A basic problem in the physics of fractals(1,2) is to understand the essential elements for the generation of these structures. This implies the formulation of models for fractal growth based on physical phenomena and the subsequent understanding of their mathematical structure in the same sense as the Renormalization Group (RG) has allowed to understand Ising-type models(3).

The first part of this program is reasonably accomplished since a few years with the formulation of the models of Diffusion Limited Aggregation (DLA) (4) and the Dielectric Breakdown Model (DBM) (5). These models consist of simple iterative processes based on the Laplace equation and a stochastic field and their dynamical evolution leads spontaneously to complex structures with a well defined fractal dimension. The relation to physical processes is quite clear and for this reason they have acquired a crucial role in the understanding of fractal growth, similar to that of the Ising model for phase transitions (6).

Until recently most of the work has been based on computer simulations (2). From a theoretical point of view these models, despite their apparently simple formulation, have eluded all approaches based on standard methods(7). Only very recently some extensions of Real Space Renormalization methods have given rise to interesting results (8-10) even though several basic questions remain unclear.

We have followed a different path. Instead of trying to adapt to this problem methods that where formulated for phase transitions we have analyzed the problem from the beginning by focusing on its invariance properties and the irreversible nature that are qualitatively different from phase transitions. This led us to introduce a new theoretical framework that appears especially suitable for irreversible fractal growth (11,12). It clarifies the origin of fractal structures in these models and provides a systematic method for the calculation of the fractal dimension. In particular, given a certain growth model, one can, in principle, predict whether it will give rise to a fractal or to a compact structure. This possibility does not seem to be present in the approaches based on renormalization (8-10).

As mentioned the models that have aquired a crucial importance in understanding the physics of fractal structures are DLA and DBM (4,5). They are based on iterative processes governed by the Laplace equation and a stochastic field. From the point of view of DBM one assumes that the already grown pattern at a given time is equipotential. It is possible then to compute the local field around this structure by solving Laplace equation

$$\nabla^2 \Phi = 0 \tag{1.1}$$

with the boundary condition of constant potential on the grown structure and a different value of the potential at infinity. The growth probability p_j for each bond (j) connected to the structure is then related to the local field

$$p_j = \frac{|\nabla\phi|_j^{\eta}}{\sum_j |\nabla\phi|_j^{\eta}} \qquad (1.2)$$

where η is a parameter that modulates the randomness of the process. This probability distribution is then used to select one bond that becomes part of the pattern. The process continues by iterating this procedure and the result is a spontaneous generation of a random fractal structure. Laplacian fields are common ingredients in diverse physical processes and realistic models for these processes often incorporate stochasticity. For these reasons these models are believed to capture the essental features of pattern formation in seemingly different phenomena like electrochemical deposition, dendritic growth, dielectric breakdown, viscous fingering in fluids, fracture propagation and others (2,6).

From computer simulations we have learned that these models generate structures of great complexity whose fractal dimension $D(\eta,d)$ depends continuously on the parameter η and on the euclidean dimension d of the space in which the structure is embedded (2). With respect to the formulation of an analytical theory one should note that the process consists of an irreversible dynamics with long range couplings both in space and in time. None of the known mathematical methods seems to apply to this situation. The absence of a Hamiltonian, in the sense that the statistical weight of a configuration depends on its entire history, gives rise to serious conceptual difficulties if one tries to adapt to this problem the RG methods developed for phase transitions (3). In addition these growth models do not show an upper critical dimension and therefore ε-expansion methods cannot be defined.

In this paper we dicsuss the basic points of our new method and briefly report about some recent developments. In particular:

In Sect. 2 we dicuss the definition of the iterative scheme.

In Sect.3 the invarince properties of the system are analyzed and the Fixed Scale Transformation is introduced.

In Sect.4 we dicuss the void distribution and the problem of the fluctuations of boundary conditions.

In Sect.5 we show some explicit results and discuss the freezing condition and the Eden limit.

In Sect.6 we discuss the nature of the approximations and the features that provide a degree of systematicity to this approach.

In Sect.7 we briefly describe the relations with the multifractal spectrum.

In Sect.8 we describe the application of this method to compute the fractal dimension of the percolating cluster.

In Sect.9 we summarize the situation and point out possible developments.

2. Search for an Iterative Equation

The growth dynamics is irreversible and it leads spontaneously to an asymptotic structure with well defined statistical fractal properties that are independent on the initial conditions. The fractal structure can be seen therefore as the **attractor** of a dynamical system and this suggests to look for iterative equations whose **fixed point** should correspond to the **fractal structure**. The first important problem is therefore to define an appropriate **subject** that should appear in these iterative equations.

It is useful in this respect to consider the two dimensional case with boundary conditions consisting of two parallel lines (11-13). The discussion is easily generalizable to more dimensions. This geometry has the conceptual advantage of defining a unique growth direction. The intersection of a given fractal struture of dimension D with a line perpendicular to the growth direction gives rise to a set of points of dimension D' = (D-1) as shown in Fig 1. By analyzing this set of points with a procedure of box covering we assign a black dot to a box if this contains some point of the set and a white dot otherwise. (Note that this procedure is appropriate also for a self-affine structure that indeed seems to be the correct scaling structure for this problem(13)). The elementary process by which a black box is subdivided into two leads to two possible configurations indicated as type 1 (one black and one white sub-box) and type 2 (both sub-boxes black). The corresponding probabilities in this process of fine graining are indicated by C_1 and C_2 respectively. The average number of black sub-boxes that appear at the next level of fine graining from one black box is

$$\langle n \rangle = \sum_i n_i C_i = C_1 + 2 C_2 \tag{2.1}$$

It is easy to show that the fractal dimension of the whole structure is related to the values of C_1 and C_2 by (8)

$$D = 1 + \frac{\ln \langle n \rangle}{\ln 2} \tag{2.2}$$

It is clear therefore that the natural subject for the iterative fixed point problem should be the **distribution of elementary configurations** $\{C_i\}$ that appear from one scale to the next in the process of fine graining. Note that this concept is easily generalizable to other fractal problems and even to fully developed turbulence (14,15). It is natural therefore to look for an iterative equation of type

$$\{C_i\}^{(k+1)} = T\{C_i\}^{(k)} \tag{2.3}$$

where k is the index of the iteration and T represents a suitable transformation based on some invariance property of the system. The fixed point of this iteration should then correspond to the fractal properties of the system.

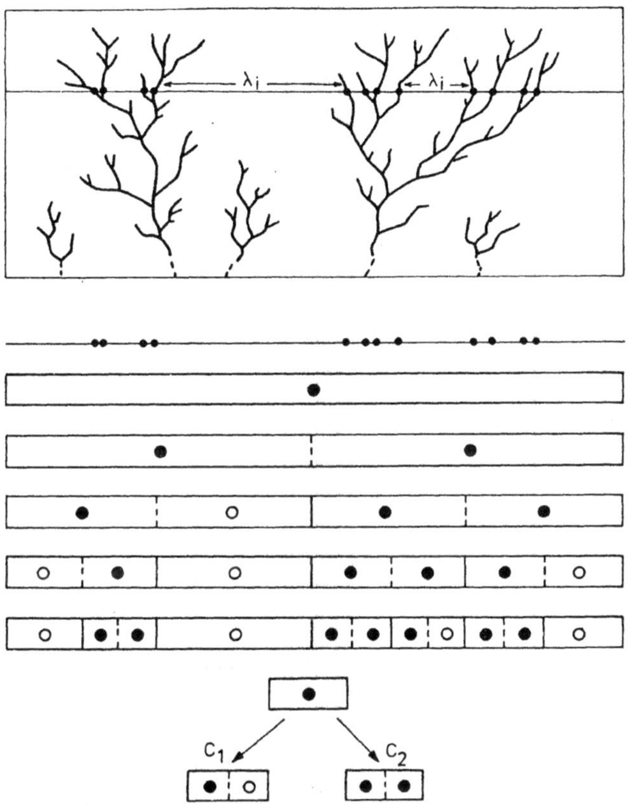

Fig. 1. Schematic picture of the process of box covering for the set of points given by the intersection of the fractal structure with a line. Bottom: elementary process of fine graining for a box (black) that contains some elements of the set.

3. Invariance Properties and Fixed Scale Transformation

We have now to define the appropriate iterative equations for the distribution $\{C_i\}$. From the point of view of the analogy with critical phenomena one would attempt to define the iteration via a renormalization scheme. The present problem however has the

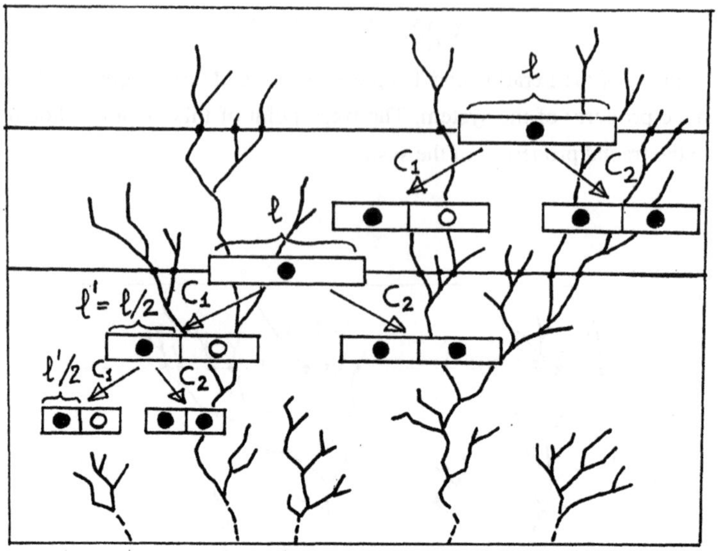

Fig. 2. Schematic picture of the invariance properties of the system. The distribution of elementary configurations (defined by a coarse or fine graining process) is invariant with respect to scale transformation but also with respect to dynamical evolution at the same scale.

peculiarity of being **intrinsically critical**; namely there is no order parameter that leads to scale invariance only for a particular value of it. The growth rules are scale invariant by construction and this gives rise to the possibility of using an alternative transformation. In particular:

i. The structure is invariant by **scale transformation** in the sense that the values of (C_1, C_2) that are obtained via a fine graining from scale ℓ to scale $\ell/2$ are the same as those from scale ℓ' to scale $\ell'/2$.

ii. In addition there is also an invariance with respect to the **dynamical evolution at the same scale** (See Fig.2). Namely if one considers two different sections of the original structure and performs a fine graining analysis at the same scale for the two different sets one obtains the same distribution (C_1, C_2) that should also be identical to the case i.

Note that this discussion holds for a homogeneous as well as a self-affine structure (13). We have now a choice for the definition of the iterative process: One can use a renormalization transformation based on the invariance property (i), or one can define the iteration from the dynamical evolution at the same scale (ii) and then use the fixed point value of the (C_1, C_2) distribution at all other scales via Eqs.(2,1-2). This second possibility is more convenient for the present problem (11,12).

We define a **Fixed Scale Transformation** (FST) that corresponds to the dynamical evolution at the same scale. This gives rise to an iterative equation of type

$$\begin{pmatrix} C_1^{(k+1)} \\ C_2^{(k+1)} \end{pmatrix} = \begin{pmatrix} M_{1,1} M_{2,1} \\ M_{1,2} M_{2,2} \end{pmatrix} \begin{pmatrix} C_1^{(k)} \\ C_2^{(k)} \end{pmatrix} \tag{3.1}$$

where the matrix element $M_{i,j}$ defines the conditional probability to have a configuration of type i followed by one of type j in the growth direction. Note that this refers to a **frozen structure** that has already grown to its asymptotic state and in which no more growth will occur in the future.

The practical calculation of $M_{i,j}$ can be done by starting with a configuration of type i and considering the growth processes that can lead to a subsequent configuration j. For example

$$M_{1,2} = \sum(\text{growth processes leading from 1 to 2}) = p_\alpha + (1 - p_\alpha)\, p_\beta + \ldots \tag{3.2}$$

where p_α represents in this case the probability that the first non trivial growth process leads to a configuration of type 2, while p_β corresponds to the second order term and so on. A detailed discussion for the explicit construction of Eq.(3,2) can be found in Ref. (12). Once the matrix elements are defined the fixed point condition corresponding to our iteration is

$$C_1 = \left(1 + \frac{M_{1,2}}{M_{2,1}}\right)^{-1} \tag{3.3}$$

and from this, via Eqs.(2,1-2) one obtains the fractal dimension D.

The **mathematical condition for the generation of fractal structures** can be now given by studying the value to which the series of Eq.(3,2) will converge. If this value is less than one this implies that there is a finite probability that the growth process will leave sites asymptotically empty. In view of the scale invariance of the Laplace equation and of the whole growth process, this conclusion holds at any scale and therefore **holes of all scales** will be generated.

As we will also see later in more detail, the screening properties of Laplace equation guarantee that the convergence of this series is quite fast and indeed to a number smaller than one. Only in the limit $\eta \rightarrow 0$ the screening is eliminated, the convergence is then slower and the series converges to one, leading to a compact structure with dimension 2 (12).

4. Fluctuations of Boundary Conditions and Void Distribution

In order to compute explicitly the matrix elements one has to specify the boundary conditions for the process of conditional growth. This is a problem that usually does not appear in the Renormalization Group method in which one integrates over the internal degrees of freedom and boundary conditions play no role. In our problem the boundary conditions instead have an important effect. In fact the growth of a structure will be very different if it is isolated or surrounded by other structures. In principle therefore one has to take into account all these possibilities, each with its own probability.

Given the probability distribution (C_1,C_2) it is possible to derive explicitly the void distribution $P(\lambda)$ which is the conditional probability that, given an occupied box of unit size, it is neighboured at the right by a void of size λ. In Ref.(12) we have presented an approximate calculation but one can actually do it exactly for all the values of the void size as shown recently by Siebesma and Tremblay(16). The result is given in an iterative form

$$P(\lambda = 0) = \frac{C_2}{\left(1 + \frac{1}{2}C_1\right)\left(C_2 + \frac{1}{2}C_1\right)}$$

$$P(\lambda = 2\ell + 1) = \frac{(1 - C_2)}{2} P(\lambda = \ell) \tag{4.1}$$

$$P(\lambda = 2\ell) = \frac{(1 + C_2)}{4} P(\lambda = \ell) + \frac{(1 - C_2)^2}{4(1 + C_2)} P(\lambda = \ell - 1)$$

where a unit length is assigned to the size of the smallest box considered. It is easy to check that the integrated void distribution has the expected behaviour (1,16)

$$P(\lambda \geq \Lambda) = F\Lambda^{-D} \tag{4.2}$$

where F is the lacunarity and D' the fractal dimension of the intersection set.

With respect to the use of this distribution as defining the boundary conditions of our elementary growth processes there is an additional fact to consider. Our basic configurations correspond to pairs of sites of which at least one is black, so that at the next higher level of coarse graining they correspond necessarily to a black site. To this site we can directly apply the above void distribution. However if we ask for the probability that a pair of sites is immediately followed by a black (occupied) site the answer is sligthly more complicated. In fact with probability $P(\lambda = 0)$ this pair is followed by another pair in which at least one of the two sub-sites is black. So if we consider the probability that the site immediately following the considered pair is black this will require the extra condition that the pair configuration on the right is of type 2 or of type 1 but with the black site on the left. This gives rise to an additional factor $(C_2 + (1/2)C_1)$ and therefore the probability (for example for $\lambda = 0$) to be used in the calculation of the matrix elements is

$$P'(\lambda = 0) = \frac{C_2}{\left(1 + \frac{1}{2} C_1\right)} \tag{4.3}$$

Note that in Ref.(12) the discussion of this distribution is not very clear but the actual calculation is finally correct and in agreement with the present discussion.

The probability distribution for the size of voids fixes the probability distribution for having a certain boundary condition in the elementary growth process. This implies that each matrix element $M_{i,j}$ should be replaced by the convolution over all possible boundary conditions (see also next section)

$$M_{i,j} \Rightarrow \sum_n P(\lambda_n ; C_1, C_2)\, M_{i,j}(\lambda_n) \tag{4.4}$$

where $\lambda_n = 2^n$. Therefore these matrix elements become nonlinear functions of the variables (C_1, C_2). The iterative equation acquires then the following structure

$$\begin{pmatrix} C_1^{(k+1)} \\ C_2^{(k+1)} \end{pmatrix} = \sum_n P(\lambda_n; C_1, C_2) \begin{pmatrix} M_{1,1}(\lambda_n) & M_{2,1}(\lambda_n) \\ M_{1,2}(\lambda_n) & M_{2,2}(\lambda_n) \end{pmatrix} \begin{pmatrix} C_1^{(k)} \\ C_2^{(k)} \end{pmatrix} \tag{4.5}$$

and the corresponding fixed point equation

$$C_1 = \left[1 + \frac{\sum_n P(\lambda_n; C_1, C_2)\; M_{1,2}(\lambda_n)}{\sum_n P(\lambda_n; C_1, C_2)\; M_{2,1}(\lambda_n)} \right]^{-1} \tag{4.6}$$

is now a nonlinear system of equations of infinite order. As we are going to see in the next section this can be solved by suitable truncation schemes.

Finally it should be remarked that the spirit of the present calculation is rather different from Real Space Renormalization not only because one uses a transformation at fixed scale. In fact the size and the number of basic configutations is **fixed** and the calculation is improvable in a systematic way by adding more terms in the series that define the matrix elements of the transformation. In addition growth processes outside the considered cell must be included up the desired level of convergence and the fluctuations of boundary conditions play an important role. These concepts appear natural and necessary in all problems of irreversible growth.

5. Practical Implementation and Convergency of the Results

In this section we describe the explicit calculation of the matrix elements $M_{i,j}$ and therefore of the fractal dimension D. Most of the discussion refers to the two dimensional case, but we will also mention some results for three dimensions.

(a) Simplest Method with Periodic Boundary Conditions

As we have seen in the previous sections these matrix elements refer to the conditional probability that a frozen cell of type i is followed, in the growth direction, by a frozen cell of type j. We begin by discussing a very simple approximation that does not take into account the fluctuations of boundary conditions. This consists in using periodic boundary conditions, that from the point of view of the void distribution would correspod to assume $P'(\lambda=0)=1$ instead of using the value of Eq.(4.3). The matrix elements can then be computed according to the scheme shown in Fig.3 in which one starts with an initial frozen cell of type 1 (circled by a box) and considers the various processes that may lead to a configuration of type 1 or 2 in the cell that follows it in the growth direction. For the calculation of the potentials the outer boundary condition can be located very close to the considered structure because we are only interested in the relative probabilities within this structure. For the same reason we do not consider growth outside the column on top of the initial frozen cell. This however may become an excessive simplification if one includes high order processes. Later we will see how this effect can be estimated quantitatively. The lateral boundary conditions are assumed to be periodic in the sense that also the growth processes are idential to those that occurr in the considered column.

The relevant growth processes are indicated by the small arrows in Fig.3. The first site to be occupied is necessarily the one above the occupied site of the initial cell, therefore this is already included in the starting diagram. In principle this is not strictly true because, if one does not restrict growth to occurr in one column, the growth of nearby sites may take place before and eventually screen completely our structure so that a pair

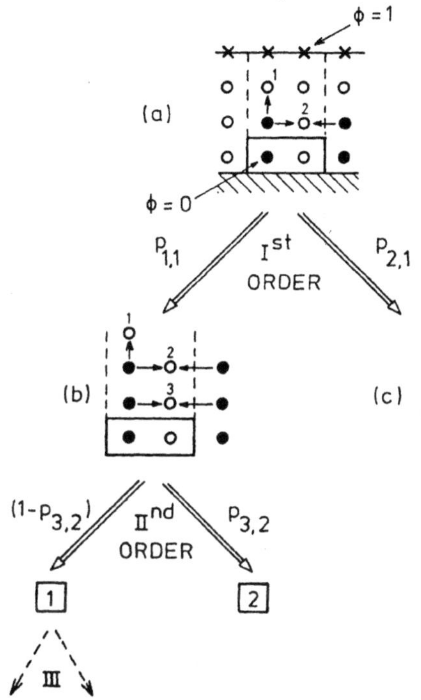

Fig. 3. Starting from a frozen cell of type 1 (encircled) we consider the growth processes that define the asymptotic probability for the next cell in the growth direction to be of type 1 or 2. Periodic boundary conditions are used with the period defined by the dashed lines. Note that the growth is not considered within the initial cell because this is conditionally frozen. The first site to be occupied will be the one on top of the occupied site of the initial cell, so this is already included in the starting diagram.

of empty sites would be left. This is a point that we will also consider later by showing that this effect corresponds to higher order contributions that have only a small effect in the results.

In Fig.3 the probabilities corresponding to the growth processes are indicated by $p_{i,j}$ where the first index (i) refers to the site that is going to be occupied and the second one (j) to the order of the process that gives the number of particles that have been added to the structure (except the first trivial one). Note that these site probabilities correspond to the sum of the various bond probabilities leading to the considered site. The explicit calculation of the growth probabilities requires the knowledge of the potential corresponding to a few relevant configurations. These can be found in the appendix of Ref.(12).

The first order growth probabilities corresponding to Fig.(3) are given by

$$p_{2,1}(\eta) = \frac{2\phi_2^{\eta}}{\phi_1^{\eta} + 2\phi_2^{\eta}} = \frac{2\,(0.1463)^{\eta}}{(0.5244)^{\eta} + 2\,(0.1463)^{\eta}} \tag{5.1}$$

$$p_{1,1}(\eta) = 1 - p_{2,1}(\eta) \tag{5.2}$$

where the potentials refer to the configuration 2 of Fig.A1 in Ref.(12).

If the event defined by $p_{2,1}(\eta)$ takes place, site 2 of Fig. 3a gets occupied at first order and the cell following the initial one will be of type 2 asymptotically (Fig. 3c). If instead $p_{1,1}(\eta)$ occurs this cell remains of type 1 but higher order processes may still lead to the occupation of its second site. For the second order process we have

$$p_{3,2}(\eta) = \frac{2\,\phi_3^{\eta}}{\phi_1^{\eta} + 2\,\phi_2^{\eta} + 2\,\phi_3^{\eta}} = \frac{2(0.0392)^{\eta}}{(0.5245)^{\eta} + 2(0.1471)^{\eta} + 2(0.0392)^{\eta}} \tag{5.3}$$

for the occupation of this second site. The potentials in this case refer to the configuration 3 of Fig A1 in Ref.(12). The total probability for this site to be occupied **after infinite growth** gives the matrix element $M_{1,2}$ corresponding to the conditional probability of having a frozen cell of type 1 followed by a frozen cell of type 2. This can be written as

$$M_{1,2}(\eta) = p_{2,1}(\eta) + \left[1 - p_{2,1}(\eta)\right] p_{3,2}(\eta) + \text{higher order terms} \tag{5.4}$$

and in principle the series should be continued until the probability of occupation of the site 2 in Fig.3a is virtually negligible (freezing condition). It is important to note however that higher order terms in the series correspond to configurations in which the site is strongly screened by growth that has occurred at other sites (see Fig.3b in which site 3 is the original site 2 of Fig.3a). This is because the penetration length for the potential given by the Laplace equation is of the size of the structure one considers. Such a fact is crucial because it allows rapid convergence of the series given by Eq.(5.4) to a number smaller than one (except for the case $\eta \to 0$). This is the key point for the formation of fractal structures. In fact, if Eq.(5.4) converges to a number smaller than one this implies that

$$M_{1,1}(\eta) = 1 - M_{1,2}(\eta) > 0 \tag{5.5}$$

asymptotically. Therefore there is a finite probability that growth will leave empty sites (holes) even asymptotically. In view of the scale invariance of the Laplace equation this conclusion holds at any scale and therefore holes of all scales are generated.

In a similar way one can consider the growth conditional to the existence of a frozen cell of type 2 in order to compute the matrix elements $M_{2,1}$ and $M_{2,2}$. From these matrix elements one can finally compute the fixed point distribution of configurations and the fractal dimension. More details about this calculation can be found in Ref.(12). The results of this method with periodic boundary conditions (λ_0) are shown in Table I for first and second order. It is not difficult to compute also higher order terms. By going up to fifth order one observes a rapid convergency (with respect to the order) to about $D = 1.55$ for DLA ($\eta = 1$). This value is rather low with respect to the computer simulations results. (These give $D = 1.70$ for circular geometry and $D = 1.60 \div 65$ for cylindrical geometry (13); this small but non negligible discrepancy may actually be intrinsic and due to the anisotropic scaling of the system). The fact that this result is only a lower bound can be easily understood by considering that the use of lateral periodic boundary conditions implies that the growing structure is immediately followed by another branch and this produces an excessive screening for the internal points as soon as a tip begins to develop.

(b) Inclusion of Boundary Condition Fluctuations

A correct treatment of the fluctuations of the boundary conditions is the natural way to improve on this point. This leads to the use of Eqs.(4.5) and (4.6) with the full λ distribution. This means that the same growth process can occur in different enviroments as schematically shown in Fig.(4). In practice one should therefore compute the values of the various matrix elements for each enviroment considered. In this respect one may notice that the series appearing in the fixed point equation (4.5) involve all powers of the distribution (C_1,C_2) but the higher order terms give rise to exponentially decreasing contributions so that suitable truncation schemes can be defined.

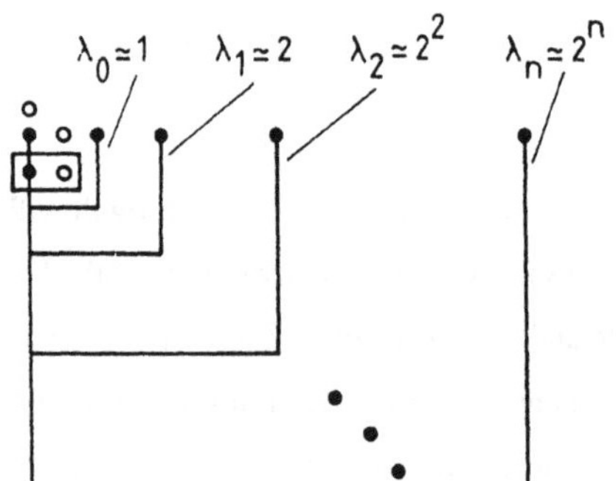

Fig. 4. Schematic representation of the different boundary conditions that can give rise to growth processes with different properties. Note that the growth process is always at the same scale while the boundary condition can fluctuate.

Here we will discuss the simplest non-trivial method to include the boundary conditions fluctuations. This consists in assuming that as soon as λ is equal or larger than the size of the considered configuration (a pair of sites), the boundary condition is essentially open ($\lambda \to \infty$), while for $\lambda = 0$ it is closed as in the case discussed before (periodic boundary conditions). This allows one to consider only two possibilities: closed configurations with probability

$$P_0 = P'(\lambda = 0) = \frac{C_2}{\left(1 + \frac{1}{2} C_1\right)} \tag{5.6}$$

and open configurations with probability

$$P_\infty = \sum_{n=1}^{\infty} P(\lambda_n) = 1 - P'(\lambda = 0) \tag{5.7}$$

The basis for this approximation is in the fact that since we will only consider a few terms with respect to the order of the calculation, the scale of the structure considered does not change much. This implies that a large value of λ or an infinite value play essentially the same role in defining relative probabilities within the considered (much smaller) structure.

The fixed point equation is then drastically simplified because from infinite order it becomes of second order. By calling $M^{cl}_{i,j}$ and $M^{op}_{i,j}$ the matrix elements corresponding respectively to closed and open configurations, we obtain

$$C_1(\eta) = \left\{ 1 + \frac{P_0[C_1(\eta)]\, M^{cl}_{1,2}(\eta) + P_\infty[C_1(\eta)]\, M^{op}_{1,2}(\eta)}{P_0[C_1(\eta)]\, M^{cl}_{2,1}(\eta) + P_\infty[C_1(\eta)]\, M^{op}_{2,1}(\eta)} \right\}^{-1} . \tag{5.8}$$

By using Eqs. (5.6), (5.7) the explicit solution of this equation is

$$C_1 = \frac{\left\{ M^{cl}_{1,2} + 2 M^{cl}_{2,1} - \frac{3}{2} M^{op}_{2,1} - \left[\left(\frac{3}{2} M^{op}_{2,1} - M^{cl}_{1,2} - 2 M^{cl}_{2,1} \right)^2 - 4 A M^{cl}_{2,1} \right]^{1/2} \right\}}{2A} \tag{5.9}$$

where the index η has been omitted for simplicity. The matrix elements with closed boundary conditions are just those computed previously. Those with open boundary conditions require instead a new calculation whose details can be found in Ref.(12).

The results of the open-closed approximation are also reported in Table I for calculations up to second and third order. By comparing them with the value D=1.55 (for DLA) corresponding to the asymptotic result (with respect to order) of the calculation with only closed configurations one can see that the self-consistent treatment of boundary conditions fluctuations improves the results substantially. In addition one may note that the agreement with the computer simulations is very good for large values of η and less accurate for $\eta \to 0$. The origin of this effect becomes clear if one considers the freezing condition in relation to the truncation of the series of Eq.(8) and similar ones. In the limit $\eta \to 0$ it is not enough to consider only a few terms in these series because the screening effect is essentially suppressed. We are now going to consider in some detail what happens in this limit.

TABLE I

Values of the fractal dimension as a function of the parameter η for the DBM model in two dimensions computed with the various schemes and compared with the results of computer simulations.

	Fractal dimension $D(\eta)$			
Present theory	$\eta=0.$	0.5	1.(DLA)	2.
(λ_0); I[st] order	1.7885	1.6465	1.4747	1.1885
(λ_0); IInd order	1.8990	1.7515	1.5418	1.1997
$(\lambda_0, \lambda_\infty)$; IInd order	1.8896	1.7549	1.6080	1.3956
$(\lambda_0, \lambda_\infty)$; IIIrd order	1.9039	1.7830	1.6406	1.4190
(any λ); ∞ order	2.	–	–	–
Computer simulations	2.	1.92	1.70	1.43

(c) The Eden Limit ($\eta \to 0$)

In order to clarify what happens in this limit it is useful to consider a specific case. Let us look for example at the growth process shown in Fig.(5) and consider the probability that the site indicad by 2 does not get occupied during the growth process. At first order the probability for this to occurr is 1/2, at second order it is 2/3. It is easy to show that at the n-th order growth process this probability is at most n/(n+1). We obtain therefore an upper limit for the matrix element

$$M_{i,j}(\eta=0) \leq \prod_{n=1}^{N} \frac{n}{(n+1)} = \frac{1}{2}\frac{2}{3}\frac{3}{4} \cdots \frac{N-2}{N-1}\frac{N-1}{N} = \frac{1}{N} \quad (5.10)$$

One can see therefore that the matrix element $M_{1,1}$ converges to zero and $M_{1,2}$ to one

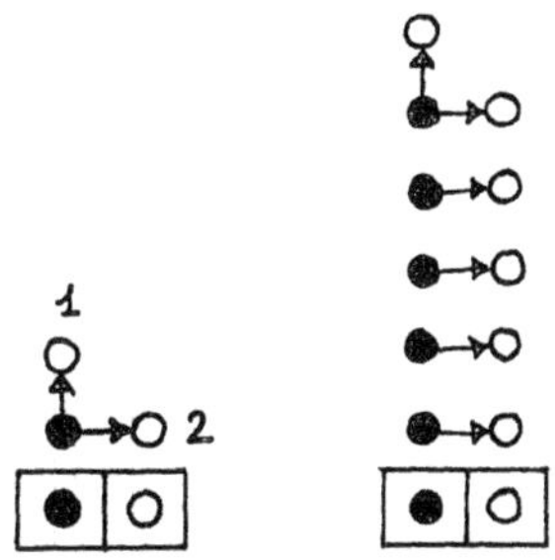

Fig. 5. Schematic picture of the growth process considered for the analysis of the Eden limit and the calculation of Eq.(5.10).

for $N \to \infty$ but only as a power law with respect to the order. The fractal dimension converges therefore to the euclidean value D=2. The fact that this limiting case is correctly reproduced is far from trivial. One may note in fact that in order to achieve this result it is necessary to go to infinite order in the evaluation of the series. From a Renormalization point of view this would imply to consider cells of infinite size. In fact the methods based on Real Space Renormalization (8-10) cannot reproduce this limit correctly.

(d) Results for Three Dimensions

It is stragthforward to apply this method also to the three dimensional version of DLA and DBM (17). The intersection in this case is done with a plane and the basic configurations are five and consist of two by two square cells. The calculation can be performed along lines similar to those we have discussed for two dimensions. The only serious difference is that the inclusion of boundary condition fluctuations is substantially more complex. The preliminary result for the fractal dimension of DLA is D=2.4 (17) to be compared with the numerical value D=2.5. (2).

6. Nature of the Approximation Scheme

In this section we discuss the scheme of approximations of the method, how it can be controlled and in wich sense it can be considered as systematic.

(a) Choice of Elementary Configurations

The first step is the choice of the configurations that define that define the coarse (or fine) graining process and that are finally related to the fractal dimension by Eq.(2.1). The choice is not unique and the one we use is the simplest but still it can reproduce any structure to any required degree of detail, so there is no approximation in this point. The situation is different when we try to construct the matrix elements for conditional growth because in this case we separate the processes that occurr above the considered structure, that we treat in detail, from those that occurr on the sides that only play the role of boundary conditions.

With respect to the void probability distribution one should note that this is derived within a scheme that assumes the fragmentation process as uncorrelated. This approximate analytical structure is then used variationally within a scheme that instead includes the correlations of the growth process.

A crucial point is the freezing condition for the evaluation of the series the define the matrix elements for conditional growth. The scheme we use to evaluate these series can be analyzed systematically to include as many terms as necessary. This brings in information that corresponds to the properties of very large cells (in the sense of the Renormalization Group) and by computing the various elements of the series one can actually control which size is large enough with respect to the vertical direction. The fluctuation of boundary conditions plays a similar role for the lateral direction. So finally we can include in a schematic but controllable way also features of extremely large configurations. This cannot be achieved with the methods based on Real Space Renormalization(8-10) and it is fot this reason, for example, that these cannot reproduce the Eden limit correctly.

(b) Empty Configurations

From the way we have defined the basic configurations that appear in the iterative equation it is clear that they should not contain the completely empty configuration. In fact this cannot be generated in the process of fine graining. For this reason we have not included this possibility in the growth dynamics that gives rise to the matrix elements. The idea is that the empy sites of the configurations of type 1 already generate voids of all sizes. However the conditional growth we consider for the definition of the matrix elements can, in principle, lead to the direct generation of a pair of empty sites. This is due to the fact that nearby branches could grow faster than the one considered and it is therefore possible that the pair of sites above the initial configuration remains empty. In order to study this effect one has to include this possibility explicitly in the Fixed Scale Transformation but then consider only the ratio at the fixed point of the two usual configurations. This is also a more general test for the validity of the description of the lateral effects only in terms of boundary conditions. For DLA in two dimensions the inclusion of this effect is to reduce the value of the fractal dimension by about one per cent (17), justifying therefore the previous conjecture that this is a higher order effect and, in general, it can be neglected.

(c) Use of the Same Growth Rules at All Scales

Another basic assumption we make is to use the same growth rules at all scales. In fact the growth rules are defined at the smallest scale considered and it is not obvious that exactly the same growth rules hold also for coarse grained variables. The two basic configurations we consider are in fact defined to describe the system at any scale and, in order to study their conditional evolution, we use the original growth rules that are originally defined only at the lowest scale. To clarfy the origin of this problem it is useful to look at Fig.6. On the left we have the smallest scale and the relative probability of growth into the cells 1 or 2 corresponds to a single growth event and it is directly related to the ratio of the potential at the two sites. On the rigth instead our cells correspond to coarse graining with boxes of size ℓ. In this case the ratio of the potentials in the two cells is the same as before in view of the scale invariance of the Laplace equation. However the growth process that leads to the cell occupation consists now of many steps and it is not obvious that in the end the relative occupation probabilities for the coarse grained cells will be the same as those corresponding to the smallest scale.

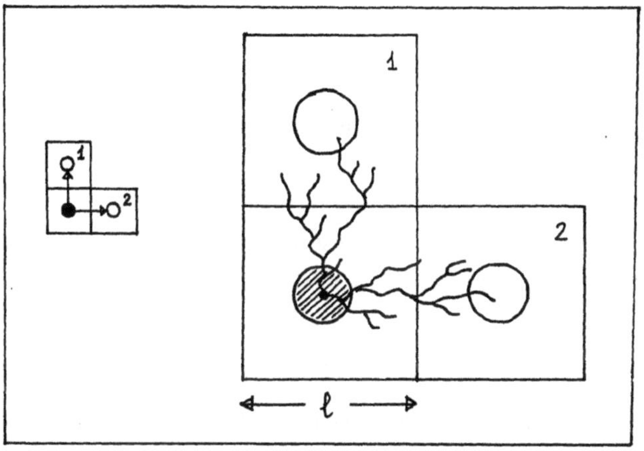

Fig. 6. Illustration of the growth process at the smallest scale and at a generic level of coarse graining.

This problem can be discussed at two levels. On the one hand one may consider that the growth process leads to a scale invariant structure. Now if we use for coarse graining the same type of objects on which the growth applies at the smallest scale (just a black or white point without introducing gray or more complex elements) it must follow that the same growth process applies to these coarse grained variables otherwise one would run into inconsistencies.

A more microscopic understanding of how this happens can be achieved by reconsidering the discussion of Fig.6. For the coarse grained cells on the rigth a full branch has to develop in order to reach the next cell. This branch will also be characterized by the fractal dimension D, so for a box of size ℓ one has to add a number of points of order

$$n(l) \approx l^{D} \tag{6.1}$$

before the adjacent cell can be considered as occupied. This corresponds in practice to the introduction of a noise reduction effect (19). From the studies of noise reduction it is known that this introduces a characteristic length

$$\xi(\ell) \approx A \log\left[n(\ell)\right] + B \tag{6.2}$$

below which the structure is essentially compact, while for much larger lengths the effect of noise reduction disappears and the original process is recovered. Therefore by using the same growth process also for coarse grained configurations we automatically eliminate the effect of this noise reduction effect. In this way the properties at small relative scales become identical to the correct asymptotic ones. Note that from a renormalization point of view it is not clear how to control this effect properly, because by going to a larger cell and then rescaling it, one will always include features of this noise reduction effect in a transformation that should instead refer to the asymptotic scaling regime.

As a consequence of this discussion one can also predict some consequences with respect to the analysis of numerical data. In fact if the box size considered is not much smaller than the total size of the system the results shoud be affected by this effect and show an anomalously larger value of C1 with respect to C2. This is exactly what can be observed in the actual analysis (See Ref. (13), p. 197).

7. Multifractal Spectrum of Growth Probability

There have been several numerical studies concerning the multifractal spectrum of the growth probability for these systems. After the initial enthusiasm it is now becoming clear that there are serious conceptual difficulties with this approach. The question that up to now has been most discussed is the probable spuriousness of all the negative moments (20). There is however another basic problem that concerns also the positive moments. The fact is that the present formulation of multifractals in terms of box counting (14) assumes a homogeneous fractal as the support of the measure while in these models the support consists of a self-affine structure (13). It is difficult therefore to judge the results of this studies. The only quantity that appears reasonably well defined seems to be the strongest singularity strength that seems to have a direct relation to the fractal dimension (2). However even for this quantity the scaling behavior form which it is derived shows deviations from linearity that are probably due to the self-affinity problem (13).

From the point of view of the present theory it is clear that the growth probabilities we use are those that should appear in the generators of the multiplicative process that corresponds to the multifractal spectrum. But here we use them directly in the growth process and within a framework that is fully compatible also with a self-affine structure. It is not clear that casting them in a multifractal scheme based on box counting would be of any advantage or even mathematically well defined.

Hovever if one neglects the above problems (as it is usually done in numerical analysis) the multifractal spectrum can also be computed analytically as a byproduct of the present theory. In practice one defines suitable square configurations that contain the probabilities used in the process of conditional growth and consider these as the generators of a multiplicative process. The resuts for the strongest singularity strength of DLA in two dimensions give values of 0.6÷0.7 depending on the particular scheme used (18).

8. The Percolating Cluster as a Fractal Growth Problem

The present theory requires that the system is critical by construction and that the structure is generated by a dynamical process. In principle therefore we can consider to apply it to phase transition-type problems to compute exponents that are defined only at the critical point like, for example, the anomalous dimension η of the Ising problem. This of course, provided that one can define a growth process that finally reproduces to the correct statistical weigth of the problem in question. This point of view is useful also to understand the meaning of a mean field theory for this problem. In fact the Landau theory for Ising gives rise to a nonzero value for exponents of type ν that describe the deviations from the critical point, but it gives a value zero for the anomalous dimension. Loosely speaking this is the analogous to the codimension for the present problem. So it is not surprising that mean field type approximatons cannot describe these fractal structures in the sense that they lead to the trivial result $D = d$.

The equilibrium transition for which the present ideas apply more naturally is the fractal dimension of the percolating cluster. It is possible in fact to generate percolation clusters with a growth algoritm. From this point of view the properties of percolation at the critical point can be described by the present theory. This is an important test because the fractal dimension of the infinite cluster in two dimensions is known exactly: $D = 1.8958$ (21). The formulation of the theory for this problem is similar to the case of DLA in the sense that one studies the fixed point corresponding to the dynamical evolution of the two elementary cofigurations etc. The difference is in the growth rules that now are those corresponding to percolation (22).

Using a very simple scheme with only two terms in the series and no fluctuations of the boundary conditions we obtain $D = 1.8231$ for only open configurations. Inclusion of the fluctuations of the boundary conditions gives instead $D = 1.8768$. A more refined scheme with analytic resummation of certain classes of terms in the series gives finally $D = 1.8931$. The agreement with the exact value is therefore excellent. This test provides an important support to the validity of the present approach as a general method to describe the properties of intrinsically critical systems.

9. Summary and Conclusions

In summary we have described a new theoretical framework for problems of irreversible fractal growth like DLA and DBM. The method is based on the following steps:

- Identification of the elementary configurations necessary to define a coarse or fine graining process on the system.
- Analysis of the invariance properties and definition of the Fixed Scale Transformation with respect to dynamical evolution and the corresponding fixed point problem.
- Definition of the matrix elements for conditional growth in terms of convergent series that define the freezing condition. This clarifies in a mathematical way the origin of fractal structures.
- Inclusion of the fluctuatins of boundary conditions in the fixed point equation.

One can see that this scheme provides a practical tool to understand the origin of fractal structures and compute their fractal dimension in a systematic way. The reason for this possibility can be appreciated by considering that the last two points describe features corresponding to structures of variable complexity, the effective size of which can be controlled by studying the convergency of the corresponding series. This possibility cannot be included in methods based on Real Space Renormalization and it is for this reason that these methods do not give the correct Eden limit while the present one does. In addition all the approximation schemes of the new approach can be easily tested in practice as we have discussed in some detail.

In addition to the standard problems of fractal growth we have also shown the applicability of these ideas to the fractal dimension of the percolating cluster that provides an important, independent test.

In principle the method can be applied to all problems in which a fractal structure is generated by a dynamical growth mechanism and at the moment we are considering various other examples.

References

1. B.B. Mandelbrot, 'The Fractal Geometry of Nature", Freeman, New York (1983).
2. L. Pietronero and E. Tosatti Eds. "Fractals in Physics", North-Holland, Amsterdam, New York (1986). H.E. Stanley and N. Ostrowsky Eds. "On Growth and Form", Nijhoff, Dordrecht (1986).
3. See for example: D.J. Amit, "Field Theory, the Renormalization Group and Critical Phenomena", McGraw Hill Int., New York (1978).

4. T.A. Witten and L.M. Sander, Phys. Rev. Lett. 47, 1400 (1981).
5. L. Niemeyer, L. Pietronero and H.J. Wiesmann, Phys. Rev. Lett. 52, 1033 (1984). L. Pietronero and H.J. Wiesmann, J. Stat. Phys. 36, 909 (1984).
6. H.E. Stanley, Phil. Mag. B 56, 665 (1987).
7. L.P. Kadanoff, Physics Today, p.6 (Feb. 1986).
8. T. Nagatani, J. Phys. A 20, L381 (1987); Phys. Rev. A36, 5812 (1988).
9. X.R. Wang, Y. Shapir and M. Rubinstein, Phys. Lett. A118, 274 (1989).
10. A. Stella, to be published.
11. L. Pietronero, A. Erzan and C. Evertsz, Phys. Rev. Lett. 61, 861 (1988).
12. L. Pietronero, A. Erzan and C. Evertsz, Physica A 151, 207 (1988).
13. C. Evertsz, "Laplacian Fractals", Thesis, Univ. of Groningen (1989), unpublished.
14. G. Paladin and A. Vulpiani, Phys. Rep. 156, 147 (1987).
15. A.P. Siebesma, R.R. Tremblay, A. Erzan and L. Pietronero, Physica A 156, 613 (1989).
16. A.P. Siebesma and R.R. Tremblay, Phys. Rev. B, in print.
17. A. Vespignani and L. Pietronero, to be published.
18. M. Marsili and L. Pietronero, to be published.
19. J. Nittmann and H.E. Stanley, Nature 321, 663 (1986).
20. R. Blumenfeld and A. Aharony, Phys. Rev. Lett. 62, 2977 (1989).
21. See for example: D. Stauffer, "Introduction to Percolation Theory", Taylor and Francis, London-Philadelphia (1985).
22. L. Pietronero and A. Stella, to be published.

CONTINUUM DESCRIPTION OF ACTIVE ZONES

Zoltán Rácz

Institute for Theoretical Physics
Eötvös University
Budapest 1088, Puskin u. 5-7, Hungary

ABSTRACT

Reaction-diffusion equations are used for studying the scaling properties of active zones formed in $A + B \to C$ type chemical reactions, in diffusion-limited aggregation, and in the Eden process. It is shown that conservation laws play an important role in determining the scaling behavior.

I. INTRODUCTION

Growth phenomena can often be described in terms of particle aggregation[1]. A common feature of these processes is that growth occurs in an outer region, in the so called active zone of the aggregate[2]. The active zone moves outward and leaves behind a frozen structure which may possess remarkable scaling properties (as an example, one might think of diffusion-limited aggregation[3]). Since we are interested in the frozen structure which is related to the dynamics of the process through the active zone, it is clear that we should study the properties of this zone and, furthermore, we should find a way of relating its properties to those of the bulk.

Although aggregation processes are conceptually simple, their mathematical description is rather involved. Given the difficulty of the problem, one tries to make some advance by developing models which are mathematically transparent but at the same time retain the basic feature of the phenomena which, in our case, is the presence of a moving, active zone. Since aggregation can be viewed as a process of reaction of two or more fields, natural candidates for such mathematical models are the reaction- diffusion equations. In the simplest case of two fields they take the following form:

$$\dot{a} = D_a \Delta a - f(a, b) \qquad (1)$$

$$\dot{b} = D_b \Delta b - g(a, b) \qquad (2)$$

where D_a and D_b are the diffusion coefficients of the fields $a(\mathbf{r}, t)$ and $b(\mathbf{r}, t)$, and the

Fractals' Physical Origin and Properties
Edited by L. Pietronero
Plenum Press, New York

reaction terms f and g are arbitrary functionals of the fields and their spatial derivatives. Of course, this form of the equations is too general. The interaction between the diffusion and the various reaction terms gives rise to an extremely rich phenomenology with applications in physics, chemistry, and many other fields. A feature of equations (1,2) which is significant for our purposes, is the fact that, by adding appropriate noise terms, they become the Langevin equations which have been succesfully used to describe critical dynamics in equilibrium systems[4]. This connection to critical phenomena becomes important if we note that the usefulness of the reaction-diffusion equations in the equilibrium case is due to the universality of the scaling behavior. The critical exponents depend only on the symmetry and dimensionality of the long wavelength fluctuations and on the conservation laws satisfied by the dynamics of those fluctuations. This universality then leads to simplifications since it allows one to extract the correct scaling behavior from (1) and (2) by expanding f and g and retaining only the lowest order terms with the right symmetries and conservation laws.

Aggregation resembles relaxation at a critical point in the sense that it is a process of approach towards a scale-invariant final state. Thus, assuming some kind of universality, one might try to follow the strategy outlined for the equilibrium case. This is what we shall do by considering equations (1,2) with reaction terms which are simple but nevertheless describe processes of current interest. The examples examined below ($A+B \rightarrow C$ type chemical reactions, diffusion-limited aggregation, and the Eden model) are characterized by different local and global conservation laws and, as we shall see, these conservation laws strongly influence and in some cases determine the scaling of the active zone.

It should be noted that, except for the case of the Eden model, we shall not discuss the effect of noise. Thus the results are of mean- field nature with all the shortcomings of a mean-field theory at a critical point.

II. DIFFUSION-CONTROLLED $A + B \rightarrow C$ TYPE CHEMICAL REACTION

An elementary example where the motion of an active zone can be followed in detail is a chemical-reaction type process, $A + B \rightarrow C$, in which the reagents are transported by diffusion and the reaction kinetics is of second order. In this case, the concentrations of the diffusing particles a and b play the role of the fields and the reaction terms are choosen to be $f = g = -kab$ where k is the reaction-rate parameter. Thus the mathematical description is given by the following equations

$$\dot{a} = D\Delta a - kab \tag{3}$$

$$\dot{b} = D\Delta b - kab \tag{4}$$

where, for simplicity, we assumed $D_a = D_b = D$. Note that since the A and B particles react in pairs the difference in their numbers is a conserved quantity. In terms of the densities this means that the spatial integral of $a - b$ is constant unless there are particle sources at the boundaries.

In order to have a localized active zone (or reaction front as it is called in chemistry), we must prepare an initial state with the reagents separated. For example, we may use $a = a_0$ and $b = 0$ for $x < 0$ while $a = 0$ and $b = b_0 < a_0$ for $x > 0$. For this choice of initial state, the solution of (3) and (4) depends only on the spatial coordinate x at all times t, i.e. the system becomes one-dimenisional. The time-evolution of the densities can be easily obtained on a computer and, as one can see from Figure 1, the reaction front where the particles C are produced is well defined.

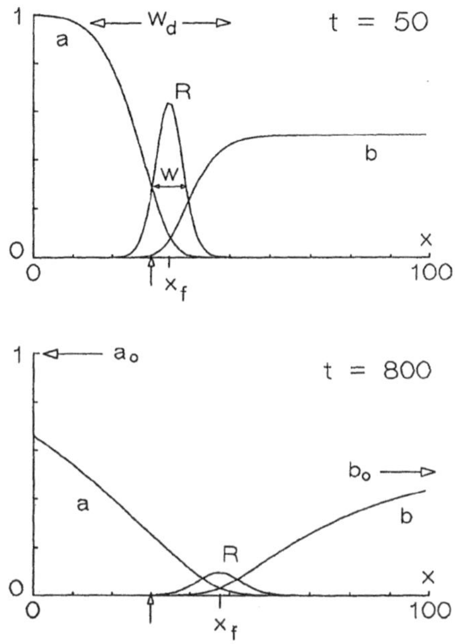

Figure 1. Formation of a reaction zone as observed by solving equations (3) and (4) numerically. The width (W_d) of the region where significant depletion of the reagents occur (depletion zone) can be seen to increase with time much faster than the width of the reaction zone (w). Length (x), time (t), the densities (a, b) of the reagents (A, B), and the production rate ($R = kab$) of C are measured in units of $l = \sqrt{D/ka_0}, \tau = (ka_0), a_0$, and $ka_0{}^2$ respectively (R is multiplied, however, by a factor 100 for better visibility). As an initial condition, we used: $a = 1$, $b = 0$ for $x < 30$ and $a = 0$, $b = 0.5$ for $x > 30$ (the $t = 0$ position of the center of the front, x_f, is shown by an arrow).

Quantitatively, the reaction zone may be characterized by the spatial distribution of the production rate of C which is given by

$$R(x,t) = ka(x,t)b(x,t). \tag{5}$$

The long-time limit of this function can be calculated analytically and the result[5] is the following scaling form:

$$R(x,t) \sim t^{-\beta} F\left(\frac{x - x_f}{t^\alpha}\right) \tag{6}$$

where the position of the center of the front, x_f, scales with time as $x_f \sim \sqrt{t}$, the width of the reaction front is proportional to t^α with $\alpha = 1/6$, the scaling exponent of the production rate of C at $x = x_f$ is $\beta = 2/3$, and the scaling function, $F(z)$, is a fast decreasing function for $z \to \pm\infty$.

The result $x_f \sim \sqrt{t}$ is rather obvious. It is just the consequence of the fact that the surplus concentration $(a - b)$ of the the majority particles diffuses freely thus the position of the reaction front $(a \approx b)$ should shift as $\sqrt{t}$. The other two exponents, α and β, are more interesting and below we show how to obtain their numerical value from a simple physical argument[5]. The basic ingredients used in the derivation are as follows:

i) The difference in the number of particles is a conserved quantity.
ii) a and b are smooth functions of their arguments.
iii) The particles diffuse to the reaction zone thus the width of the depletion zone (see Figure 1) scales as $W_d \sim \sqrt{t}$.
iv) The width (w) and the 'height' $R_f = R(x_f, t)$ of the reaction zone scale with time as $w \sim t^\alpha$ and $R_f \sim t^{-\beta}$, and $\alpha < 1/2$ i.e. $w \ll W_d$.

The values of α and β are calculated by deriving two scaling laws connecting these exponents. The first one follows from the conservation law: the number of particles C produced in the reaction zone is equal to the number of A and B particles entering the zone. The number of C particles produced in a unit of time can be estimated as $wR_f \sim t^{\alpha-\beta}$, while the number of A and B particles entering the reaction zone in a unit time is given by their currents $j_a = -D\partial a/\partial x$ and $j_b = -D\partial b/\partial x$ towards the reaction zone. Since a and b decrease from their initial value to zero in a distance which is proportional to W_d (Figure 1), we can estimate j_a and j_b to be proportional to the inverse of W_d i.e. $j_a \sim j_b \sim t^{-1/2}$. Thus, comparing the exponents in $wR_f \sim j_a$ we have the following scaling relation:

$$\alpha - \beta = -1/2 \quad . \tag{7}$$

The second scaling law is obtained by noting that the $j_a \sim \partial a/\partial x \sim j_b \sim \partial b/\partial x \sim t^{-1/2}$ relation can be used to estimate the average values of a and b in the reaction front: $a \sim b \sim w/t^{1/2}$. Thus the production rate of C particles can be obtained as $R_f \sim t^{-\beta} \sim ab \sim w^2/t \sim t^{2\alpha-1}$ and comparison of the exponents leads to the scaling relation

$$2\alpha - 1 = -\beta \quad . \tag{8}$$

The solution of equations (7) and (8) is $\alpha = 1/6$ and $\beta = 2/3$ thus the analytical results are recovered.

We would like to finish this chapter by just repeating the key words of the above argument: conservation law, smoothness, diffusion, and scaling.

III. DIFFUSION-LIMITED AGGREGATION (DLA)

DLA has been discussed extensively so I will assume the reader is familiar with the problem. Those who would like to be introduced to the topic may consult Meakin's contribution in this book or they may read Witten and Sander's original paper[3].

The active zone of DLA clusters may be characterized by the so called growth probability measure, $\hat{P}(\mathbf{r}, N)d\mathbf{r}$, which gives the probability that the Nth particle sticks to the existing cluster in the neighborhood of site $\mathbf{r}$. This probability has a multifractal structure[6] thus its description in terms of reaction-diffusion equations seems to be a rather hopeless task. The situation looks more promising, however, if the spherically averaged probability, $P(r, N)dr$, is considered[2] (Figure 2).

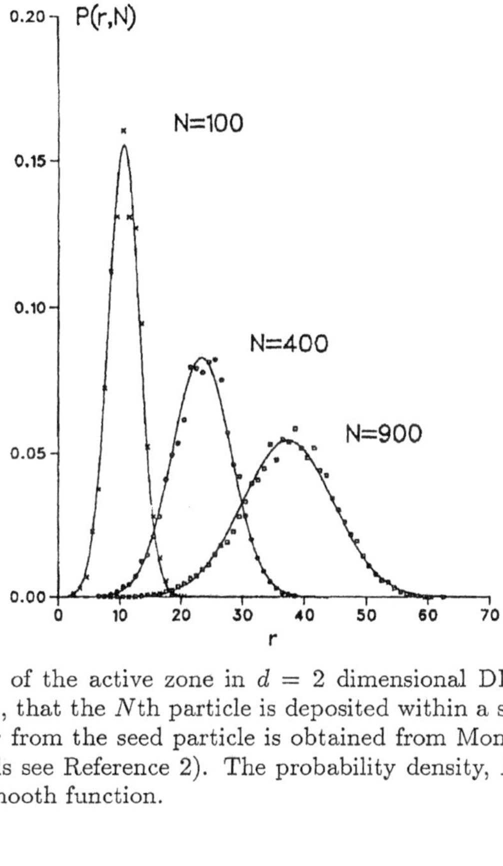

Figure 2. Evolution of the active zone in $d = 2$ dimensional DLA. The probability, $P(r, N)dr$, that the Nth particle is deposited within a shell of width dr at a distance r from the seed particle is obtained from Monte Carlo simulations (for details see Reference 2). The probability density, $P(r, N)$, can be seen to be a smooth function.

Actually the simulation results for $P(r, N)$ are very well fitted by Gaussians (solid lines on Figure 2)

$$P(r, N) = \frac{1}{\sqrt{2\pi} w_N} \exp\left[-\frac{(r - \bar{r}_N)^2}{2w_N^2}\right] \quad , \tag{9}$$

and one can conclude that the active zone can be characterized by just two parameters, the mean deposition radius $\bar{r}_N$ and the width of the active zone w_N. Since $\bar{r}_N$ is practically the radius of the cluster, its scaling for large N ($\bar{r}_N \sim N^{1/D}$) is determined by the fractal dimension (D) of the frozen structure. The exponent, $\bar{\nu}$, of the width $w_N \sim N^{\bar{\nu}}$ is not related to D in any obvious way. For small clusters[2] $\bar{\nu} < 1/D$ but as the cluster grows $\bar{\nu}$ increases and there is some evidence[7] that it may reach the value $1/D$.

Thus the spherically averaged properties are rather simple so it is not unreasonable to expect that the picture discussed above may emerge from a continuum theory.

A mean-field type continuum theory based on reaction-diffusion equations has been constructed by Ball et.al.[8] In this theory, field $a(\mathbf{r},t)$ is choosen to represent the immobile cluster ($D_a = 0$) while the other field, $b(\mathbf{r},t)$, is designated as the diffusing field of incoming particles. The reaction terms describing the interaction of the fields may be constructed using the following argument. In the particle version of DLA the field b is zero on the cluster and its gradient at a surface site is proportional to the probability of growth at that site. On a lattice, this means that the probability of attachment at a site ($\mathbf{i}$) neighboring the cluster is proportional to $b(\mathbf{i},t)$. Since the field $a(\mathbf{j},t)$ may be interpreted as the probability that site $\mathbf{j}$ is occupied by the cluster, the reaction rate $f(\mathbf{i},t)$ which is proportional to the probability of growth of a at site $\mathbf{i}$ may be approximated as

$$f(\mathbf{i},t) \sim \sum_{\mathbf{l}} a(\mathbf{i}+\mathbf{l},t)b(\mathbf{i},t) = \left\{ za(\mathbf{i},t) + \sum_{\mathbf{l}} [a(\mathbf{i}+\mathbf{l},t) - a(\mathbf{i},t)] \right\} b(\mathbf{i},t) \tag{10}$$

where the summation over $\mathbf{l}$ means summation over the z nearest-neighbors of site $\mathbf{i}$.

Since the growth of a is equal to the depletion of b we have $g = -f$ and the reaction-diffusion equations can be obtained by using the continuum limit of (10). The sum on the right-hand side of equation (10) is the discretized version of Δa thus after rescaling time and space variables we have

$$\dot{a} = (a + \Delta a)b \quad , \tag{11}$$

$$\dot{b} = D\Delta b - (a + \Delta a)b \quad . \tag{12}$$

Usually these equations are considered in the quasistationary approximation ($\dot{b} = 0$). The underlying physical assumption is that the growth of a is so slow that the field b has time to adjust to its stationary value. For our purposes this quasistationary approximation may be considered as the definition of the continuum version of DLA[8].

The appropriate boundary conditions for a spherically symmetric solution of equations (11,12) with $\dot{b} = 0$ follow from the presence of a constant particle source at infinity [$b(\infty,t) = b_\infty$], and from the fact that no current flows through $r = 0$ [$(\partial b/\partial r)_{r=0} = 0$]. The initial condition is given by specifying a cluster density $a(r,0) = a_0(r)$ which is localized near $r = 0$.

The continuum version of DLA has been studied analytically[8] and the results show that the active-zone picture does emerge in the long-time limit. In particular, the following points have been shown. 1) The effective radius of the *cluster* increases with time as $\bar{r} \sim t$ i.e. the active zone moves with constant velocity. 2) The density of the *cluster* left behind the active zone scales with r as $a(r,t) \sim r^{-1}$ which is a characteristics of fractal objects of dimension $d-1$. 3) The width of the active zone, w, scales with the radius of the *cluster* as $w \sim \sqrt{\bar{r}}$.

Below we would like to show how the above results may be obtained from simple considerations in which the use of a conservation law, the assumptions of scaling and smoothness, and the solution of diffusion equation figure prominently.

The assumption of scaling is introduced as a requirement that the frozen part of the cluster had a density of the form

$$a(r,t) \sim r^{D-d} \qquad (r < \bar{r}) \quad , \tag{13}$$

where $\bar{r}$ was the radius characterizing the position of the active zone. The diffusion equation enters the problem once it is noted that the reaction term in equation (12) is negligible for $r \gg \bar{r}$ thus the field b in that region satisfies the stationary diffusion equation. Since the field b is zero inside the cluster, the approximate boundary conditions for b are given as $b(r \approx \bar{r}, t) = 0$ and $b(\infty, t) = b_\infty$, consequently $b(r,t)$ can be written as

$$b(r,t) \approx b_\infty \left[1 - \left(\frac{\bar{r}}{r}\right)^{d-2}\right] \qquad (r > \bar{r}) \quad . \tag{14}$$

Assuming smoothness, the above functional forms (13, 14) are continued into the active zone ($r \sim \bar{r}$) where the fields a and b react. The last ingredient of the argument is the conservation law inherent in the process: the A particles entering the active zone turn into B particles i.e. the sum of their numbers is conserved. This can be used to relate the width of the active zone to the size of the cluster. We just have to calculate the current of B particles entering the active zone

$$j_b \sim \left.\frac{\partial b}{\partial r}\right|_{\bar{r}} \sim \frac{1}{\bar{r}} \tag{15}$$

and compare it with the production rate of A particles

$$abw\big|_{\bar{r}} \sim a\frac{\partial b}{\partial r}ww\big|_{\bar{r}} \sim \bar{r}^{\,2\alpha+D-d-1} \quad . \tag{16}$$

The comparison yields a relationship

$$w \sim \bar{r}^{\,(d-D)/2} \tag{17}$$

which shows that the scaling of the active zone may be directly related to the fractal dimension of the frozen part. The numerical value of the exponent $(d-D)/2$ itself is not satisfactory since it should be near 1 which happens only if $D \approx d-2$. It is known[9], however, that $D \geq d-1$. In principle, this discrepancy is not surprising since the continuum theory of DLA is a mean-field theory. It becomes more of a problem if we notice that the derivation of (17) is rather robust. It is not easy to see which of the assumptions underlying (17) may break down when the fluctuations are taken into account. A distinct possibility is that some nonlinear terms which have been neglected in the derivation of (11) and (12) are actually relevant for obtaining the correct DLA behavior.

Next we calculate the fractal dimension D. Again, we start with the conservation law by noting that the amount of a deposited in a unit time is approximated as $j_b(\bar{r}) \approx 1/\bar{r}$. This amount is spread over a distance w thus the density of a deposited in the active zone is given by $j_b(\bar{r})/w$. The deposition in a shell of radius $\bar{r}$ lasts while the active zone moves across so the time of deposition may be calculated as $\tau \approx w/\dot{\bar{r}}$. Thus the density of a in the frozen part is obtained in the following form

$$a(\bar{r}, t \to \infty) \sim \frac{j_b(\bar{r})}{\dot{\bar{r}}} \sim (\bar{r}\dot{\bar{r}})^{-1} \quad . \tag{18}$$

The inequality $D \geq d-1$ follows already from the above equation since $\dot{\bar{r}}$ can either decrease or stay constant as the size of the cluster grows. In fact, the active zone moves with constant velocity. In order to see this we note that the front of the cluster ($r \gg \bar{r}$) is in a constant $b = b_\infty$ field thus the equation governing its motion is given by

$$\dot{a} = b_\infty(a + \Delta a) \quad . \tag{19}$$

The solution of this equation may be written in the form

$$a(r,t) \sim t^{-d/2} \exp\left[b_\infty(t - \frac{r^2}{4t})\right] \tag{20}$$

and one can see that the exponential determines the time dependence of the radius r_1 at which the growth of a becomes nonnegligible at large distances. Clearly, the characteristic radius of the active zone must be proportional to r_1 so we have $\bar{r} \sim t$ and equation (18) yields

$$a(r, t \to \infty) \sim r^{-1} \tag{21}$$

with the consequence that $D = d-1$. Using this result, we obtain the time dependence of w from (17)

$$w \sim t^{1/2} \tag{22}$$

and so the value of exponent α defined in equation (6) is found to be 1/2. The other exponent β can also be calculated by noting that the rate of production of a at $\bar{r}$ may be approximated as $a(\bar{r},t)b(\bar{r},t) \sim a(\partial b/\partial r)w \sim t^{-3/2}$ and consequently $\beta = 3/2$.

We have now completed our task of recovering the results of the analytical theory[8] from simple physical arguments. A final observation is that the two systems considered so far are different mainly in their conservation laws (the diffusivity of A particles is not a relevant parameter since the exponents in the problem of chemical reaction do not change if we set $D_a = 0$). Thus we believe the change in the exponents must be attributed to the change in the conservation laws.

IV. EDEN MODEL

The Eden process[11] is a model of cluster growth which was originally introduced in biology and later generalized[12] and used in physics. Actually, all these processes are slight variations of the following local growth rule: the probability of growth is equal at every site of the surface. The clusters grown by these rules are compact[13] ($D = d$) and only their surface properties are nontrivial. Describing the surface in terms of the probability density $P(r,N)$ (for definition see Figure 2) one finds[2] that an 'active-zone' picture similar to that obtained for DLA emerges. The Gaussian fits to $P(r,N)$ are remarkably accurate again and thus the active zone can be characterized by two parameters. The average deposition radius scales as $\bar{r}_N \sim N^{1/d}$ which is an obvious consequence of the compactness of the cluster. The scaling of the active zone $w \sim N^{\bar{\nu}}$ is more interesting. It yields an exponent $\bar{\nu}$ which is definitely different from $1/d$.

The problem of the exponent $\bar{\nu}$ has been much studied[2,12,14–20]. Although the results of Monte Carlo simulations[12,14,17–19] in $d = 2$ agree with those obtained from the stochastic Burgers' equation[16], there seems to remain some discrepancy between the simulations and the continuum description in $d = 3$. Since it is not quite clear which growth rules lead to Burgers' equation in the continuum limit[20] it may be useful to consider alternative descriptions of the Eden process. Below we shall examine such an alternative approach based on reaction-diffusion equations. From our point of view, this example is interesting because of the contrast between the local conservation law present in the Eden model and the global conservation laws discussed in the previous sections.

The derivation of the continuum model is based on the observation that the Eden model may be considered as the following limit of DLA: the B particles are not allowed to diffuse ($D_b = 0$) and their initial density is set to 1 at every site not occupied by the seed cluster of A particles. In the continuum limit this means that we have to put $D = 0$ in equation (12) and as an initial condition we should use $b_0 = 1$ and $a_0 = 0$ everywhere except in a small region around a seed particle ($r \approx 0$) or a $d-1$ dimensional substrate ($x \approx 0$) where $b_0 = 0$ and $a_0 = 1$ should be set. Thus the reaction-diffusion approach yields the following set of equations for the Eden model

$$\dot{a} = \quad (a + \Delta a)b \tag{23}$$

$$\dot{b} = -(a + \Delta a)b \quad . \tag{24}$$

The conserved quantity in the above process is the sum of the number of A and B particles. This sum is conserved at every lattice sites i.e. we have a local version of the conservation law associated with the DLA. Unfortunately, this local conservation law is not helpful in producing exponent estimates from simple arguments. It may be used, however, for reducing the number of equations to one. Since $a + b$ is a constant and the initial conditions fix the actual value of the constant at 1, equation (24) may be eliminated and we obtain

$$\dot{a} = (a + \Delta a)(1 - a) \quad . \tag{25}$$

This equation has solutions which describe uniformly translating localized fronts

$$a(x, t) = G(x - vt) \quad , \tag{26}$$

and it can be shown[21] that the selected velocity of the front is $v = 2$. It follows then from (26) that the function characterizing the active zone $[R(x,t) = a(x,t)b(x,t)]$ can be written in the form

$$R(x, t) = F(x - vt) \tag{27}$$

and a comparison with equation (6) yields the mean-field exponents $\alpha = 0$ and $\beta = 0$. Thus we can see that the change from DLA to the Eden process which can be interpreted as a change from global to local conservation of $a + b$ has radically changed the value of the exponents.

Of course, one expects that the 'flat' active zone described by (27) becomes unstable to long wavelength transverse fluctuations in dimensions $d > 2$. We have not yet investigated this instability but we can present some arguments which indicate that the scaling properties which emerge as a result of the instabilities are similar in nature to those of an interface whose motion is governed by Burgers' equation[22].

In order to find a connection to Burgers' equation let us introduce $\mathbf{v} = \nabla a$ and take the gradient on both sides of equation (25):

$$\dot{\mathbf{v}} = -(\mathbf{v}\nabla)\mathbf{v} + (1 - 2a)\mathbf{v} + (1 - a)\Delta\mathbf{v} \quad . \tag{28}$$

Assuming now that the intrinsic width of the active zone is small we can define an interface between the regions rich in A or B by requiring $a = b = 1/2$. It follows then from (28) that near the interface $\mathbf{v}$ satisfies Burgers' equation:

$$\dot{\mathbf{v}} + (\mathbf{v}\nabla)\mathbf{v} = \frac{1}{2}\Delta\mathbf{v} \quad . \tag{29}$$

Kardar et.al.[16] studied this equation in connection with the Eden model. They added a noise term and found that the scaling of the solution of (29) implies the following form for the width of the active zone:

$$w \sim t^{1/3} \quad . \tag{30}$$

This result is exact for $d = 2$ and there is a suggestion that it may be valid even for $d > 2$ (Monte Carlo simulations[17,19], however, do not support such an extention to higher dimensions).

The above derivation thus yields $\alpha = 1/3$ for the reaction- diffusion version of the Eden model. It also illustrates the effect of fluctuations on the exponents. We would like to emphasize, however, that these were not the main points of our arguments in this section. Our aim here was to demonstrate how the exponents change as a global conservation law is changed into a local one.

CONCLUDING REMARKS

Conservation laws are known to be relevant factors in determining the dynamic universality classes in equilibrium critical phenomena. In this lecture I tried to demonstrate that they may play an equally important role in classifying nonequilibrium growth processes.

References

1. See for example *Fractals in Physics*, L.Pietronero and E.Tosatti eds., (North-Holland, Amsterdam, 1986).
2. M.Plischke and Z.Rácz, Phys.Rev.Lett.**53**,415(1984).
3. T.A.Witten and L.M.Sander, Phys.Rev.Lett.**47**,1400(1982).
4. P.C.Hohenberg and B.I.Halperin, Rev.Mod.Phys.**49**,435(1977).
5. L.Gálfi and Z.Rácz, Phys.Rev.A**38**,3151(1988).
6. T.C.Halsey, P.Meakin, and I.Procaccia, Phys.Rev.Lett.**56**,854(1986).
7. P.Meakin and L.M.Sander, Phys.Rev.Lett.**54**,2053(1985).
8. R.C.Ball, M.Nauenberg, and T.A.Witten, Phys.Rev.**A29**,2017(1984).
9. R.C.Ball and T.A.Witten, Phys.Rev.**A29**,2966(1984).
10. Y.Kantor, T.A.Witten, and R.C.Ball Phys.Rev.**A33**,3341(1986).
11. M.Eden, *Proceedings of the Fourth Berkeley Symposium on Mathematical Statistics and Probability*, F.Neyman ed. (University of California, Berkeley, 1961) Vol.4. p.223.
12. R.Jullien and R.Botet, J.Phys.A**18**,2279(1985).
13. D.Dhar, Phys.Rev.Lett.**54**,2058(1985).

14. M.Plischke and Z.Rácz, Phys.Rev.**A32**,3825(1985).
15. P.Freche, D.Stauffer, and H.E.Stanley, J.Phys.A**18**,L1163(1985).
16. M.Kardar, G.Parisi, and Y.C.Zhang, Phys.Rev.Lett.**56**,889(1986).
17. P.Meakin, P.Ramanlal, L.M.Sander, and R.C.Ball, Phys.Rev.**A34**,5091(1986).
18. M.Plischke, Z.Rácz, and D.Liu, Phys.Rev.**B35**,3485(1987).
19. D.E.Wolf and J.Kertész, Europhys.Lett.**4**,651(1987).
20. J.Krug and H.Spohn, Phys.Rev.**A38**,4271(1988).
21. A.Juhász and Z.Rácz, unpublished.
22. J.M.Burgers, *The Nonlinear Diffusion Equation* (Riedel, Boston, 1974).

MULTIFRACTALITY, SCALING, AND DIFFUSIVE GROWTH

Thomas C. Halsey

The James Franck Institute and the Department of Physics
The University of Chicago
Chicago, Illinois

I. INTRODUCTION

The formation of branched, ramified, fractal structures in pattern formation limited by diffusion was first pointed out by Witten and Sander in 1981.[1] In the intervening years, the study of such patterns has blossomed into a major area of non-linear physics. We have gradually learned, and are still learning, the correct concepts in which to couch quantitative discussion of the problem. One of the key such concepts is the multifractal structure of the growth probability distribution of a diffusion-limited pattern.[2,3] In this contribution, I shall argue that this structure, as encoded in the $f(\alpha)$ function of the distribution, provides not merely a rich phenomenological description of the patterns, as has been widely realized. It also gives the foundation on which a more physical scaling picture of diffusion-limited growth may be built.

This contribution is organized in six sections. In section II, I will give a description of the most widely used diffusive growth model, diffusion-limited aggregation (DLA). I will briefly discuss its physical relevance, and I will introduce a useful electrostatic analogy for this growth process. This electrostatic analogy in turn suggests a continuous family of generalized DLA models, the $\eta-$models. In section III, I will review the multifractal formalism, with emphasis upon its application to diffusive growth. In sections IV and V, I will discuss two physical approaches, one due to Turkevich and Scher, and one due to this author, that lead to scaling relations amongst the multifractal exponents. The Turkevich and Scher approach concentrates on the behavior of the fastest growing regions of the structure, that of this author exploits the electrostatic analogy of section II. In section VI, I conclude with some comments on needed research in this challenging field, with particular reference to the need for more complete methods of describing the scaling structure of diffusive growth models.

Fractals' Physical Origin and Properties
Edited by L. Pietronero
Plenum Press, New York

II. DIFFUSION-LIMITED AGGREGATION

DLA was originally introduced as a physically motivated computer algorithm for the generation of clusters. One starts with a seed particle, and introduces into the system sufficiently far away a randomly walking particle, which walks until it first touches the seed. At this point, it sticks permanently, and another particle may be introduced to the system. There are numerous variants of this simple model, in which the dimensionality of space is varied, the random walker or the clustered particles are restricted to a lattice, the particle sticks a probability less than one on each contact with the cluster, or other alterations are made in the rules.[1,4] The clusters generated by this method are highly ramified, presenting a strongly branched appearance (Figure 1). They are also fractal. The scaling of the radius r of the cluster with the number of particles n is

$$n \sim r^D, \qquad (II.1)$$

where the cluster dimension D is, in general, less than d, the dimensionality of space. For two dimensional off-lattice DLA, $D = 1.71$, while for three-dimensional DLA, $D = 2.5$.[4]

DLA can also be defined using an electrostatic analogy.[5] Suppose that the cluster is considered as a conductor at a fixed potential, say $\phi = 0$, and that there is a distant conductor (arbitrarily close to ∞) at a different potential, say $\phi = 1$. Then the probability that a random walker arriving from ∞ will first touch the cluster at the surface point w is proportional to the local electric field at w, given the boundary conditions mentioned. If we call this electric field $P(w)$, then we can write the growth probability $G(w)$ at w as

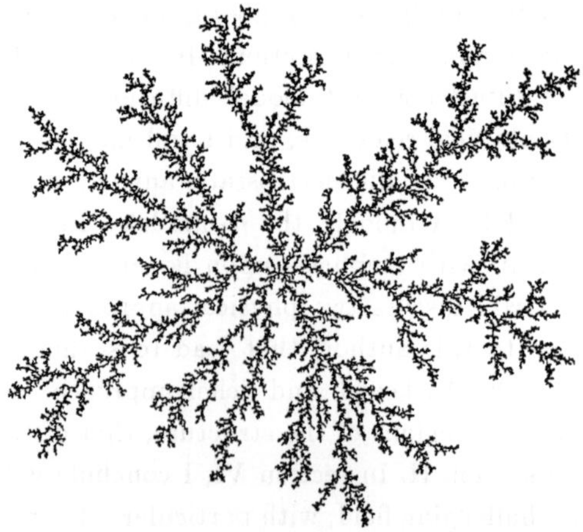

Figure 1. An off-lattice DLA cluster of 35,000 particles (grown by M. Leibig).

$$G(w) = \frac{P(w)}{\int_S dw P(w)}, \qquad (II.2)$$

where the integral is over the entire surface S of the cluster.

This electrostatic analogy can also be used to define a class of related models, termed the η-models. These models were first introduced by Niemeyer, Pietronero, and Wiesmann as candidate models for the dielectric breakdown of insulating media.[6] In the η-models, the boundary conditions at the cluster and at ∞ are identical to those described above, but the growth probability is proportional to some power of the electric field,

$$G(w) = \frac{P^\eta(w)}{\int_S dw P^\eta(w)}. \qquad (II.3)$$

This relation defines a different growth model for every value of the parameter η. The case $\eta = 1$ is simply DLA. The case $\eta = 0$ is another well-known growth model, the Eden model.[7] Various η-models (with $\eta \geq 0$) have been studied; qualitatively they are quite similiar to DLA, though the dimension D decreases monotonically with η.

The clusters grown using the DLA algorithm are very similiar to those observed in a variety of natural growth processes. Notable examples include colloidal aggregation, viscuous fingering, and electrodeposition.[8-10] Only in the first of these cases is the diffusion of particles literally the limiting factor in growth. In viscuous fingering the pressure field, and in electrodeposition the electric potential, approximately obey the Laplace equation, so that these problems are mathematically analogous to DLA. Of course, in none of these problems is diffusion (or its analog) the only physical effect. In the absence of a general theory of DLA, it has proven difficult to predict theoretically which physical perturbations will destroy the ramified, fractal structures characteristic of DLA, and which will not. Nevertheless, the numerous observations of DLA-like structures in nature suggests that DLA should be robust against many possible variations in the underlying microscopic physics.

III. MULTIFRACTALITY

"Multifractality" is a fancy word for a relatively simple concept. The growth probability distribution $G(w)$ defined in the above is a probability measure defined upon a fractal support, the surface of the DLA cluster. It has become clear over the past years that frequently such "fractal measures" can be characterized by the scaling of their moments, with the scaling exponents of different moments being non-trivially related. Suppose that the size of a particle in a DLA cluster is a, and the scale of the cluster itself is r. Since these are the only length scales in the problem, it is natural to define a moment exponent function $\tau(q)$ by[2,11]

$$\int dw G^q(w) = \frac{\int dw P^q(w)}{[\int dw P(w)]^q} \equiv a^{1-q}(\frac{a}{r})^{\tau(q)}. \qquad (III.1)$$

The factors of a insure that this relation is dimensionally correct. It is clear that for $q = 0$, $\tau(q) = -D_s$, the fractal dimension of the surface of the cluster. However, for $q \to \infty$ the integral will be more and more dominated by the regions of large $G(s)$, and $\tau(q)$ will be primarily determined by the growth measure scaling in these regions. Conversely, for $q \to -\infty$ the integral will be dominated by the regions of especially small $G(s)$. Let us explore this point in more detail. Since the integrand in Equation (III.1) will be slowly varying over length scales of a, the integral may be approximated by a sum over regions of size a. If the total growth measure in the i'th such region is G_i, then we may write

$$\sum_i G_i^q = (\frac{a}{r})^{\tau(q)}. \qquad (III.2)$$

Now we wish to break the set $\{G_i\}$ into classes with the same measure. The G_i vary quite widely over the cluster; the growth probability at a tip is considerably larger than that deep inside one of the "fjords" apparent in Figure 1. In fact, at a tip, the local growth probability density diverges (a divergence that is cut off at the scale of a), while in an indentation, the probability density goes to zero (again, this is cut off at the length scale of the particle). Thus it is natural to write

$$G_i \equiv (\frac{a}{r})^{\alpha_i}, \qquad (III.3)$$

defining the local growth measure scaling exponent α_i. The behavior of the number of regions with scaling exponent between α and $\alpha + d\alpha$, $N(\alpha)d\alpha$, defines a second exponent $f(\alpha)$,

$$N(\alpha)d\alpha = (\frac{a}{r})^{-f(\alpha)}. \qquad (III.4)$$

Thus we have that

$$\sum_i G_i^q = \int d\alpha (\frac{a}{r})^{q\alpha - f(\alpha)} = (\frac{a}{r})^{\tau(q)}. \qquad (III.5)$$

The integral over α may be approximated using a saddlepoint technique, provided that (a/r) is sufficiently small. The value of α dominating the integral will be that for which

$$\frac{df(\alpha)}{da} = q, \qquad (III.6)$$

defining implicitly the functions $\alpha(q)$ and $f(\alpha(q))$. Then we obtain immediately that

$$\tau(q) = q\alpha(q) - f(\alpha(q)), \qquad (III.7)$$

and, taking the derivative with respect to q of both sides of Equation (III.7), and using Equation (III.6),

$$\frac{d\tau(q)}{dq} = \alpha(q). \qquad (III.8)$$

Equations (III.6-8) are the equations of a Legendre transform.[3,12] Using them, one can pass from the moment scaling function $\tau(q)$ to the local scaling density function $f(\alpha)$ and back.

Typically, there will be minimum and maximum values of α characterizing the scaling of the most concentrated and the most disperse regions of probability on the measure. If $\tau(q)$ is an analytic function of q, as seems to be the case for almost all physical systems of interest, then one can draw some further conclusions regarding the form of $f(\alpha)$.[3] In the first place, $f(\alpha)$ must be concave downwards, with $d^2f/d\alpha^2 < 0$. Furthermore, $df/d\alpha$ must go to $+\infty$ at the minimum value of α, α_{min}, and must go to $-\infty$ at the maximum value of α, α_{max}. This leads qualitatively to the type of $f(\alpha)$ function seen in Figure 2.

Some special points on this curve possess particularly simple interpretations. At $q = 0$, $\tau(q) = -D_s$, the dimension of the surface of the cluster, as remarked above. But $\tau(q = 0) = -f(\alpha(q = 0)$, with $\alpha(q = 0)$ defined implicitly by $df/d\alpha = 0$. Thus, the maximum value of $f(\alpha)$ corresponds to the dimension of the cluster surface.

If $f(\alpha_{min,max} = 0)$, as is the case in Figure 2, then the minimum and maximum values of α correspond to at most a finite number of points on the surface of the cluster, i.e., to a number of points that does not scale with the ratio of the cutoff a to the size of the cluster r. (This, again, appears to be the case for almost all systems of physical interest.) Furthermore, the maximum probability region or regions on the surface

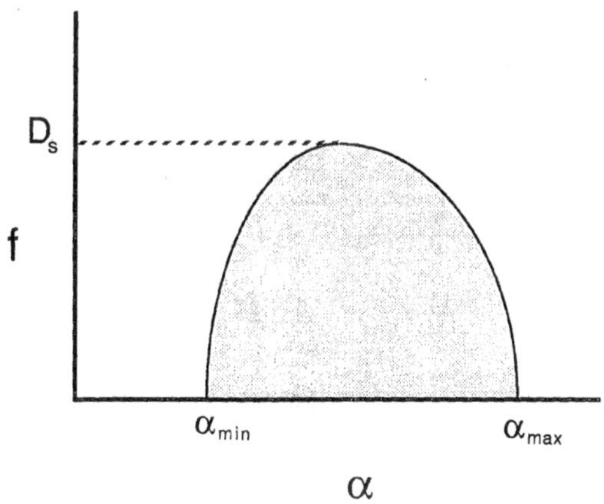

Figure 2. A typical $f(\alpha)$ curve. The maximum of the curve is the dimension of the surface, the minimum and maximum values of α determine the maximum and minimum growth probabilities.

have a growth probability of $(a/r)^{\alpha_{min}}$, and the minimum probability region or regions have a growth probability of $(a/r)^{\alpha_{max}}$. Note that the smallest value of α corresponds to the largest probability, and vice versa.

The $f(\alpha)$ function for the growth probability for DLA, and for various of the other η-models, has been studied numerically by several authors.[2,13] The most comprehensive work, by Hayakawa et al., is clearly in agreement with the above phenomenology.

DLA clusters are stochastic objects, so some averaging is necessary to define the function $\tau(q)$, or $f(\alpha)$, as an ensemble property. If brackets $\langle\rangle$ refer to averaging over a probabilistic ensemble of DLA clusters, then one can choose to define either an "annealed" $\tau(q)$, $\tau_a(q)$, or a quenched $\tau(q)$, $\tau_q(q)$, respectively by the relations

$$\langle\sum_i G_i^q\rangle = (\frac{a}{r})^{\tau_a(q)}, \qquad (III.9a)$$

$$\langle\log(\sum_i G_i^q)\rangle = \tau_q(q)\log(a/r). \qquad (III.9b)$$

Most computer studies have relied upon annealed averaging, but quenched averaging probably yields a more physical result. In averaging over the entire ensemble of possible clusters, some clusters will appear, such as a perfectly linear cluster, or a cluster with a "tunnel" of exponentially declining probability, that might alter an annealed average, despite their very low probability.[14] Quenched averages should prove more robust against these effects. In averaging over a relatively small number of stochastically generated clusters, these questions are probably academic, as only rather typical members of the ensemble will appear.

IV. THE SCALING ARGUMENT OF TURKEVICH AND SCHER

Turkevich and Scher have recently proposed a simple physical idea, which can be used to yield a scaling relation between the exponent α_{min} and the dimension of the cluster as defined by Equation (II.1).[15] The radius r that appears in Equation (II.1) can be defined in different ways, as the maximum radius of the cluster, the radius of gyration of the cluster, or in some other manner. If the clusters are truly self-similiar, then they are characterized by no length scale aside from the size of the cluster and the size of the individual particles. Then these different methods of defining the radius should be equivalent, in the sense that for any cluster they will be proportional to each other, with the constants of proportionality independent of the size of the cluster.

It is convenient to take the maximum radius of the cluster r_M as our definition of radius. Now, the maximum radius of a cluster will grow upon the addition of a new particle only if that particle lands at the position that was previously at the maximum radius. If it does so, then the radius will grow by some quantity of order a. Thus, writing the probability of landing upon the maximum radius particle as G_{max}, we have

$$\langle\frac{dr_M}{dn}\rangle \approx aG_{max}. \qquad (IV.1)$$

Now we know from section III above that $G_{max} \leq (a/r_M)^{\alpha_{min}}$. Observing the scaling with r_M of both sides of Equation (IV.1), we obtain

$$D \geq 1 + \alpha_{min}. \tag{IV.2}$$

If we further make the plausible assumption that the maximum radius point also corresponds to the maximum probability point, then we obtain

$$D = 1 + \alpha_{min}. \tag{IV.3}$$

Unfortunately, this relation is not quite in agreement with the numerical evidence. Typical measurements of α_{min} for DLA in two dimensions give $\alpha_{min} \approx .65$, while the exponent $D \approx 1.71$.[13] Note that these values are still in accord with the inequality (IV.2). This discrepancy may be a consequence of the relation holding only as an inequality, or it may be the result of systematic errors in the calculation of $f(\alpha)$, which remain rather poorly understood.

For other values of η, it is sometimes convenient to write this scaling relation in terms not of the $f(\alpha)$ function for the growth measure, but rather in terms of the $f(\alpha)$ function for the electric field.[16] Recall that $P(w)$ is the normal electric field at the surface point w, given that the cluster surface is at a potential $\phi = 0$, and that a distant conductor (say, at a distance R from the center of the cluster, $R >> r$) is at a potential $\phi = 1$. The total electric field absorbed by the cluster will, in two dimensions, scale logarithmically in (r/R). In fact, this can be used to define an "electrostatic" radius of the cluster, r_E, which will presumably behave in the same way as r_M above,

$$\int dw P(w) \equiv 2\pi[\log(R/r_E)]^{-1}, \tag{IV.4}$$

so that the flux absorbed by a cluster is the same as that absorbed by a circular conductor of radius r_E inside an outer circular conductor of radius R. Now the growth measure for the η-model is defined by the η'th power of the electric field. Defining $\sigma_\eta(q)$ by

$$\int dw[G_\eta(w)]^q \equiv a^{1-q}(\frac{a}{r})^{\sigma_\eta(q)}, \tag{IV.5}$$

and using for $\tau(q)$ the normalized electric field measure,

$$\frac{\int dw[P(w)]^q}{[\int dw P(w)]^q} \equiv (\frac{a}{r})^{\tau(q)}, \tag{IV.6}$$

we have immediately the relation between $\sigma_\eta(q)$ and $\tau(q)$,

$$\sigma_\eta(q) = \tau(\eta q) - q\tau(\eta). \tag{IV.7}$$

The Turkevich and Scher relation should clearly be as valid for arbitrary η as it is for $\eta = 1$, provided that α_{min} for the growth measure is used. Thus a simple calculation shows that, in terms of α_{min} for the electric field measure, the Turkevich-Scher relation (in its strong form) is

$$D = 1 + \alpha_{min}\eta - \tau(\eta). \tag{IV.8}$$

These relations may be easily generalized to arbitrary dimensionality; one finds that the Turkevich-Scher law (Equation (IV.8)) is independent of dimensionality.[16]

V. THE ELECTROSTATIC SCALING RELATION

A further scaling relation can be derived using an energetic argument based upon elementary electrostatics.[16,17] A system with two conductors held at fixed potential is a capacitor, whose energy ϵ is simply related to the potential across the capacitor and the charge Q stored therein. Since the potential across this capacitor is $\Delta\phi = 1$, we have

$$\epsilon = +\frac{1}{2}Q = \frac{1}{8\pi}\int dw P(w). \tag{V.1}$$

Of course, this energy can also be expressed as the volume integral of the electric field squared,

$$\epsilon = \frac{1}{8\pi}\int_V dv(\vec{\nabla}\phi)^2. \tag{V.2}$$

Now suppose we move the cluster surface point w normal to the surface by a distance $f(w)$ (Figure 3), while holding its potential, and that of the distant surface, constant. The work performed in this operation will be determined by the change in the charge of the surface. This work is performed by an external charge reservoir at fixed potential upon the system; its value is

$$\delta w = \delta Q = \frac{1}{4\pi}\delta\int dw P(w). \tag{V.3}$$

This work must be equal to the change in the energy stored in the system, so that

$$\delta\int dw P(w) = \frac{1}{2}\delta\int_V dv(\vec{\nabla}\phi)^2. \tag{V.4}$$

The change in the integral on the right-hand side is due to two effects: the exclusion of a shell of thickness $f(w)$ from the volume, and the change in $\vec{\nabla}\phi$. To zeroth order in f, $(\vec{\nabla}\phi)^2$ near the surface may be replaced by $(P(w))^2$, an elementary calculation then shows that

$$\delta\int dw P(w) = \frac{1}{2}\delta\int_V dv[P(w)]^2 f(w). \tag{V.5}$$

Now suppose that $f(w)$ is the change in the surface of the cluster arising from the addition of a particle at w'. Of course, $f(w)$ will be localized to within a particle size a about w', and its total area $\int dw f(w)$ will be simply the d-dimensional particle volume $k_d a^d$. Since $P(w)$ is slowly varying on scales of a, we may immediately average over the probability $G_\eta(w')$ of a particle accreting at any position upon the surface, to obtain

$$\langle \frac{d}{dn} \int dw P(w) \rangle = \frac{k_d a^d}{2} \langle \frac{\int dw [P(w)]^{2+\eta}}{\int dw [P(w)]^\eta} \rangle, \tag{V.6}$$

where the brackets indicate averages over the ensemble of clusters.

To pass from this identity to the electrostatic scaling law, some assumptions are needed. First, the order of differentiation and averaging on the left-hand side of Equation (V.6) must be interchanged. Second, the average of the ratio on the right-hand side must be replaced by the ratio of the averages. For $\eta = 1$, this should not pose any problems, as the denominator will not fluctuate significantly, since it depends only upon the logarithm of r_E. For other values of η, correlated fluctuations between the numerator and denominator could invalidate this assumption. Of course, if one restricts the ensemble on both sides of the equation to "typical" (i.e., well-behaved) clusters, one can still average the numerator and denominator separately. In two dimensions, these assumptions, in concert with the multifractal form for the moments of $P(w)$, yield immediately

$$\frac{dr}{dn} \propto (\frac{a}{r})^{\tau(2+\eta)-\tau(\eta)}. \tag{V.7}$$

Thus the electric field moments in an η model will obey

$$D = \tau(2+\eta) - \tau(\eta). \tag{V.8}$$

This relation can be as easily generalized to other dimensionalities as that discussed in section IV above.

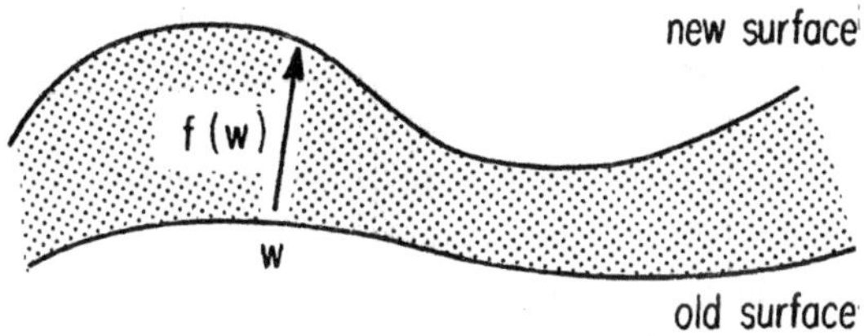

Figure 3. The shaded area represents the volume excluded from free space in the growth of the surface. The normal change in the surface position at w is $f(w)$.

Table 1. The definition of $\tau(q)$, and the Turkevich-Scher and electrostatic scaling laws. α_{min} refers to $f(\alpha)$ for the electric field measure.

$$\frac{\int dw[P(w)]^q}{[\int dw P(w)]^q} \equiv (\frac{a}{r})^{\tau(q)}$$

$$D = 1 + \alpha_{min}\eta - \tau(\eta)$$

$$D = \tau(2+\eta) - \tau(\eta) + (2-d)$$

This relation is in excellent agreement with currently available numerical results. Thus, for two dimensional off-lattice DLA, Halsey, Meakin and Procaccia give $\tau(3) = 1.71 \pm .01$, in excellent agreement with $D = 1.71$.[2] ($\tau(1) = 0$ for a normalized measure). For other values of η, there is also good numerical agreement.[18] This electrostatic scaling law, and that of Turkevich and Scher, are listed (in the form appropriate for arbitrary dimensionality) in Table 1.

VI. CONCLUSION

The $f(\alpha)$ function gives not only an extensive phenomenological characterization of the growth properties of diffusively growing clusters, it also gives an appropriate characterization. The existence of scaling laws for $f(\alpha)$ strongly suggests that the scaling of moments of the growth distribution will be one of the key objects in our eventual quantitative understanding of this problem. Unfortunately, there are many physically relevant properties of the structure of DLA clusters for which $f(\alpha)$ is too crude a measure. One of the most glaring such properties is the hierarchical structure of a DLA cluster, which recreates branches with roughly the same proportions, and containing roughly the same angles between stems, at every length scale of the cluster. While this structure is encoded in a rough way in $f(\alpha)$, its subtleties must escape such a simple function.

In fact, this hierarchical structure is reminiscent of the structure of strange attractors at the onset of chaos. These phase space objects possess asymptotically an exact hierarchical structure, which may be described by the scaling function for the strange attractors.[19] Unfortunately, it is not at all clear how to extend such a scaling function description to a system that possesses, at best, only a hierarchical structure "averaged" over stochastic fluctuations. Nevertheless, such a "stochastic" scaling function would seem to be a necessity for any comprehensive description of the structure of a DLA cluster, and thus for any comprehensive theory of diffusive growth. One measure of the intrinsic interest of a scientific problem is its ability to force us to create new tools; by this measure, diffusive growth has been, and remains, one of the most fascinating scientific problems of recent years.

ACKNOWLEDGEMENTS

The work reported in this contribution has been performed in collaboration with M.H. Jensen, L.P. Kadanoff, P. Meakin, I. Procaccia, and B. Shraiman. I am also grateful for discussions with C. Amitrano, J. Cardy, P. Jones, T.A. Witten, Jr., and other colleagues too numerous to mention. This work has been supported by the National Science Foundation through individual grants and through the Materials Research Laboratory of the University of Chicago. Some of the work was made possible by the hospitality of the Service de Physique Théorique, C.E.N. Saclay, France.

REFERENCES

1. T.A. Witten, Jr. and L.M. Sander, Phys. Rev. Lett. **47**, 1400 (1981).

2. T.C. Halsey, P. Meakin, and I. Procaccia, Phys. Rev. Lett. **56**, 854 (1986).

3. T.C. Halsey, M.H. Jensen, L.P. Kadanoff, I. Procaccia, and B. Shraiman, Phys. Rev. **A 33**, 1141(1986).

4. P. Meakin, Phys. Rev. A **27**, 1495 (1983).

5. L. Pietronero and H.J. Wiesmann, J. Stat. Phys. **36**, 909 (1984).

6. L. Niemeyer, L. Pietronero, and H.J. Wiesmann, Phys. Rev. Lett. **52**, 1033 (1984).

7. M. Eden, in *Proceedings of the Fourth Berkeley Symposium on Mathematical Statistics and Probability, Vol. 4*, J. Neyman, ed. (University of California Press, Berkeley, 1961) p. 223.

8. S.R. Forrest and T.A. Witten, Jr., J. Phys. A **12**, L109 (1979).

9. D. Bensimon, L.P. Kadanoff, S. Liang, B. I. Shraiman, and C. Tang, Rev. Mod. Phys. **58**, 977 (1986), and references therein.

10. R. Brady and R.C. Ball, Nature (London) **309**, 225 (1984); M. Matsushita, M. Sano, Y. Hayakawa, H. Honjo, and Y. Sawada, Phys. Rev. Lett. **53**, 286 (1984).

11. P. Meakin, H.E. Stanley, A. Coniglio, and T.A. Witten, Jr., Phys. Rev. A **32**, 2364 (1985).

12. U. Frisch and G. Parisi, in *Turbulence and Predictability in Geophysical Fluid Dynamics and Climate Dynamics, Proc. of Int. School of Physics "Enrico Fermi" LXXXVIII*, M. Ghil, R. Benzi, and G. Parisi, eds. (North-Holland, Amsterdam,1985) p. 84.

13. C. Amitrano, A. Coniglio, and F. di Liberto, Phys. Rev. Lett. **57**, 1016 (1986); Y. Hayakawa, S. Sato, and M. Matsushita, Phys. Rev. A **36**, 1963 (1987).

14. J. Lee and H.E. Stanley, Phys. Rev. Lett. **61**, 2945 (1988).

15. L. Turkevich and H. Scher, Phys. Rev. Lett. **55**, 1026 (1985); Phys. Rev. A **33**, 786 (1986).

16. T.C. Halsey, Phys. Rev. A **38**, 4749 (1988). Note that the generalization of the Turkevich-Scher law to arbitrary η, Equation (IV.8), is different from that originally proposed in Reference 15.

17. T.C. Halsey, Phys. Rev. Lett. **59**, 2067 (1987).

18. C. Amitrano, unpublished.

19. See, e.g., M.H. Jensen, L.P. Kadanoff, and I. Procaccia, Phys. Rev. A **36**, 1409 (1987).

IS THERE A PHASE TRANSITION IN THE MULTIFRACTAL SPECTRUM OF DLA?

Jysoo Lee, Preben Alstrøm and H. Eugene Stanley

Center For Polymer Studies and Department of Physics
Boston University, Boston, MA 02215 USA

I. INTRODUCTION

The diffusion-limited aggregation[1] (DLA) model has been found to describe a remarkably large number of interesting physical systems such as fluid flow in porous media, colloidal aggregation, and electrodeposition.[2–17] Although DLA is one of the most important models of fractal growth phenomena, and is described by a quite simple set of rules, we do not understand DLA as completely as we do, say, the two-dimensional Ising model. For example, even the existence of the fractal dimension in the large-cluster limit is not clear. The situation becomes more complicated, since the fractal dimension alone is not sufficient to characterize the growth process.[4–6] Furthermore, in order to *fully* characterize the growth process, one needs an infinite number of independent exponents, which is usually called the multifractal spectrum.[7–9]

There have been enormous efforts using various techniques such as real-space renormalization[10] numerical simulations[5,6,13], phenomenological arguments[11,14], conformal mapping[15–16], and a field-theoretical method.[12] Most recently, Pietronero *et al.*[17] have presented a novel theory of fractal growth which includes DLA as a notable example. Owing to these efforts, valuable information for some part of the spectrum has been obtained. Especially for the region corresponding to the 'tip' of the cluster, most of the methods give similar results. However, the exact solution for the multifractal spectrum has not been determined at present.

In particular, there has been essentially no reliable information for the part of the spectrum corresponding to the 'fjord' of the DLA cluster. The origin of this difficulty is the fact that this region is characterized by *extremely* small growth probabilities. Therefore, numerical simulation cannot give reliable results due to numerical accuracy (the smallest growth probability for a large DLA cluster is much smaller than the numerical accuracy). Furthermore, different methods seem to give different results and also disagree with the experiments, a fact that has plagued investigators in this field.[18]

We have been studying the multifractal spectrum of DLA based on an exact-enumeration approach, which means we *must* consider every possible cluster configuration up to a certain size. This exact enumeration follows the general procedure outlined by Nagatani[19] in connection with a position-space renormalization-group formulation for DLA. Since we find the minimum growth probability to a high numerical accuracy, we can determine the 'fjord' part of the multifractal spectrum.

Fractals' Physical Origin and Properties
Edited by L. Pietronero
Plenum Press, New York

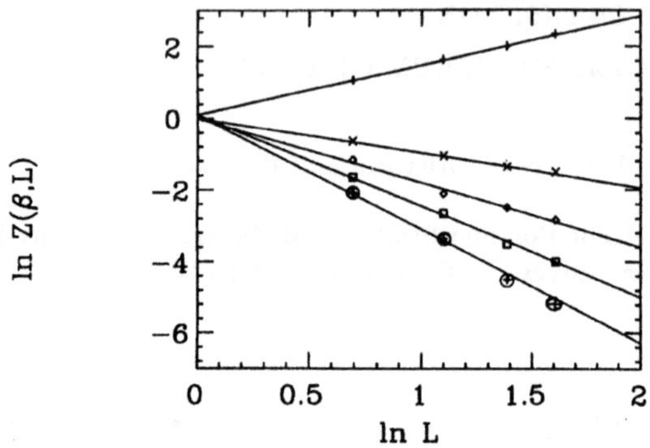

Fig. 1. Dependence of $\ln Z_A(\beta, L)$ on $\ln L$ for $\beta \geq 0$. $(+)$, $(\times)$, $(\diamond)$, $(\square)$ and $(\oplus)$ means $\beta = 0, 2, 3, 4, 5$, respecively.

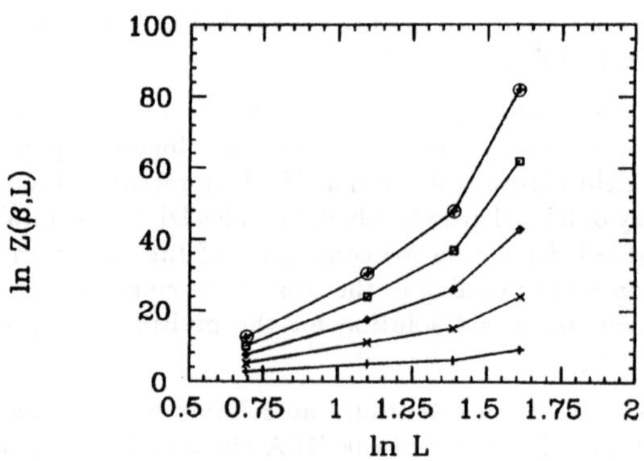

Fig. 2. Dependence of $\ln Z_A(\beta, L)$ on $\ln L$ for $\beta < 0$. $(+)$, $(\times)$, $(\diamond)$, $(\square)$ and $(\oplus)$ means $\beta = -1, -2, -3, -4, -5$, respectively.

We consider clusters of size L, where $L = 2,3,4,5$. We find out that we have to consider 3.0×10^{17} different cluster configurations for $L = 5$. By finding symmetries in the system, we are able to reduce them to 9361 configurations, which indicates there are enormous number of symmetries in the system.

Furthermore, we find evidence suggesting the existence of a phase transition[20,21] in the multifractal spectrum. In other words, the 'free energy' of the system develops a singularity near a certain critical 'temperature'. We also find that this transition has several interesting consequences. For example, the free energy is not defined below the critical temperature β_c, the large energy part of the 'entropy' function is a straight line of slope β_c, and there are large fluctuations of energy near the critical temperature.

This paper is organized as follows. In Sec. II, we describe the exact enumeration method used here to obtain the multifractal spectrum. In Sec. III we summarize the key results forming a possible phase transition. Section IV discusses the behavior of the smallest growth probability. The Section VII summarizes some open questions.

II. METHOD

For configuration α, we determine its weight C_α, i.e., the probability of getting that configuration, and all its growth probabilities $p_{i,\alpha}$ with very good accuracy. One must take care to distinguish two different averages. The first, which we call the *annealed* average, calculates

$$Z_A(\beta, L) = <\zeta>_{conf} = \sum_\alpha C_\alpha \zeta_\alpha, \tag{1}$$

where $\zeta_\alpha = \sum_i p^\beta_{i,\alpha}$. For the *quenched* average we calculate

$$\ln Z_Q(\beta, L) = <\ln\zeta>_{conf} = \sum_\alpha C_\alpha \ln \zeta_\alpha. \tag{2}$$

We also defined the annealed free energy $F_A(\beta, L)$, energy $E_A(\beta, L)$ and specific heat $C_A(\beta, L)$ by

$$F_A(\beta, L) = -\frac{\ln Z_A(\beta, L)}{\ln L}, \tag{3a}$$

$$E_A(\beta, L) = \frac{\partial F_A(\beta, L)}{\partial \beta}, \tag{3b}$$

and

$$C_A(\beta, L) = -\frac{\partial E_A(\beta, L)}{\partial \beta}. \tag{3c}$$

The corresponding thermodynamic quantities for the quenched average can be defined in a similar way.

III. RESULTS

1a. For $\beta > 0$, we find both Z_A and Z_Q scale as power laws in the variable L (Fig. 1). Accordingly, we find an excellent convergence with L of both $F_A(\beta, L)$ and $F_Q(\beta, L)$ (Fig. 3).

1b. As β is decreased below 0, $Z_A(\beta, L)$ deviates from a power law behavior, and becomes exponential (Fig. 2). For Z_Q we find only a slight deviation from a power law, compared to Z_A. This exponential behavior leads to a divergence with L of the $F_A(\beta, L)$ curves (Fig. 3).

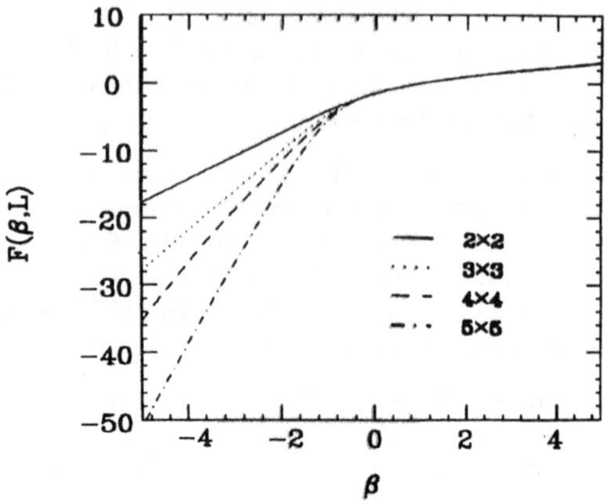

Fig. 3. Dependence of $F_A(\beta, L)$ on β for $L = 2 \sim 5$. One can see the 'knees' developing around $-2 < \beta < 0$.

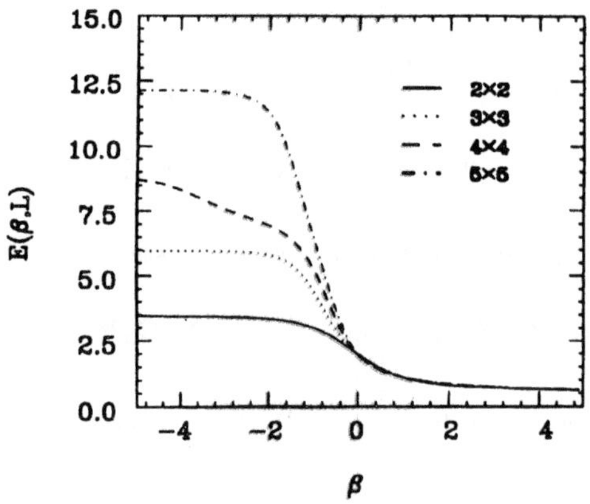

Fig. 4. Dependence of $E_A(\beta, L)$ on β for $L = 2 \sim 5$. One can notice the sharp change for $-2 < \beta < 0$.

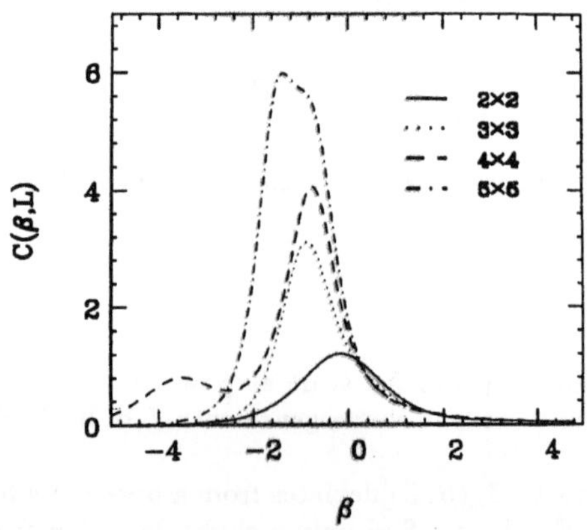

Fig. 5. Dependence of $C_A(\beta, L)$ on β determined for $L = 2 \sim 5$. One can notice that the maximum value of the specific heat increases as L increases.

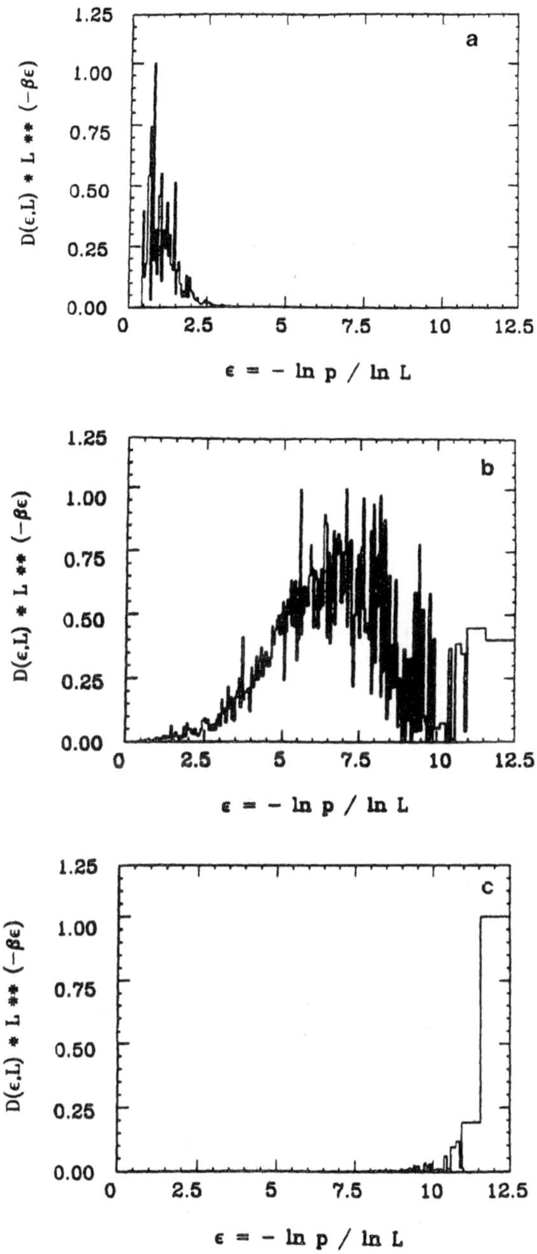

Fig. 6. Energy fluctuations above, near and below the phase transition. Shown is the density of states multiplied by 'Boltzmann factor' $L^{-\beta\epsilon}$ for the case of $L = 5$ and (a) $\beta = 1.0$, (b) $\beta = -1.0$, and (c) $\beta = -2.0$.

2. As L increases, we find that $F_A(\beta, L)$ develops a 'kink' in the region $-2 < \beta < 0$ (Fig. 3). This behavior can be seen more clearly in $E_A(\beta, L)$ and $C_A(\beta, L)$ plots, which show that the kinks become sharper as L increases (Figs. 4 and 5).
3. For $-2 < \beta < 0$, there are contributions to $Z_A(\beta)$ from a wide range of probabilities, a sign of 'cooperative effect' – see Fig. 6, reproduced from Fig. 13 of Ref. 23(b). For the definition of the density state function, see Ref. 23(b).

If the kinks become ever sharper as $L \to \infty$ limit, it implies a singularity in the free energy curve, analogous to a thermodynamic system which shows a phase transition. Hence it is tempting to refer to the apparent breakdown of power law scaling in $Z_A(\beta, L)$ as a 'phase transition'.

If this is a *phase* transition, what are the 'phases'? Since for $\beta > 0$ the behavior is dominated by the large growth probabilities associated with the tips, while for β sufficiently negative ($\beta < -2$) it is dominated by the very small growth probabilities in the fjords, we shall use the term *tip phase* for $\beta > \beta_c$ and the term *fjord phase* for the $\beta < \beta_c$. In tip phase, the behavior is dominated by growth-site probabilities which scale. However in fjord phase, it is dominated by the probabilities which do not scale (Fig. 7). At present, it is not clear whether these two distinct phases become indistinguishable in $L \to \infty$ limit.

For completeness, we now discuss the possibility of a phase transition for the quenched case. It is natural to assume that the quenched case corresponds to the results for a *typical* cluster. The reason is that the quenched case emphasizes the configurations themselves (i.e., the C_α), not the ζ_α. Our study of the quenched case , based on the exact-enumeration data, shows a weak deviation from the power law behavior, and the kink in $F_Q(\beta, L)$ seems to be sharpening as L increases to $L = 5$, the largest value studied by our exact enumeration approach. Recently, we have used the quenched approach to study masses up to $M = 100$. Again, we find that $Z_Q(\beta, L)$ has a weak deviation from a power law behavior, and the kinks in F_Q, E_Q, and C_Q seem to be sharpening as M increases. From these studies, we cannot make a definite statement if there exists a phase transition, even though we averaged over 2500 clusters. For large mass ($M \gg 100$), it is very difficult to calculate the very small p_i accurately, so at present the results are not conclusive. However, recent work by Havlin *et al*[24] on a single DLA cluster of mass 10^3 seems to suggest there is a kink in F_Q. If this preliminary finding is corroborated by additional work, it would be possible to answer whether there is a phase transition even in the quenched case.

IV. THE BEHAVIOR OF THE SMALLEST PROBABILITY

In addition to the thermodynamic functions F_A, E_A, and C_A, we also studied the behavior of $p_{\min}(L)$, the smallest growth probability among *all the possible* DLA configurations of linear size L. We find that well below the transition 'temperature' ($\beta < -2$), $Z(\beta, L)$ is dominated by the contribution from $p_{\min}(L)$. However, in the $L \to \infty$ limit, it is possible that growth probabilities different from $p_{\min}(L)$ dominate the moments for small β (e.g., for $\beta \sim -2$).

This $p_{\min}(L)$ comes from configurations that are topologically the same as tunnel configurations (Fig. 8). For these non-typical configurations (the fractal dimension of these configurations is 2), one can show $p_{\min}(L) \sim \exp(-AL^2)$[23(c)].

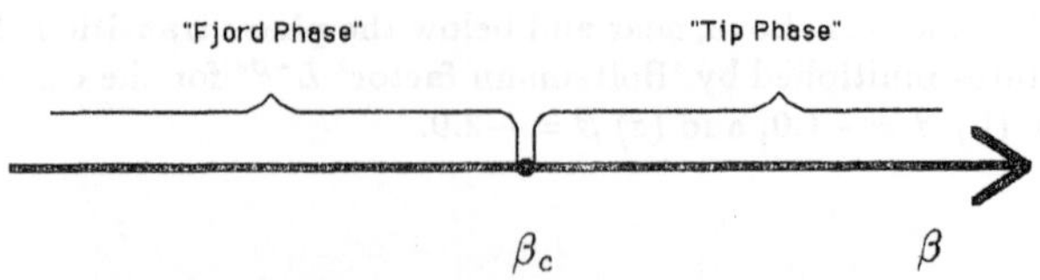

Fig. 7. Schematic 'phase diagram' showing the fjord and tip phases.

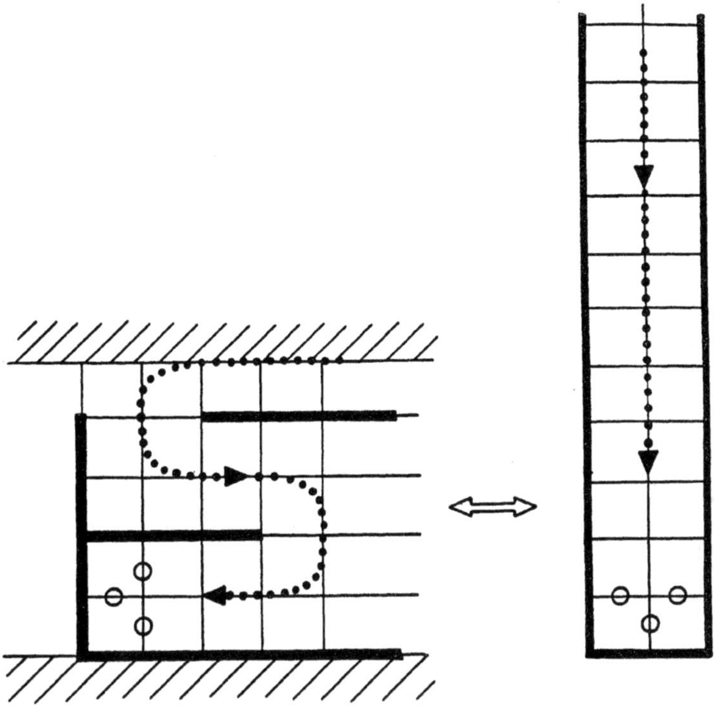

Fig. 8. One of the configurations, which have $p = p_{\min}(L = 5)$. Here, we apply periodic boundary conditions in the horizontal direction. The bottom line is a line of seed particles. The light lines are unoccupied bonds, the heavy lines are occupied bonds. The broken line indicates the path of a random walker to reach the bond with $p = p_{\min}$. The open circles indicates the bonds with minimum growth probability $p = p_{\min}$.

We now discuss a point that has led to some confusion in the literature. We want to emphasize that $p_{\min}$ is not *alone* giving rise to the phase transition. Actually, around the transition temperature, the system can not even 'see' $p_{\min}(L)$. Rather, this transition is the 'cooperative effect' of the p_i's which are sufficiently small. The role of $p_{\min}(L)$ is simply setting up $E_{\max}(L)$, the 'cut off' of the system.

In order to estimate the contribution of $p_{\min}(L)$, one must also estimate $C_{\min}(L)$, the *sum of the weights of all the configurations* which have $p_{\min}(L)$. The analytic estimation of $C_{\min}(L)$ is quite difficult, our exact enumeration study (up to $L = 5$) seems to suggest

$$C_{\min}(L) \sim \exp(-BL^{x}), \tag{4}$$

where x is close to 2. Using this information, it is possible to argue that the behavior of $Z_A(\beta, L)$ for sufficiently negative β.

One can divide the sum $Z_A(\beta, L)$ into $\sum_{\min}$ (the contribution from $p_{\min}(L)$) and $\sum'$ (from the other p_i's)

$$Z_A(\beta, L) = \sum{}' + \sum_{\min} \geq C_{\min}(L) \times p_{\min}^{\beta}(L) \sim \exp(-BL^{x} - A\beta L^2).$$

(i) If $x < 2$: in the $L \to \infty$ limit and $\beta < 0$, $Z(\beta, L) \geq \exp(-A\beta L^2)$. Therefore, $Z(\beta, L)$ increases exponentially with size L, implying a phase transition at $\beta = 0$.

(ii) If $x = 2$: in the $L \to \infty$ limit and $\beta < -B/A$, $Z(\beta, L)$ increases exponentially with size L, implying a phase transition at $\beta = \beta_c > -B/A$.

(iii) If $x > 2$: in the $L \to \infty$ limit, $\sum_{\min}$ gives an exponentially small contribution.

Because of the limited data ($L = 2, 3, 4, 5$), it is very difficult to estimate the asymptotic behavior of the system. Our estimated value of $x \sim 2$, which makes very difficult to conclude.

In cases (ii) and (iii), the simple argument does not give a definite answer. One has to consider not only the $p_{\min}(L)$ but also all the other p_i's to reach any conclusion. For a more careful argument, see Sec. V of Ref. 23(b).

We want to conclude this section with mentioning one subtle consequence of this phase transition, the importance of 'rare' configurations. Since for sufficiently negative β, the $Z(\beta, L)$ are dominated by the contributions from the DLA clusters that are *not* 'typical', the multifractal spectrum of a typical DLA cluster differs from that of an annealed-averaged spectrum. Therefore, the annealed-average multifractal spectrum cannot be compared with that obtained by large mass simulation or experiment, where one sees only typical DLA clusters.

V. OPEN QUESTIONS

1. *Is there a phase transition in the annealed-average multifractal spectrum of DLA?*

The present work addresses precisely this question. Since our calculation is only for very small L, it is very difficult to predict the behavior of the $L \to \infty$ limit. Also, our numerical estimate of exponent x lies near the marginal value 2, which makes the situation more tricky. Recently, Harris and Cohen[25] presented an estimate for the weights as well as the smallest growth probability of the 'tunnel' configurations. They find that the contribution to $Z_A(\beta)$ by each of these configurations is smaller than $\exp(A\beta N - BN\ln N)$, where A and B are some positive constants, N is the mass. Therefore, Harris and Cohen conclude these configurations give negligible contribution to $Z_A(\beta)$ in $L \to \infty$ limit. However, we argue that one has to consider a whole set of configurations with same p_i to estimate the contribution to $Z_A(\beta)$. For example, the configuration shown in Fig. 8 is *just one* of the many configurations which have $p_{\min}(L)$. Although the contribution of *one* of these configurations are negligible, the sum of them may not.

2. *Is there a phase transition in the multifractal spectrum of 'typical' DLA?*

This is another interesting question recently raised by Blumenfeld and Aharony (BA)[26]. They assume

$$p'_{\min}(L) \sim \exp(-A_1 L^x), \tag{1}$$

where $p'_{\min}(L)$ is the minimum growth probability of a typical DLA cluster of linear size L, while A_1 and x are size-independent positive constants. Then, the β-th moment $Z_A(\beta, L)$ satisfies the inequality

$$Z_A(\beta, L) \equiv \sum_i p_i^\beta \;\; \geq \;\; L^{d_{\min}} \times \exp(-\beta A_1 L^x), \tag{2}$$

where $d_{\min}$ is the fractal dimension of sites with minimum growth probabilities. Thus, for negative β, the moment $Z_A(\beta, L)$ should increase at least exponentially. BA thus conclude that there is a 'breakdown' of power law scaling for $\beta < 0$. The validity of this interesting argument is based on the key assumption (1), which needs further investigation.

We thank A. Aharony, R. Blumenfeld, M. Jensen, S. Redner and, especially, T. C. Halsey for helpful discussions, and G. Huber for critical reading of the manuscript. We also acknowledge support from the National Science Foundation, Office of Naval Research and Boston University Academic Computing Center.

REFERENCES

1. T. A. Witten and L. Sander, Phys. Rev. Lett. **47**, 1400 (1981); Phys. Rev. B **27** 5686 (1983).

2. Applications are described in many recent review articles. See, e.g., P. Meakin, in *Phase Transitions and Critical Phenomena* (eds. C. Domb and J.L.Lebowitz), Vol. 12 (Academic, Orlando, 1988).

3. For general background, see the recent books J. Feder, *Fractals* (Pergamon, NY, 1988); H.E. Stanley and N. Ostrowsky, eds. *Random Fluctuations and Pattern Growth: Experiments and Models* (Kluwer Academic Publishers, Dordrecht, 1988); T. Vicsek, *Fractal Growth Phenomena* (World, Singapore, 1989) and references therein.

4. T. C. Halsey, P. Meakin, and I. Procaccia, Phys. Rev. Lett. **56**, 854 (1986).

5. C. Amitrano, A. Coniglio, and F. di Liberto, Phys. Rev. Lett. **57**, 1016 (1986).

6. P. Meakin, H. E. Stanley, A. Coniglio, and T. A. Witten, Phys. Rev. A **32**, 2364 (1985); P. Meakin, A. Coniglio, H. E. Stanley and T. A. Witten, Phys. Rev. A **34**, 3325 (1986).

7. B. B Mandelbrot, J. Fluid Mech. **62**, 331 (1974). See also the recent review B. B. Mandelbrot, H.E. Stanley and N. Ostrowsky, eds. *Random Fluctuations and Pattern Growth: Experiments and Models* (Kluwer Academic Publishers, Dordrecht, 1988).

8. H. G. E. Hentschel, and I. Procaccia, Physica **8D**, 435 (1983); P. Grassberger, Phys. Lett. A **97**, 277 (1983);D. Schertzer and S. Lovejoy, in *IUTAM Symposium on Turbulence and Chaotic Phenomena in Fluids, Kyoto, Japan* 141 (1983); P. Grassberger and I. Procaccia, Physica **13D**, 34 (1984); P. Grassberger, Phys. Lett. **107A**, 101 (1985); R. Benzi, G. Paladin, G. Parisi, and A. Vulpiani, J. Phys. A **17**, 3521 (1984); *ibid.* **18**, 2157 (1985); U. Frisch, and G. Parisi, in *Turbulence and Predictability in Geophysical Fluid Dynamics and Climate Dynamics*, Proc. Int. School of Physics Enrico Fermi, Course LXXXVIII, eds M. Ghil, R. Benzi, and G. Parisi (North-Holland, Amsterdam, 1985); S. Lovejoy and D. Schertzer, Bull. Am. Met. Soc. **67**, 221 (1986); S. Lovejoy, D. Schertzer, and A. A. Tsonis, Science **231**, 1036 (1987).

9. T. C. Halsey, M. H. Jensen, L. P. Kadanoff, I. Procaccia, and B. I. Shraiman, Phys. Rev. A **33**, 1141 (1986).

10. H. Gould, F. Family and H. E. Stanley, Phys. Rev. Lett. **50**, 686 (1983).

11. R. C. Ball, R. M. Brady, G. Rossi, and B. R. Thompson, Phys. Rev. Lett. **55**, 1406 (1985).

12. G. Parisi and Y. C. Zhang, J. Stat. Phys. **41**, 1 (1985).

13. Y. Hayakawa, S. Sato and M. Matsushita, Phys. Rev. A **36**, 1963 (1987).

14. T. C. Halsey, Phys. Rev. Lett. **59**, 2067 (1987).

15. I. Procaccia and R. Zeitak, Phys. Rev. Lett. **60**, 2511 (1988).

16. T. Bohr, P. Cvitanović and M. H. Jensen, Europhys.Lett. **6**, 445 (1988).

17. L. Pietronero, A. Erzan, and C. Evertsz, Phys. Rev. Lett. **61**, 861 (1988).

18. See, e.g., the discussion on this point in K.J. Måløy, F. Boger, J. Feder and T. Jøssang, in *Time Dependent Effects in Disordered Materials* [eds. R. Pynn and T. Riste], Plenum, NY 1987; J. Nittmann, H. E. Stanley, E. Touboul and G. Daccord, Phys. Rev. Lett. **58**, 619 (1987); P. Alstrøm, Phys. Rev. A **37**, 1378 (1988).

19. T.Nagatani, Phys. Rev. A **36**, 5812 (1987); J. Phys. **A20**, L381 (1987).

20. The concept of a phase transition in multifractal spectra was found in the study of dynamical systems, such as Julia sets [D. Katzen and I. Procaccia, Phys. Rev. Lett. **58**, 119 (1987); M. Jensen, P.Cvitanović, T. Bohr, Europhys.Lett. **6**, 445 (1988)]. In particular, based on a study of Julia sets, Bohr et al. conjectured the existence of a phase transition for aggregates generated by probabilistic diffusion. This conjecture has been supported further from a description of stochastic growth phenomena as a dynamical critical state (see, e.g., P. Alstrøm, preprint; P. Alstrøm, P.Trunfio, and H. E. Stanley, in Ref. 3).

21. (a) Regarding the moments of the distribution of voltage drops across the bonds of a random resistor network, L. de Arcangelis, S. Redner, and A. Coniglio [Phys. Rev. B **34**, 4656 (1986)] observed a change in the relative importance of the contribution of the hottest and coldest bonds to the moments, suggesting the possibility of a transition point. (b) R. Blumenfeld, Y. Meir, A. Aharony, A. B. Harris [Phys. Rev. B **35**, 3524 (1987)] proved for a 'ladder model' of the random resistor network that exponentially small currents appear, leading to a transition where the multifractal description breaks down and the moments diverge. (c) A phase transition has also been observed for the voltage drops across the bonds of the Sierpinski gasket family of deterministic fractals.

22. L. Niemeyer, L. Pietronero and H. J. Wiesmann, Phys. Rev. Lett. **52**, 1033 (1984).

23. (a) J. Lee and H. E. Stanley, Phys. Rev. Lett. **61**, 2945 (1988). (b) J. Lee, P. Alstrøm and H. E. Stanley, Phys. Rev. A **39**, 6545 (1989). (c) J. Lee, P. Alstrøm and H. E. Stanley, Phys. Rev. Lett. **62**, 3013 (1989).

24. S. Havlin, A. Bunde and B. Trus, preprint.

25. A. B. Harris and Michael Cohen, preprint.

26. R. Blumenfeld and A. Aharony, Phys. Rev. Lett. **62**, 2977 (1989).

Part 4

Application of Fractal Growth Models to Physical Phenomena

FRACTALS AND PATTERNS IN ELECTRODEPOSTION

Leonard M. Sander and David G. Grier

Department of Physics
The University of Michigan
Ann Arbor, MI, 48109-1120, USA

INTRODUCTION

Of the most common sources of complex (and fractal) patterns in nature is unstable growth. For example, growth limited by *diffusion* (e.g., chemical precipitation, crystallization, etc.) is very familiar and is intrinsically unstable. The fundamental process is known to metallurgists as the Mullins-Sekerka instability (Mullins and Sekerka, 1957). It is the result of the fact that when an object grows because it is being fed by matter diffusing from outside, the tip of a bump on its surface will collect more matter than a neighboring flat portion; the bump protrudes into the region where the density of diffusers is higher. The tip grows quickly as a result and screens the flat surface. Plane surfaces are unstable.

As a result, an astonishing variety of shapes occur in this type of growth depending on conditions. Among these are disorderly fractal patterns, such as the well-known DLA clusters (Witten and Sander, 1981, 1983; Sander, 1986, 1987). These clusters have a fluctuating number of competing, splitting tips which may be viewed as the result of the proliferation and interaction of instabilities . Much of the evidence about these patterns comes from computer simulations, since an analytic theory of DLA has, thus far, proved elusive. It is also possible for diffusion-limited growth in the presence of anisotropy to stabilize into a special non-trivial steady state with complex spatial order, known in this context as a dendrite (Langer, 1980, Kessler, Koplik and Levine, 1988). For our purposes, we can think of a dendrite as being characterized by a single parabolic tip which is prevented from splitting by anisotropy, and which may shed sidebranches as it advances. This steady state case of diffusion-limited growth has been analyzed with a good deal of success in recent years.

Both of these cases are known to occur in the laboratory (see Figures 1 and 2). The most famous example of a dendrite is a snowflake, which is known to everyone, and which has challenged theorists since the days of Kepler. More recently, it has become clear that disorderly crystals (for example, on an amorphous substrate) can be fractals with scaling over a large range (Radnoczi, et al.1987). In fact, as we will see below, some recent experiments (Dougherty, et al., 1987, Grier, et al., 1987) have shown patterns (such as the dense radial pattern) which are neither fractal, nor dendritic, but have some of the properties of both. In this chapter we will attempt to give a kind of guide to the various patterns which have been encountered. We will see what circumstances give rise to fractal patterns, and how they relate to orderly dendrites. We will show that a minor extension of the pure diffusion-limited growth model can account for the dense radial regime. We will use, a rich example of the processes, electrochemical deposition.

Fractals' Physical Origin and Properties
Edited by L. Pietronero
Plenum Press, New York

THE STEFAN PROBLEM

In this section we state the problem of diffusion-limited growth in continuum terms; this is known as the Stefan problem (see Langer, 1980). We will briefly discuss below the relationship of this formulation to discrete models (such as DLA). To fix our ideas, consider a primitive model of electrodeposition from a solution onto a cathode. Imagine that ions in an electrolyte with density u(**r**,t) diffuse until they reach the cathode, where they deposit. Then we have:

$$\nabla^2 u = B\partial u/\partial t \tag{1}$$

$$\partial u/\partial n \propto v_n. \tag{2}$$

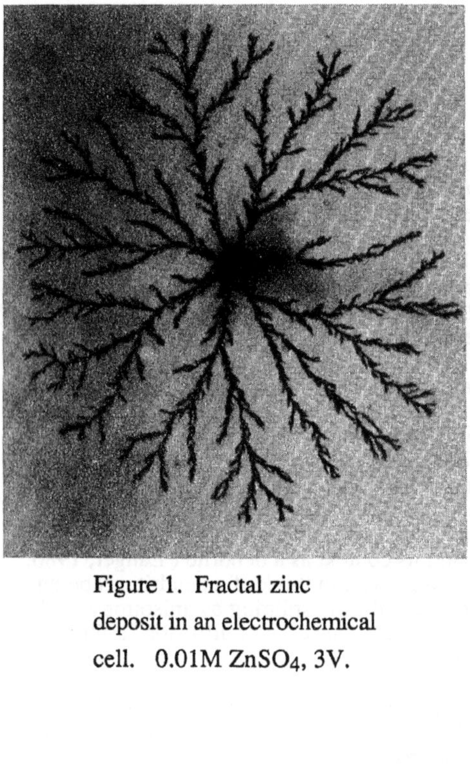

Figure 1. Fractal zinc deposit in an electrochemical cell. 0.01M $ZnSO_4$, 3V.

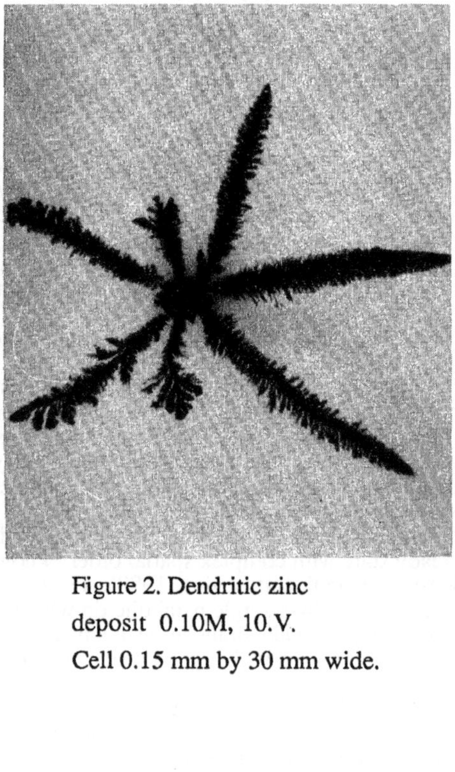

Figure 2. Dendritic zinc deposit 0.10M, 10.V. Cell 0.15 mm by 30 mm wide.

That is, u should obey the diffusion equation; B is the diffusion constant. The normal growth velocity of the interface of the metal deposit is proportional, on the average, to the flux of ions onto the surface, $\partial u/\partial n$.

If the left-hand side of equation (1) can be neglected, then we are said to be in the quasi-static regime. This occurs for slow growth, and in this case, the diffusion equation becomes the Laplace equation. As we will see, this is, in fact the relevant regime for the electrochemical experiments which we will describe and for other physical situations, as well. It is rarely the appropriate approximation for crystallization limited by the diffusion of latent heat, however.

The remaining equation necessary to describe the Stefan problem is a boundary condition on the field, u, at the interface of the growing object, and far away. The latter value can be scaled out of the problem (in the quasi-static regime), but the exact form of the condition on the interface tunes the pattern through its various forms. It is the purpose of this chapter to try to explicate how this tuning happens and how, at least in some situations the transition between regimes occurs. The most usual form adopted for the boundary condition is:

$$u_s = d_0 \kappa \tag{3}$$

where d_0 is a length related to the surface tension, and κ is the curvature of the surface. In fact, it is necessary have some cutoff such as surface tension in the problem. If we were to try to set $u_s = 0$ as we might be tempted to do to represent an absorbing surface, we would find that the interface (the cathode, in our gedanken experiment version of electrochemistry) would develop unphysical cusps in finite time.

It is now known through the work of many groups (see Kessler, Koplik and Levine, 1988 for a review) that these equations in themselves cannot give rise to an ordered dendrite. In fact, the surface tension, and thus the parameter d_0, must be taken to be a function of the angle between the surface and, say, crystal axes in order to stabilize a tip. With anisotropy snowflake patterns resembling the tip of each branch of Figure 2 are the solutions to Equations (1) - (3).

How then, do fractals arise? In the absence of anisotropy, tips are not stable: they grow for a time, and then split. A proliferation of such tip-splittings should give rise to a disorderly pattern of some sort. Whether that pattern is fractal or not, however, is controversial. Certainly, if the growth is not quasi-static, we would not expect fractals to arise because it is difficult to see how the diffusion equation with its short-range propagator could allow the power-law correlations of a fractal to develop.

We will argue, however, that in the quasi-static case without anisotropy, or when the anisotropy is averaged out by external noise, the generic case of diffusion-limited growth, and the generic solution to the Stefan problem, is fractal growth. Our argument rests mainly on experimental and numerical evidence, to which we now turn, since we still have no tractable theory for this regime.

REALIZATIONS OF DIFFUSION-LIMITED GROWTH

The best-known example of fractal patterns in diffusion-limited growth come from the body of numerical evidence surrounding the diffusion-limited aggregation (DLA) model (Witten and Sander, 1981,1983; see Sander, 1986 for a review). This computer model, in which random walkers wander, one at a time, until they attach to a growing cluster, may be viewed as a noisy version of the Stefan model. The probability density for finding a walker is certainly given by equation (1), and a cutoff (albeit not of the form of surface tension) is given by the finite size of the walkers. However, instead of equation (2), we have the condition that the *probability* of growth of a point is given by $\partial u/\partial n$. The patterns seem to be self-similar fractals with fractal dimension of 1.7 in two dimensions and strongly resemble Figure 1.

The most direct implementation of the relationship between fractal growth and the Stefan problem was given by Niemeyer, et al. (1984), who introduced a model of the DLA type now called the dielectric breakdown model. In this technique, equation (1) is solved by relaxation (instead of by Monte Carlo, which is what random walkers amount to) and a cluster is grown by again thinking of equation (2) as giving the probability of growth of a point on the edge of the cluster. All of this can be visualized by thinking of u as the electrostatic potential, and $\partial u/\partial n$ as the electric field at a point on the edge of a dielectric which is about to break down. The cluster is the breakdown pattern.

In fact, in this case, there is no reason why the breakdown probability should not be proportional to some arbitrary function of the electric field, e.g., $(\partial u/\partial n)^{\eta}$. When this is used, fractals different from DLA are produced; DLA should correspond to $\eta = 1$, and simulations of the model show this to be so. Experiments on real breakdown patterns may or may not correspond to $\eta = 1$, depending on the microscopic physics of the process.

However, there is a large class of systems which automatically give $\eta = 1$, and DLA-type kinetics, including quasi-static thermal crystallization, viscous fingering, and, in some limits, electrochemical growth. These will be good candidate systems to look for DLA fractals, and possibly other patterns. These are systems with a *conserved current*, **j**. In quasi-static conditions,

$$\nabla \cdot \mathbf{j} = 0. \tag{4}$$

If this current obeys a generalized Fick law:

$$\mathbf{j} = - c \nabla u \tag{5}$$

and the flux of **j** gives rise to growth

$$v \propto \mathbf{n} \cdot \mathbf{j} \tag{6}$$

Then the analogy is complete because Equation (6) is the same as (2), and from (4) and (5) we get $\nabla^2 u = 0$, the Laplace equation, which is the quasistatic version of Equation (1).

An important example of this sort of realization of is the case of viscous fingering (Paterson, 1984; see Bensimon, et al., 1986, for a review). A viscous fluid trapped between narrowly spaced plates (a Hele-Shaw cell) or in a porous medium usually obeys D'Arcy's law, an example of a generalized Fick law:

$$v = -k/\mu \nabla u$$

Here k is the permeability of the medium, μ the viscosity, and u the pressure in the viscous fluid. This is of the form of Equation (5). If we pump an inviscid fluid into the system, it will displace the original one in an unstable way -- the instability is identical in form to the Mullins-Sekerka instability and is controlled at short scales either by surface tension or the pore size. The complex pattern of fingering is, at least in some porous media (Nittmann, et al., 1985) to a good approximation a fractal of the DLA type, as we expect.

It is now natural to ask if a viscous fingering experiment can exhibit a crossover to orderly dendritic growth. This question was answered in the affirmative by Ben-Jacob et al. (1985), who introduced anisotropy into a Hele-Shaw cell by inscribing grooves onto the plates. At low flow rates the patterns were disorderly, and seemed to be approaching the fractal regime. At higher flows (when the grooves presumably are more effective in directing the fluid) orderly patterns resembling snowflakes were easily observed.

ELECTROCHEMICAL DEPOSITION

In recent years a number of groups have taken up the study of electrochemical deposition as a model system for studying fractals, dendrites and the transitions between them. It has been known since the time of Faraday that dendrites can be produced by depositing from solution. And, in recent years very beautiful experiments have shown how to produce well-characterized fractals both in three-dimensional (Brady and Ball, 1984) or essentially two-dimensional (i.e. very thin, Matsushita, et al., 1984, Kaufman, et al., 1986) cells. Several groups including ours then turned to the study of the transitions between various sorts of patterns in the formation of zinc deposits (Sawada, et al., 1986, Grier, et al., 1986). In more recent experiments our group has also looked at other metals such as copper.

Our cells consist of plates of plastic spaced by about 0.1 mm between which a film of electrolyte is confined. The deposits typically are made on a small cathode in the center of the cell and the anode is in a form of a ring a few centimeters in diameter.

It may, at first glance seem that electrochemical growth cannot be treated as diffusion-limited because in real electrochemical cells the ions rarely move under the influence of a density gradient alone. If the electric fields in the system are not screened out, there is a drift current in addition to the diffusion current. In particular, the electrical characteristics of our apparatus is ohmic, indicating that there are very definitely electric fields in the solution.

In fact, as pointed out by Brady and Ball (1984), Sander (1987) and Kessler, et al. (1988) this is quite misleading because in the quasi-static limit *both* the electrostatic potential and the density obey the same equation, the Laplace equation. In fact, we can think of u as representing the electrochemical potential of the chemically active species, say the zinc, and for the moment assume that the SO_4 acts as a uniform background. Now, for a dilute solution:

$$\begin{aligned} u &= k_B T \ln(c) + q\phi + X(T) \\ &\approx k_B T\, \delta c / c_o + q\phi + X(T) \end{aligned} \tag{7}$$

Here we have linearized the concentration, c, of the zinc with respect to its spatial average, c_o (which we can do at very low voltages, $qV/k_BT < 1$); q is the charge on the zinc. X(T) is a function of temperature alone. Now, using the Nernst-Einstein relation, we have for the current density:

$$\mathbf{j} = -(qc_oB/k_BT)\,\nabla u.$$

Since the current is conserved, in the quasi-static regime, we recover $\nabla \cdot \mathbf{j} = 0 = \nabla^2 u$. Even though there is both diffusion and drift in the system in this case, as long as the gradients have time to relax, there is a problem of the Stefan form. In fact, in our experiments, we believe that we are in the Laplacian growth regime even at large voltages because there is substantial small-scale convection in the cell, which we observe by watching the transport of ground glass. It is likely, and we intend to check this by direct measurement, that the density is completely mixed, leading once more to the Laplace equation, this time from the drift current alone.

As we have already seen (Figures 1 and 2) by changing growth conditions we can pass from fractal to dendritic growth. In the fractal regime (which is the case of very slow growth in our case) the patterns have been carefully measured and have a fractal dimension close to that of the DLA simulations, about 1.7. The dendritic regime (Figure 2) is occurs for high voltages and concentrations, i.e., for fast growth. It seems clear, from the discussion above, that these zinc leaves are being stabilized by some sort of anisotropy, which seems to be kinetic in origin. This effect is special to zinc; we have not produced any similar pattern in copper or other metals that we have looked at. Its origin in the physics and electrochemistry of zinc surfaces is presently under investigation.

However, and this was the surprise in the original work (Sawada et al., 1986, Grier et al., 1986), for intermediate growth rates we find a pattern that we did not see in the viscous fingering experiments. It has many tip-splittings like a fractal, but its overall outline is stably round in a round cell, and its average density is constant (see Figure 3). We call this the dense radial pattern In the next section we will see how it fits in to the overall picture.

THE DENSE RADIAL PATTERN

The pattern illustrated in Figure 3 is ubiquitous in deposition experiments. We find it in deposition from salts of zinc, copper, cadmium, and other metals. It was found by

Hibbert and Melrose (1987) in a deposition experiment of copper in a filter paper support. It is, however, extremely puzzling.

The main thing that puzzled us and other workers in the field was that this pattern seems to be immune to the Mullins-Sekerka instability. The outline is round, and appears to become rounder as the pattern grows. But, in terms of the considerations at the beginning of this paper, its seems that a round shape should be unstable: one of the filaments should get ahead of the others, by a fluctuation, and then grow unstably because it is then in a region where the voltage is higher; and the electic field at the surface is bigger This does not happen, however. Instead, the pattern typically grows rounder as it gets larger.

There have been a series of explanations in the literature of this phemonenon (Voss and Tomkiewicz, 1985, Ben-Jacob, et al., 1986; Sander, 1987; Grier et al., 1988). We will present here our arguments for discarding all but the last explanation, which is based on a consideration of the resistance of the metal deposit itself. That is, we think that because the longer filaments which fluctuate ahead have an extra voltage drop because they are longer, they do not grow faster, but mor slowly than the others.

Before we go into the details of our explanation, it might bewell to explain what the dense radial pattern is not. It is not, as one might first guess (because electric fields are present), a result of straight-line motion in the fluid, i.e., ballistic aggregation, which makes compact clusters (see Sander 1986 and references therein). In a fluid the mean free path of an ion is very short, and ions move at terminal velocity. That is, they follow electric field lines and diffuse down density gradients which are very complex because of the complex boundary conditions at the cathode.

We do not believe that we are out of the quasi-static regime, as we previously suggested (Sander, 1987). The simulations of Voss and Tomkiewicz (1985), multiparticle DLA, amount to the same assumption, as has been shown theoretically (Nauenberg, et al., 1984). Our quarrel with this view is experimental: if we were really in the regime of the full diffusion equation, Equation (1), then the pattern would be independent of what happens beyond a certain length, the diffusion length. In that case, the patterns would not depend on the shape of the electrode at distances large compared with some short length. However, a glance at Figure 4 shows that this is not so: the pattern follows what look to be electric field lines, and we have a Laplacian growth problem. We are somehow contriving to integrate the Laplacian growth stably, which should not be possible, because of the Mullins-Sekerka instability.

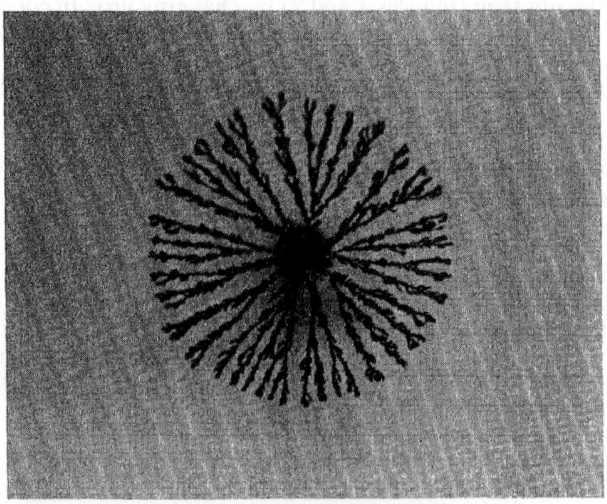

Figure 3. A dense radial deposit of zinc.

Figure 5 shows another example of the long-range effects of the electrodes, the mysterious Hecker effect (Sander, 1987), which is an abrupt change in density of a copper electrodeposit half-way between the anode and cathode that occurs over a large range of conditions within the dense radial regime. We do not know why this occurs, but it certainly reflects the fact that long-range fields are present in the cell.

The work of Ben-Jacob, et al. (1986) appeals only to a kinetic term in the boundary condition. It is easy to see that this will not give stable growth by itself, but it is not very different from our view, the essentials of which are in Grier, et al. (1987). In this treatment, we suggested that the metal deposit has an appreciable resistance compared to the electrolyte. If we model the pattern of Figure 3 as a disk, then we may associate with the disk an effective resistivity, ρ_d Note that this may be a rather large number, even if the metal which forms it is a good conductor, because the pattern is composed of a number of very fine branches (in our case, about 0.05mm in diameter.) In fact, we can directly measure ρ_d by measuring the dependence of the total resistance of the cell on the fraction occupied by metal. We find that the ratio of ρ_d to ρ_e, the resistivity of the electrolyte, is about 0.1. This is within a factor of 2 of what we estimate from the geometry of the pattern.

Now the boundary condition on the potential which replaces Equation (3) (we totally neglect surface tension because the branches are disconnected) is:

$$u_s = \sigma \rho_d r_s \ln(r_s/r_o)v \tag{8}$$

This is nothing more than Ohm's law for a disk of metal of outer radius r_s and inner (cathode) radius r_o, using conservation of mass (Equation (6)) for the current

We now performed a linear stability analysis of Equations (4), (5), and (8). We found that the growth rate of a bump on the surface is negative (stable growth) if the bump

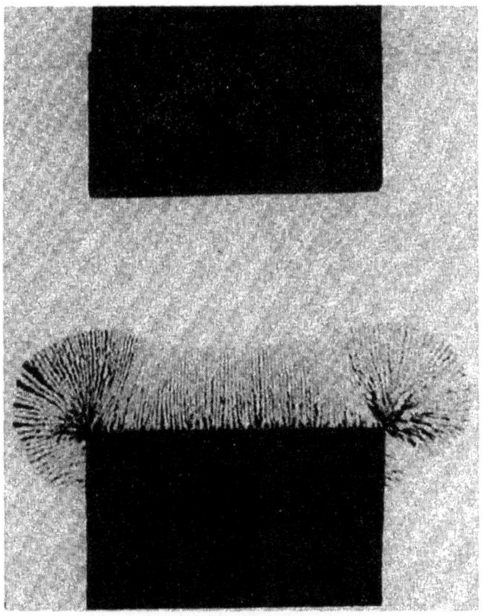

Figure 4. Copper deposit showing the effects of electrode shape.

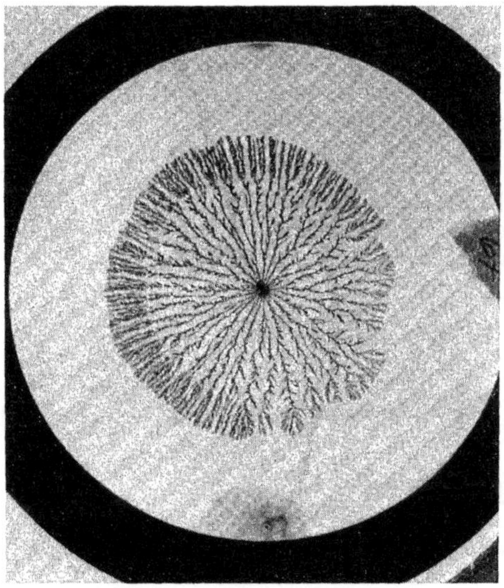

Figure 5. The Hecker effect in copper. The density change occurs half-way out.

is wide enough, even if $\rho_d/\rho_e < 1$. In our situation, our analysis shows that we have stability for long wavelength perturbations for ρ_d/ρ_e greater than about 0.05.

There is a subtlety in this analysis which we must note. We assume, in Equation (8), that the current inside the deposit flows radially, and the voltage drop is measured by the distance from the center. If the deposit were indeed a solid disk, this would not be valid, since the current could flow azimuthally inside as well as outside. We would be forced to solve two coupled Laplace equations. This can be done, of course, and it shows that the Mullins-Sekerka instability persists unless $\rho_d/\rho_e>1$. This is well-known for the case of viscous fingering, where the analogous situation is that of finite viscosity contrast. The finely divided nature of the pattern of Figure 3 is the necessary for the stabilization to occur; we have, not, in fact, linearized around a solid disk, but around the dense radial pattern itself.

All of our measurements of dense radial patterns, so far, are consistent with the picture that we have given, namely Laplacian growth stabilized by finite resistance. We are in the process of conducting a systematic study to see what controls the resistance of the deposit when we change the control parameters, voltage and concentration. For some reason that we do not understand, slow growth must correspond to low resistance, so that we see apparently fractal patterns, and faster growth to high resistance, so that we cross over to dense radial pattern formation. And we are trying to understand the effects of the convection of the electrolyte that we mentioned above.

SUMMARY

In this chapter we have tried to give some guide for the richness of diffusive pattern formation. The fundamental picture, that noisy, or isotropic conditions lead to DLA-like fractals, and that anisotropy can lead to dendrites, is consistent with all of the evidence that we are familiar with. The dense radial pattern, which is explained by a slight generalization of the basic model, is an interesting morphology in its own right.

There are two directions in which further work should be done on the matters discussed here. One is experimental: there is a good deal that we do not understand about the electrochemical system we have worked on such as the Hecker effect, what controls the crossover to dense radial, how zinc dendrites form, etc. Some of these will probably lead us into details of electrochemistry, but there are probably a number of lessons to still be learned about the general nature of the formation of complex patterns, some of them fractal, from this system.

In another vein, we should notice that the strong analogy between deposition and viscous fingering would lead us to suspect that for low viscosity contrast, a sufficiently complex pattern of fingers might stabilize into a round pattern (J. Maher, private communication). This possibility should be pursued both experimentally and theoretically.

ACKNOWLEDGEMENTS

We would like to acknowledge helpful discussions with R. Ball, N. Hecker, D. Kessler, H. Levine, and J. Maher. Supported by NSF Grant DMR-88-15908.

REFERENCES

Ben-Jacob, E., Deutscher, G., Garik P., Goldenfeld, N.D. and Lareah, Y., 1986, Phys. Rev. Lett. **57**, 1903.

Ben-Jacob, E., Godbey, R., Goldenfeld, N.D., Koplik, J., Levine, H., Mueller, T. and Sander, L.M., 1985, Phys. Rev. Lett. **55**, 1315.

Bensimon, D., Kadanoff, L.P., Liang, S., Shraiman, B., and Tang, C., 1986, Rev. Mod. Phys. **58**, 977.

Brady, R. and Ball, R. C., 1984, Nature (London) **309**, 225.

Dougherty, A., Kaplan, P.D. and Gollub, J.P., 1987, Phys. Rev. Lett. **58**, 1652.
Grier, D., Ben-Jacob, E., Clarke, R. and Sander, L.M., 1986, Phys. Rev. Lett. **56**, 1264.
Grier, D., Kessler, D., and Sander, L.M., 1987, Phys. Rev. Lett. **59**, 2315.
Hibbert, D. B., and Melrose, J. R., 1987, Phys. Rev. **A**
Kaufman, J., Baker, C., Nazzal, A., Flickner, M., Melroy, O., and Kapitulnik, A., 1986 Phys. Rev. Lett. **56**, 1932.
Kessler, D. Koplik, J. and Levine, H., 1988, Adv. in Phys., **37**, 255.
Langer, J.S., 1980, Rev. Mod. Phys. **52**, 1.
Matsushita, M. Sano, M., Hayakawa Y., Honjo, H., and Sawada, Y., 1984, Phys. Rev. Lett. **52**, 286.
Mullins, W.W., and Sekerka, R., 1957, J. Appl. Phys. **28**, 333.
Nauenberg, M., Richter, R., and Sander, L., 1983, Phys. Rev. **B28**, 1649.
Niemeyer, L., Pietronero, L., and Weismann, H., 1984, Phys. Rev. Lett. **52**, 1033.
Nittman, J., Daccord, G. and Stanley, H., 1985, Nature **314**, 141.
Paterson, L., 1984, Phys. Rev. Lett. **52**, 1621.
Radnoczi, G., Vicsek, T., Sander, L., and Grier, D., 1987, Phys. Rev. **A 35** , Rapid Communications, 4012.
Sander, L., 1986, Nature, **322**, 789.
Sander, L., 1987, in "Physics of Structure Formation", (Springer, W. Guttinger and G. Dangelmayer, eds.)
Sawada, Y., Dougherty, A. and Gollub, J.P., 1986, Phys. Rev. Lett.**56**, 1260.
Voss R. and Tomkiewicz, M., 1985, J. Electrochem. Soc., **132**, 371
Witten, T.A. and Sander, L.M., 1981, Phys. Rev. Lett. **47**, 1400.
Witten, T.A. and Sander, L.M., 1983, Phys. Rev. **B 27**, 5686.

ON THE POSSIBLE APPLICATION OF

FRACTAL SCALING IDEAS IN DENDRITIC GROWTH

R.C. Ball

Cavendish Laboratory
Madingley Road
Cambridge CB3 0HE, U.K.

This paper is concerned not with the nearly parabolic shape of dendritic growth near its forward tip, but with the eventual large scale morphology which develops as sidebranches grow and further levels of branching evolve. We focus on the ideal case, where growth is limited by the kinetics of pure diffusion in the medium ahead of the growth in competition only with the energetics of surface tension at its surface.

In practice there will always be a finite diffusion length, beyond which diffusion cannot keep up with the advance of the growing dendrite, and gravitational perturbations may also play a significant role. However it is possible in principle for the diffusion-controlled regime to give an indefinitely wide range of scales between the radius of the growing tip and the overall size of the dendrite.

There is relatively little experimental or theoretical information available directly concerning this regime for dendritic growth, but we do know a great deal about the related 'Diffusion Limited Aggregation' (DLA) model introduced by Witten and Sander[1] in which there is only diffusion control and the intrinsic instability of this process with respect to branching on all scales is limited only by the fixed lattice scale used. Here a statistically self-similar fractal structure is grown whose fractal dimension can be related to the singular probability of growth occurring at the outermost tips of the cluster.

It is widely believed that in DLA the total flux $\mu(r)$ diffusing onto the growth within a distance r from an extreme tip scales (within statistical fluctuation) as[2]

$$\mu(r) \approx \mu_{TOT}(r/R)^{\beta},$$

where μ_{TOT} is the total flux onto the growth. A simple geometric interpretation of this scaling is in terms of the tip of the cluster being as effectively screened from the incoming diffusion field as would be that of a cone[2,3,4]. This cone picture provides a useful visualisation of the argument below, but is not strictly necessary; it also puts simple bounds on β: $1/2 \le \beta \le 1$ in $d=2$ and $d-2 \le \beta \le d-1$ in $d \ge 3$.

Let us now suppose that similar scaling for $\mu(r)$ obtains in dendritic solidification; the value of b need not match DLA and most importantly we cannot take for granted the value of the tip radius which will depend on the outcome of competition between diffusion and surface tension.

Fractals' Physical Origin and Properties
Edited by L. Pietronero
Plenum Press, New York

All recent theories of dendritic solidification agree that the condition for the tip radius a is given in terms of the tip velocity v, in appropriately reduced units, by[5]

$$va^2 = \text{constant}.$$

The constant on the RHS of this equation has been of intense interest and debate, and has recently been shown to be critically dependent on the anisotropy of the surface tension (at least for unsidebranched solutions); for the present purposes it suffices that it be non-zero[6].
We can determine both a and v by using the assumed tip scaling for the flux which gives the further velocity relation

$$v \approx \mu(a)a^{1-d} \approx \mu(b)b^{\beta}a^{1-d-\beta},$$

where b is an arbitrary (but larger than a and fixed) reference lengthscale which we exploit below.

Eliminating the tip radius from the above pair of relations gives a result of the form

$$v_{tip} \approx [b^{\beta}\mu(b)]^{\eta}$$

where the new exponent η is given by

$$\eta = 2/(\beta+3-d).$$

Now imagine that we view the dendrite strucuture and the diffusion field on the coarser scale b, which we choose to be larger than the radius of any significant growing tip, including those of sidebranches. The advance of some region (of scale b) of the growth with time will follow the velocity of its own true, fastest fine scale tip which we can no longer resolve. However if we assume that our analysis above applies to each such region, we can relate its tip velocity back to the coarse scale diffusion field using the above relations and we have a closed coarse scale version of the original growth problem.

The new coarse scale model of course lacks many prefactors and details, but the scaling part of its specification matches precisely the 'Dielectric Breakdown Model' (DBM) of Niemeyer, Pietronero and Wiesman[7]. They introduced the rule of

$$\text{growth probability} \sim (\text{diffusion flux})^{\eta}$$

using a lattice of fixed scale and η as a purely phenomenological parameter. In the present interpretation η is fixed by the self-consistency condition above matching it to the strength of the singularities in the diffusion field for clusters grown using that same value of η. Numerically this is an unappealing but entirely practical specification.

In three (and higher) dimensions the selected value of η must lie between $\eta=2$ (consistent with the lowest possible value of $\beta=d-2$) and $\eta=1$ (consistent with the highest possible value of $\beta=d-1$), assuming that β is monotonic in η. In two dimensions we have similarly that $1<\eta<4/3$.

We can also find an equivalent relationship by coarse graining the other way round, from a much finer scale DBM up to the dendrite. Around each growing tip we must coarse-grain up to a local scale a such that the conditions for a stable dendrite tip are satisfied:

$$va^2 \approx \mu(a)a^{3-d} = \text{constant}.$$

This then relates the advancing tips of the dendrite to a covering of the DBM whose scale of refinement varies according to the local fluxes.

Because the true unnormalised flux enters the tip condition we have a non-negligigble choice of growing conditions or 'ensemble'. Taking the total flux μ_{TOT} to be normalised to a constant with time may seem the simplest, but this 'constant flux ensemble' corresponds to the rate of mass gain by the dendrite not increasing as it grows bigger. More typically we would have a constant difference in temperature or composition driving the growth, which leads to μ_{TOT} increasing with the radius of the growth as R^{d-2}. In what follows below we focus on the latter 'constant potential ensemble'.

We can readily find the radius-mass relationship for the dendrite as it grows although this should not be interpreted in terms of a fractal dimension because it reflects also changes in the tip radii. We have

$$dM/dt = \mu_{TOT}$$

and, using the DBM version of the growth,

$$dR/dt \sim [\ \mu_{TOT} R^{-\beta}\ ]^{\eta}.$$

Eliminating the time and integrating in the constant potential ensemble then gives the growth law

$$M \sim R^{d+1-\eta},$$

where the self-consistency condition for η and β has been used.

The distribution of growth rates in the DBM model is known to be very broad, conforming to the multifractal scaling that

$$(R/a)^{f(\alpha)} \quad \text{regions of size } a \quad \text{have} \quad \mu(a)/\mu_{TOT} \approx (R/a)^{-\alpha}.$$

As a result we will have a correspondingly broad distribution of tip radii in the dendrite and different features of the dendrite may be dominated by tips of quite different radii. The distribution of tip radii may be found by enforcing the velocity condition

$$v \approx R^{d-2}\ (a/R)^{\alpha}\ a^{1-d} \quad \approx \quad a^{-2}$$

so that for a given tip radius a we must have

$$\alpha+3-d \quad = \quad \ln(R)/\ln(R/a)$$

and the number of tips growing with radius a scales as

$$(R/a)^{f(d-3\ +\ \ln(R)/\ln(R/a)\ )} \quad = \quad R^{f(\alpha)/(\alpha+3-d)}.$$

The total number of tips is given by R^{q_t} where for $q=q_t$

$$(3-d)q + \tau(q)=0,$$

where $q=df/d\alpha$ and $\tau(q)$ is[2] the Legendre Transform of $df/d\alpha$, $\tau(q)=q\alpha-f$. In d=3 dimensions this gives the particularly simple result that $q_t=1$. Similar results obtain for the total surface area R^{d-1+q_s} and mass R^{d+q_m} of the tips where for q_s, $d-1+\ (3-d)q\ +\tau(q)=0$, and for q_m, $d+\ (3-d)q\ +\tau(q)=0$. However these results should be treated with some caution as they are dominated by parts of the tip distribution corresponding to very slow growth.

All of the above analysis assumes that tips are still stably growing and takes no account of the possibility that screening of the diffusion field might set in quickly enough to drive them into recession (negative growth). Thus it is unclear whether we can expect the mass calculated above to be dominated by slowly growing tips to agree with the mass calculated earlier by integrating the acretion.

REFERENCES

1. T. A. Witten and L. M. Sander, Phys. Rev. Lett. **47** 1400 (1981).
2. T. C. Halsey, P. Meakin and I. Procaccia, Phys. Rev. Lett. **56** 854 (1986).
3. R. C. Ball, R. M. Brady, G. Rossi and B. R. Thompson, Phys. Rev. Lett. **55** 1040 (1985).
4. L. Turkevich and H. Scher, Phys. Rev. Lett. **55** 1026 (1985).
5. J. S. Langer, Rev. Mod. Phys. **52** 1 (1980).
6. see, e.g. J. S. Langer, Physicsa **140A** 44-50 (1986).
7. L. Niemeyer, L. Pietronero and H. J. Weismann, Phys. Rev. Lett. **52** 1033 (1984).

REALISTIC MODELS OF DIELECTRIC BREAKDOWN

H.J. Wiesmann

ABB Corporate Research
CH-5405 Baden, Switzerland

INTRODUCTION

Dielectric breakdown phenomena are observed, whenever the electric field in an insulating medium exceeds a critical value. The breakdown process creates a conducting structure within the dielectric. We want to understand the structural properties of the patterns. We focus on the conditions under which they become fractal and in particular we want to clarify the nature of cut-off parameters to which real systems are subject. These specific aspects of the breakdown problem have often been neglected in the past. One of the reasons is the following: the main technical interest in electrical breakdown is motivated by the objective to construct reliable insulating systems. The consequence is a concentration on the breakdown voltage and, in a deeper context, on the underlying microscopic processes. The structural properties of breakdown are a complementary aspect of the problem and its relevance for technical systems has been realized only in the past years. The more it is remarkable that the first experiments, carried out by Lichtenberg in 1777, were done with a strong interest in the morphology of the discharge figures.

In order to understand the significance of breakdown models for real phenomena, let us point out some characteristic properties of the physical breakdown process. As a simple specific example we consider a system of two electrically conducting parallel plates with an insulating medium in between. Carrying out an experiment on this system means, to apply a voltage to the electrodes and to increase it with time. The question 'how fast' is of importance but has to be answered later. Nevertheless let us remark that most breakdown models are formulated as quasi-stationary boundary value problems. Typically we observe the formation of a spark at a *critical value* of the external voltage. It connects the electrodes in a singular path, which breaks the original symmetry of the system (translation). Apparently there is a *random element* in the system, responsible for the choice of the path. Even in a needle-plate geometry, where the starting point is a priori determined, we observe randomness in the shape of the path.

Fractals' Physical Origin and Properties
Edited by L. Pietronero
Plenum Press, New York

A more careful resolution of the experiment leads us to the distinction of at least *two phases*, concerning the time evolution of the breakdown procedure. In a first one, which should be considered as the true intrinsic process, there is no conducting path yet between the electrodes. Only in the second one this connection is established, whereupon the capacity formed by the electrodes is discharged. The discharge proceeds along a one-dimensional path which in general is selected from the previously formed structure by a criterion of 'first connection'. It is combined with a high current density, heat dissipation and luminosity. Therefore the observation of the first phase is often covered by the high intensity of the second one. Although this final discharge is the essential and often lethal effect for every technical system, it is in a more fundamental sense an artefact of the arbitraryness of boundary conditions. It is a finite-size effect. If breakdown structures can be associated with fractal properties, it is certainly the pattern which is formed during the first phase. As a remark we may add that in a Lichtenberg-type experiment (discharge along a solid-gas interface) the final electric connection of the electrodes is avoided and allows a pure observation of the first phase.

For a full understanding of breakdown processes both microscopic and global or structural aspects have to be considered. But in most cases this can be done only in a complementary way. Roughly speaking the microscopic attempt neglects the global structure and vice versa. A macroscopic theory, being able to describe global aspects will contain at least the following elements as a minimum:

a) the geometrical definition of the system, including electrodes
b) the specification of the dielectric material
c) the solution of the electrostatic field equations before and during breakdown
d) a local law for the dynamic breakdown process, based on b) and c).

Within this framework we have a large variety of possibilities to attribute random properties to the system. We mention some examples before discussing the consequences for the breakdown behavior.

α) Surface roughness of the electrodes will induce fluctuations in the field strength near the surface.

β) Quenched random properties of the dielectric material will certainly influence the breakdown process[1-3].
We have to distinguish two typical cases of different nature. An example of one type is a ceramic material with random voids[4]. Here the essential random element is the completely different breakdown condition in the solid and in the gas-filled holes. It is not the local variation of the electric field due to different values of the dielectric constant of the voids and the ceramic itself, which is only minor. An example of a different type is a metal-loaded dielectric[5] (below the percolation critical point). Here the strong field enhancement near the conductive inclusions is essential, whereas the breakdown field in the insulator will vary only weakly or even be constant.

γ) Timelike fluctuations within the dielectric initiate or affect in many cases the breakdown. Examples are fluctuations in the number of free electrons in a gas, scattering- and ionization processes in connection with radiation[6], and micro-discharges (prebreakdown) in epoxy resins[7]. We can again distinguish between effects that strongly affect the local field distribution and others that mainly affect breakdown conditions directly.

One could expect that it is possible to determine typical breakdown patterns corresponding to the nature of the random element in the system. This is not directly true. The key role for the structural properties of the discharge pattern is played by the form of the growth law governing the dynamics of the breakdown process. This becomes plausible by comparing two opposite versions of a growth law.

i) A strict threshold law assumes breakdown exactly if the local field intensity exceeds the threshold value. Therefore the degree of freedom for the local breaking processes is small, we have low or no ramification at all. The breakdown path has generically dimension one. Grosso modo, this is independent of the random properties of the material, although they may strongly influence the detailed shape of the path.

ii) In contrast to the situation i), a very smooth breakdown law will open a large number of degrees of freedom, which potentially allows much richer structures with high ramification.

Summarizing we can say that the more selective the process is, the closer we are to a one dimensional structure, the less selective it is, the closer we are to the case of diffuse breakdown. From a fractal point of view the interesting domain is between the extreme situations i) and ii). Real processes cover the whole range. If the corresponding patterns do not show true fractal properties, this is in most cases due to cut off parameters like the critical field for onset of breakdown and due to dissipative processes.

In section 2 we will discuss 'ideal' and 'realistic' models for breakdown. The ideal model is characterized by an equipotential conducting structure and zero critical field. It allows a one parameter family of fractal structures exhibiting different H-dimensions. We discuss whether there is a physical background to this mathematical fact. In addition we examine the influence of a critical field and the consequences of dissipative processes in the conducting phase. Dissipation leads to an internal field $E_i > 0$ in the discharge channels and therefore to a non constant potential distribution.

In section 3 we give numerical examples, illustrating the influence of critical and internal field strength.

In section 4 we consider gas discharges. We distinguish two types of processes. In 'leader' discharges we have thermal equilibrium between free electrons and atoms. They are an example of low dissipation with respect to the current density. 'Streamers', a process initiating the final leader discharge, are characterized by a high electron and a low gas temperature with high dissipation. We sketch a generalized breakdown model which is able to describe gas discharges in a unified way including as well equilibrium and non-equilibrium process.

IDEAL AND REALISTIC MODELS

The essential idealization made in the original NPW breakdown model[8] is the assumption of a perfect conducting phase growing in a perfect insulator ($\sigma = \infty$ and $\sigma = 0$ respectively) and the omission of a critical field ($E_c = 0$). The latter assumption is equivalent to the statement that the process is independent of the applied voltage. From a physical point of view this assumption seems to be absurd. Nevertheless the implications of the assumption on the properties of the resulting structure are less severe than a replacement of the perfect conductor by an imperfect one. This should be understood and will be explained in the following.

Let us first show that a voltage-independent process is equivalent to a power law behavior of the growth probability measure, expressed as a function of the surface field. If μ denotes the lattice growth probability from site $\underline{k}$ to $\underline{l}$ (with $|\underline{k} - \underline{l}| = 1$) depending in an arbitrary way on the surface field $(\phi_k - \phi_l)$, then μ is of the form

$$\mu(k,l) = f(|\phi_k - \phi_l|) / \sum_{(m,n)} f(|\phi_m - \phi_n|) \tag{1}$$

The sum is taken over all surface bonds. If the voltage ϕ is changed to $\lambda\phi$ then μ is not affected if f fulfils the equation

$$f(\lambda y) = h(\lambda) \cdot f(y) \tag{2}$$

for arbitrary h. This is equivalent to

$$F(\lambda y) = F(\lambda) \cdot F(y) \tag{3}$$

if we put $F(y) = f(y) / f(1)$. The only measurable solution of (3) is a power law, leading to

$$f(y) = cst \cdot y^{\eta}, \qquad y > 0 \tag{4}$$

In the case of a *perfect* conducting phase the applied voltage is the only physical parameter in the problem. Independence of the voltage means that the whole information governing growth is contained in the geometrical properties of the conductor. The solution of the boundary value problem determines local from global properties. As we know, the resulting structures are self similar fractals but their properties are different for different exponents η. In other words: we do not have one 'ideal' structure from which 'real' objects can be distinguished by several values of cutoff parameters. We have a whole family of ideal objects. If we consider the real case of a non perfect conductor, we can maintain the equivalence of voltage independence and power law. Note that this is only the case if the mechanisms leading to non uniform potential distribution on the interface are restricted to a class, for which the ratio

ϕ_{k1} / ϕ_{k2}

is independent of the electrode voltage. k_1 and k_2 denote 2 different interface points. Nevertheless, the resulting structures will no longer be true fractals, as will be shown below.

Introducing a critical breakdown field E_c, i.e. putting

$$f(y) = 0 \qquad \text{for} \qquad y < E_c , \qquad\qquad y > 0 \tag{5}$$

is not compatible with (4). But we can still consider (4) to be valid for $y > E_c$. This means that the growth law is modified (cut-off) in those points of the conductor surface where the field is low. The extension of this domain is the smaller, the larger the applied voltage is. In addition its growth probability is smaller than that of the high field domains ($\eta > 0$). This is the reason, why the power law (4) gives realistic results at least in the high voltage limit.

The remaining question is, whether the probability exponent η has a physical or only a mathematical meaning. The question may be weakened to : can we give physical reasons for having a *family* of different growth laws. A rigorous treatment of this question goes far beyond the current context and needs a detailed microscopic analysis (see also[9]). Nevertheless we want to give two possible answers. The wrong answer would be to associate η or a similar parameter, numbering different growth laws, with different quenched random properties of the dielectric material. A better answer is probably linked with the question concerning the velocity with which the boundary values are changed (voltage increase) and with the fact that ionization coefficients are strongly nonlinear in the electric field. We may notice that there is a discrepancy between the experimental situation, where we have time and space dependent boundary conditions and the 'quasi-stationary' models with a stationary boundary value on a (stepwise) moving boundary. How are the dynamic experimental situation and the quasi-stationary model related to each other? If the local potential depends linearly on the electrode voltage, and if we assume a strict non-probabilistic threshold law which causes local breakdown as soon and immediately if the increasing field E exceeds the critical one E_c, then the dynamic process is equivalent to a quasi stationary one, supposed that in the latter growth occurs according to a maximum principle. In other words: the bond with maximum field in the stationary case is identical to the one which reaches next in time E_c in the time dependent process. Within the family of ideal models this corresponds to the limit of large η. The case of a strict threshold is often assumed to be the standard case[1,2]. However, if the microscopic process which is modeled by a breaking bond needs a typical intrinsic time, then the question is relevant, whether the boundary values change fast or slow compared to this time unit. A fast increase can simultaneously increase the local field above E_c at several sites, before the conducting structure will be changed and together with it the field solution. This is an important justification for the probability-function used in the breakdown model. It does not solely reflect quenched stochastic properties of the dielectric.

Dissipative Processes

The most drastic deviations from fractal breakdown behavior are obtained, if we introduce dissipative processes in the conducting phase. It seems clear that by mutually approaching the conductivities of the conducting and the insulating domain we reach a point, where the typical instabilities with filamentary patterns disappear. Such regimes are observed in polymers[10] ('charge injection') and in gases ('diffuse corona' formation). They are also found in electrodeposition[11,12] and have been analysed and modeled in[13]. For a rigorous description of this situation we need a second system of partial difference / differential equations, which determine the state of the conducting domain. Instead of a boundary value problem we have to treat an interface problem, with continuity conditions to be fulfilled at the interface. The growth law can then be formulated in an analogous way as before on the basis of the interface field. The essential point thereby is not the study of a specific mechanism for the resistance. Many systems can not be treated as Ohmic resistances (mobility edge e.g.) Therefore we simplify the full problem. Instead of solving an equation which describes the conducting phase with its specific dissipation, we modify the original boundary value problem. We introduce a variation $\phi_o - \delta\phi$ of the original constant potential distribution ϕ_o in the conducting domain. If $-\delta\phi$ corresponds to a potential-decrease along current lines, this can always be interpreted as the consequence of a dissipative mechanism. On a lattice structure the procedure becomes particularly simple. On a tree the potential has to decrease in growth direction.

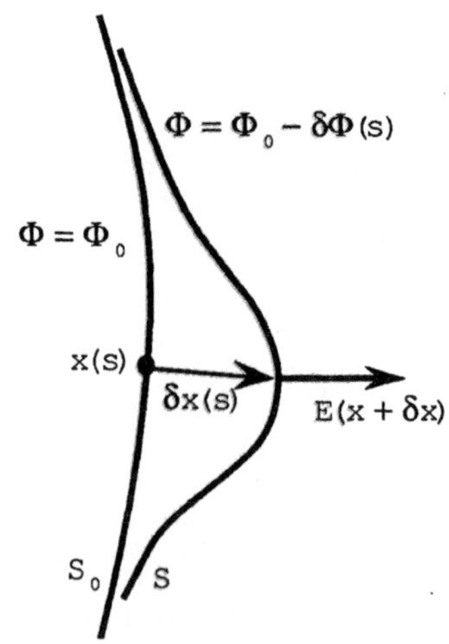

Fig. 1. Perturbation S of the growing interface S_o. Small dissipation (small $\delta\phi$) leads to an enhanced surface field E at points of increased curvature. Large dissipation compensates the increase of E and stabilizes the interface motion.

Before studying numerical examples we discuss the main influence of resistance on the stability of a growing front in the continuum picture. To this end we compare the surface $S_o = \{x(s)\}$ of a conducting domain with its perturbation $S = \{x(s)+\delta x(s)\}$ as illustrated in figure 1. In the case of constant potential $\phi = \phi_o$ on S_o *and* S we obtain an enhancement of the surface field E(x+dx) at a point of increased curvature. Linking the surface velocity v to the surface field E in a monotonous (non sublinear) way leads to the well known Mullins-Sekerka instability[14]. Dissipation reduces the potential distribution on S to $\phi_o - \delta\phi$, as compared to S_o such that the surface field E(x+dx) is also reduced. The originally unstable situation becomes stabilized if this reduction at least compensates the enhancement caused by the variation δx in the case of constant potential.

In addition we notice that the critical breakdown field E_c defines a natural unit for the internal field E_i in the conducting domain. If a surface S_t at time t is growing to $S_{t+\delta t}$ at time $t+\delta t$ under the influence of E_t, this implies that $E_t > E_c$ in the area between S_t and $S_{t+\delta t}$. Otherwise the growth probability would be zero. Between time t and $t + \delta t$ the field-energy in the same area must have *decreased* and we have $E_i < E_t$. A restriction of the potential distribution in the conducting phase to $E_i < E_c$ avoids energetically meaningless situations. In the following we measure therefore E_i by

$$\alpha = E_i / E_c \qquad \alpha < 1 \tag{6}$$

Finally we might remark, that E_i defines an upper limit for the size of the breakdown structure and therefore a length scale. The upper limit of the range, R_{max}, is given by

$$\int_o^{R_{max}} dr \; E_i = \phi_o \qquad (\phi_o \text{ applied voltage}) \tag{7}$$

NUMERICAL SIMULATIONS

We have studied the patterns resulting from a lattice breakdown model including a critical field E_c and an internal field E_i along the discharge lines for several types of geometry and different values of the probability exponent η, i.e. we have chosen

$$p = \begin{cases} (E - E_c)^{\eta} & E > E_c \\ 0 & E < E_c \end{cases} \tag{8}$$

for the growth probability p. Alternatively one could also use $p = E^{\eta}$ for $E > E_c$. The choice (8) is due to the strong non-linearity of ionization coefficients for avalanche generation (see also [9]). They exhibit a similar threshold behavior. The potential distribution on the discharge pattern is equal to the applied voltage ϕ_o in the starting point or points (conducting electrode) and decreases by E_i along each bond in growing direction. For simplicity reasons we stick in the following to euclidean dimension $d = 3$, $\eta = 1$ and $E_i = \alpha E_c$ whit α = constant < 1 for the whole structure. This is a reasonable approximation in the case of gas discharges but in other applications we might have a different behavior.

The main results are the following:

i) The influence of the critical field depends on the applied voltage. In fact E_c/ϕ_o is the only relevant parameter in the problem. In the high voltage limit we recover the fractal structures of the original idealized ($E_c=E_i=0$) model. For low voltages the critical field acts as a cut-off for growth mainly in the screened regions. In consequence the number of bifurcations is reduced and selfsimilarity is lost. The effect of increasing the ratio E_c/ϕ_o is similar to a change of η towards higher values in the ideal model. Figure 2b illustrate an increase of E_c/ϕ_o by a factor 1.5 as compared to 2a at a moderate value of $E_i = 0.14 \cdot E_c$.

ii) Introducing an internal field into the structure, simulating the effect of dissipation, has drastic consequences as soon as E_i is no longer small compared to E_c. The fractal appearance of the structure is completely lost in the case $E_i \approx E_c$. The discharge lines do no longer exhibit strong geometrical fluctuations but become aligned approximately along the initial field line distribution. In contrast to figure 2, figure 3 shows the strong influence of a high internal field $E_i \approx E_c$. This is typical for streamers in strongly electronegative gases like SF_6.

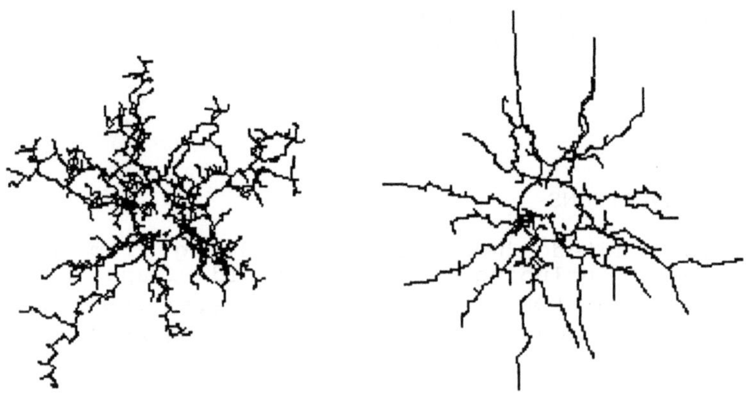

a b

Fig. 2 Influence of the critical field E_c on the lattice discharge structure for low internal field E_i. The pattern extends in 3-d space starting from a sphere of radius 5. Growth is allowed in the directions of the unit cube and its diagonals. In both cases the internal field is $E_i = 0.14 \cdot E_c$. In figure 2b E_c/ϕ_o is increased by a factor 1.5 as compared to figure 2a, where $E_c/\phi_o = 0.1$. The maximum initial field is $E_{init} = 0.17 \cdot \phi_o$. (lattice unit = 1)

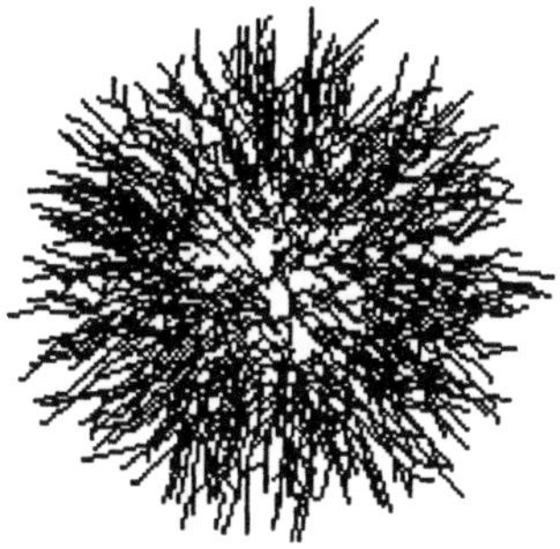

Fig. 3. Strong influence of a high internal field $E_i \approx E_c$ (dissipation) on the pattern. The fluctuations are strongly reduced and a sharp radial limitation is obtained in contrast to figure 2. The voltage corresponds to $E_c/\phi_o = 0.043$.

In all three cases growth starts from a 'spherical' electrode with a radius of 5 lattice units. This was done for comparison with a specific experimental situation.

It is interesting to compare the density of occupied lattice points as a function of radius as well as the charge per occupied point. These relations are shown in figures 4a and b. With increasing E_i the density changes from a fractal-like behavior $n \sim r^{D-3}$ to $n \sim$ constant. The fluctuations in the contour of the figure become smaller and smaller which is a direct consequence of the radial potential decrease we obtain for large E_i. At the same time the charge distribution goes over from a shape which exhibits strong screening to an other one where the charge density decreases with radius. As the density of occupied points becomes roughly constant for large E_i, the charge density per occupied point can be reinterpreted as density per volume.

The limit of large E_i with decreasing charge density therefore resembles the case of a 'diffuse corona' in gases or the homogeneous 'charge injection' in polymers. This is the simplest case of a continuous, non filamentary discharge for which in spherical geometry the internal field is radial and constant inside a sphere of radius r. Its maximum extension is given by the radius r_c at which the surface field becomes equal to the critical one. The corresponding charge distribution therefore is

$$\rho = \begin{cases} 2\varepsilon_o E_c r^{-1} & r < r_c \\ 0 & r > r_c \end{cases} \tag{9}$$

with

$$r_c^2 = r_o \cdot \phi_o / E_c \tag{10}$$

where r_o denotes the radius of the electrode with applied voltage ϕ_o against ∞.

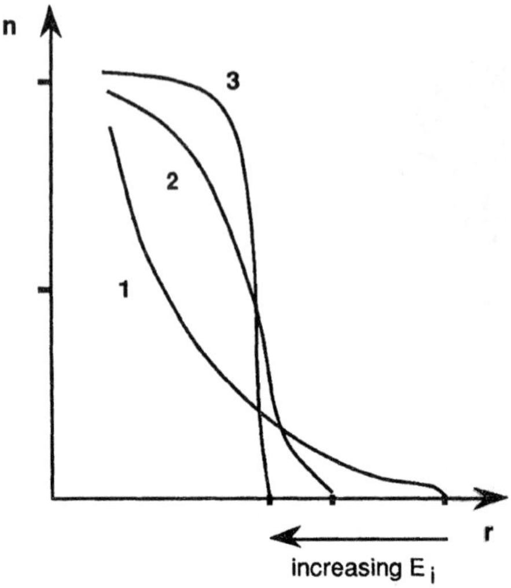

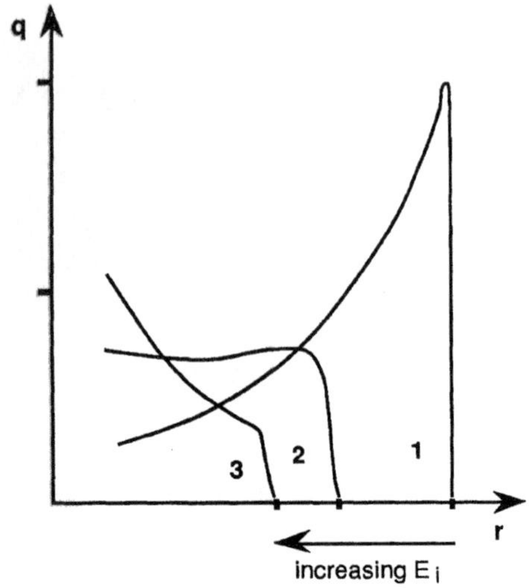

Fig. 4a. Influence of the internal field E_i on the average density n of occupied points as a function of radius. With increasing E_i the distribution changes from a fractal like $n \sim r^{D-3}$ behavior (1) to n ~ constant for $r < r_c$ (3).

Fig. 4b. Average charge of the occupied lattice sites as a function of radius. For low E_i we observe highly charged tips with a screened interior (1), whereas for large E_i the charge distribution tends to $q \sim r^{-1}$, $r<r_c$ (3).

GAS DISCHARGES

It is impossible to give a unique and coherent physical description of breakdown in gases, which could be used to judge the validity and limits of numerical models. (For general information see [15]). One reason is the asymmetry of matter with respect to the sign of charge. It requires a distinction between positive and negative polarity with different microscopic processes involved. This is obvious for asymmetric electrode configurations which a priori determine the starting point of the growth process, like a needle-plate geometry. For negative needle polarity, electron velocities have the same, whereas for positive polarity they have the opposite direction than the growth process. In the case of a symmetric configuration and a starting point in between the electrodes we may observe cathode and anode directed processes. A second reason is the fact, that we have to distinguish between nonequilibrium phenomena like streamer propagation, a fast process with high electron temperatures compared to the gas, and equilibrium processes like the leader discharge with similar temperature of all particles and full ionization of the gas in the channel. Therefore we will concentrate on two exemplary processes.

The main phenomenon which controls breakdown in insulation systems with electro-negative gases is the *leader* process[16]. The criterion for leader inception is of big practical importance. It depends mainly on the critical field E_c, the electrode geometry and the chemical composition of the gas. (Notice that in gases it is not the electric field E directly but the ratio $(E/n_{gas})_c$ which has a critical value, n_{gas} denoting the gas density. Nevertheless we omit the density dependence in the following.) The leader is a stepwise filamentary process that proceeds in steps of length l, depending on the relative local field E/E_c. Each leader step is triggered by a precursor originating from a single streamer within a streamer corona. The corona has been formed before, starting either from the previous leader tip or from the electrode. The process is then iterated, depending on the applied voltage, as can be seen in figure 6. Like E_c the leader channel field E_i depends on the gas density, but it is considerably smaller than E_c and decays with time during the discharge. Typical leader propagation times lie in the μs range.

In contrast to the leader with its high degree of ionization, high current density and low resistance, a streamer is characterized by a high channel field and low current density [17,18]. If enough current is fed into the streamer channel, then the dissipated energy leads to a local increase of the gas-temperature and finally to full ionization. The filament thus becomes a leader branch.

If we want to compare experimental structures, such as the leader discharge pattern or the streamer corona with results obtained from the numerical models, we may choose two different procedures:

First we consider both processes as separate events, omitting the fact that streamer coronas evolve at the tip of leader branches.

The two phenomena develop on completely different length scales. If we look at each process in its natural unit length, the remaining but important difference consists in a high value of E_i/E_c for the streamer ($\approx$ 0.14 for air up to $\approx$ 1 for SF_6) against a low one for the leader. On the basis of the numerical results we expect a relatively dense, radially oriented structure, becoming more pronounced with increasing electronegativity. This is shown in figure (5). The streamer in air corresponds to a weaker electronegativity than the one in SF_6. A continuous change of the structure is obtained by applying mixtures of air and SF_6. Notice that the geometry has cylindrical but not spherical symmetry. In contrast to this, leader discharges, as for example the Lichtenberg figure in [8] exhibit typical fractal properties. We may remark that this is not valid for the historical Lichtenberg figures. The reason is the slow voltage increase, leading to higher internal resistance.

Secondly we look at the combined streamer-leader system. This leads us to an additional insight concerning the length scales and the interpretation of the critical field E_c of the leader process.

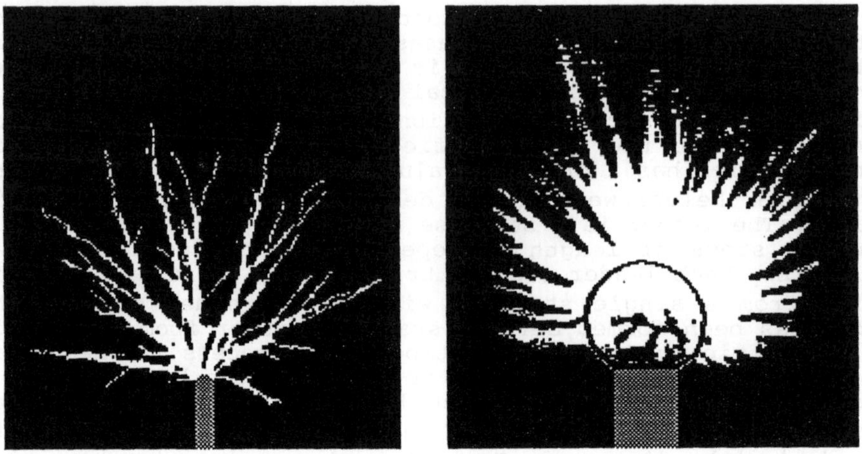

a b

Fig.5. Still photograph of experimental streamer coronas in air (fig. 5a) and in a strongly electronegative gas (fig. 5b) (80% SF_6 / 20% N_2, 0.1MPa). In air the internal field is relatively weak compared to E_c : $E_i \approx 0.14 \cdot E_c$, whereas in SF_6 it is of the same order as E_c. Scales are different.

The elementary streamer step is based on microscopic processes like photoabsorption and scattering cross sections, we do not discuss here, see [6]. The corona radius however is defined by the applied voltage ϕ_o. The potential at the streamer

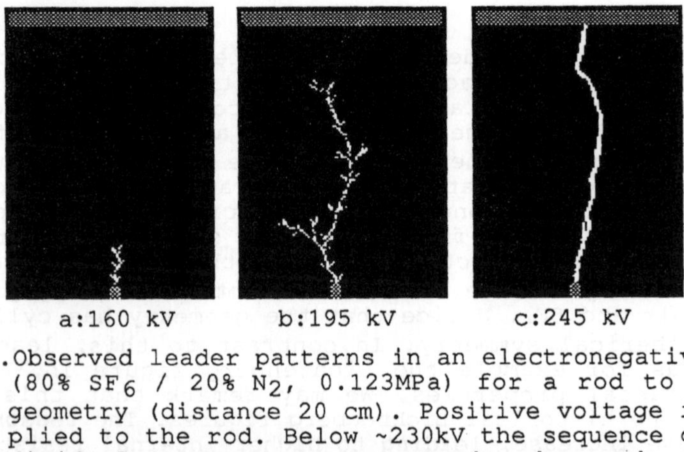

a:160 kV b:195 kV c:245 kV

Fig.6. Observed leader patterns in an electronegative gas (80% SF_6 / 20% N_2, 0.123MPa) for a rod to plane geometry (distance 20 cm). Positive voltage is applied to the rod. Below ~230kV the sequence of individual streamer coronas can be observed, out of which one branch evolves to the subsequent leader step (6a,b). After the connection of the electrodes a discharge of high intensity takes place, such that the detailed structure that evolved before is no longer observable.

tip is approximately ϕ_o - rE_i and must be large enough to maintain a tip field $E \geq E_c$. As the leader step length is correlated with the streamer corona radius, this explains the voltage dependence of the leader-step. Because of the low internal field, the leader has in general a very long range. In most cases it ends at the counter-electrode (figure 6c). Indeed it is rather difficult to produce arrested leaders experimentally as shown in figure 6a and b.

Finally we want to give a reinterpretation of the leader critical field E_c^L. This leads us to an understanding, why the simplest breakdown model, as it was introduced in [8] leads to structures that are in good qualitative agreement with real leader discharge patterns. Let us start with a streamer configuration Z_S as illustrated in figure 6 which we want to characterize by a constant internal field E_i^S along the filament of constant cross section σ. In order to find a criterion for full ionization of the channel we calculate the dissipated energy density u at time t in the point x of the streamer-channel. We obtain

$$u(t,x) = \frac{1}{\sigma} \int_{t_x}^{t} dt \;\; E_i I(t,x) \tag{11}$$

where I denotes the current in the filament at t and x and t_x the time at which x was the tip of a filament. We can express u also in terms of the total charge Q or charge density q

$$Q(t,x) = \sigma \int_{\{y|x \rightarrow y\}} ds(y)\, q(y) \tag{12}$$

carried by the part of the structure that has grown out of x : $\{y|(x \rightarrow y\}$.

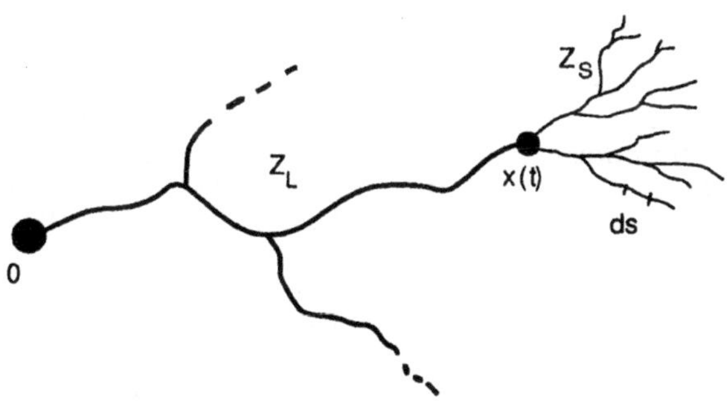

Fig. 7. Transition from a peripheral process Z_S(streamer) with high resistance to the low resistance (leader) discharge Z_L. The growth criterion for x combines the charge $Q = \int ds(y) q(y)$ with the ionization energy density u_{ion} of the channel.

Therefore we have

$$u(t,x) = \frac{1}{\sigma} E_i^s Q(t,x) \tag{13}$$

under the assumption of constant E_i^s. If we denote by u_{ion} the minimal energy-density for full ionization of the channel, then we get a charge-criterion for ionization by putting

$$Q_{ion} = \sigma/E_i^s \cdot u_{ion} \tag{14}$$

The leader tips can therefore be defined as the points

$$\{x(t) \mid Q(t,x) = Q_{ion}\} \tag{15}$$

separating the leader part Z_L (inner points with respect to x) from the peripheral streamer Z_S (peripheral points). Altogether this means that we have obtained an interpretation of the leader critical field in terms of the ionization energy density of the gas.

On the other hand Q(t,x) can be associated with the charge carried by site x in the original lattice model if applied to the leader structure. Q is equal to the sum of all field values associated with the bonds that are linked to site x. This establishes the connection with the field dependent growth probability.

REFERENCES

1. L. de Arcangelis, S. Redner, and H. Hermann, J. Phys. Lett. 46:L585 (1985).
2. P.M. Duxbury, P.L. Leath, P.D. Beale, Phys. Rev. B 36:367 (1987).
3. F. Family, Y.C. Zhang, T. Vicsek, J. Phys. A 19:L733 (1986).
4. R. Gerson, T. Marshall, J. Appl. Phys. 30:1650 (1959).
5. P.D. Beale, P.M. Duxbury, Phys. Rev. B 37:2785 (1988).
6. E. Nasser, "Fundamentals of Gaseous Ionization and Plasma Electronics", Wiley-Interscience, New York (1971).
7. E.O. Forster, IEEE Trans. Electr. Insul. EI-20:891 (1985).
8. L. Niemeyer, L. Pietronero, H.J. Wiesmann, Phys. Rev. Lett. 52:1033 (1984).
9. L. Pietronero and H.J. Wiesmann, Z. Phys. B 70:87 (1988).
10. T. Hibma and H.R. Zeller, J. Appl. Phys. 59:1614 (1986).
11. D.G. Grier, E. Ben-Jacob, Roy Clarke, and L.M. Sander, Phys. Rev. Lett. 56:1264 (1986).
12. Y. Sawada, A. Dougherty, and J.P. Gollub, Phys. Rev. Lett. 56:1260 (1986).
13. D.G. Grier, D.A. Kessler, and L.M. Sander, Phys. Rev. Lett. 59:2315 (1987).
14. W.W. Mullins and R.F. Sekerka, J. Appl. Phys. 34:323 (1963).
15. "Electrical Breakdown of Gases", J.M. Meek and J.D. Craggs, ed., John Wiley, New York (1978).

16. L. Niemeyer and H.J. Wiesmann, Modeling of Leader branching in electronegative gases, in: Proc. Vth Int. Symp. on Gaseous Dielectrics, Knoxville (1987).
17. I. Gallimberti, G. Marchesi, R. Turri, Corona formation and propagation in weakly or strongly attaching gases, in: Proc. 8th Int. Conf. on Gas Discharges, Oxford (1985).
18. L. Niemeyer and H.J. Wiesmann, Structure of the impulse corona in electronegative gases, in: Proc. IXth Int. Conf. on Gas Discharges, Venice (1988).

CLUSTER-CLUSTER AGGREGATION WITH DIPOLE-DIPOLE INTERACTIONS

R. Botet[1], G. Helgesen[2], A. T. Skjeltorp[3], P. M. Mors[4], and R. Jullien[1]

[1]Laboratoire de Physique des Solides, Université Paris-Sud, Centre d'Orsay, Bât. 510, 91405 Orsay France
[2]Department of Physics, University of Oslo 0316 OSLO 3, Norway
[3]Institute for Energy Technology, 2007 Kjeller, Norway
[4]Instituto de Fisica, Universidada Federal do Rio Grande de Sul, CP 15051, 91500 Porto Alegre, RS, Brazil

The standard Cluster-Cluster aggregation model has been introduced by Meakin (1983) and Kolb et al. (1983) to study some experimental situations where particles dispersed in a fluid medium can diffuse and aggregate by sticking. Moreover, the particles keep their individuality inside a cluster : there is no melting nor coalescence during aggregation. This can be the case for colloidal or aerosol systems.

This idea is indeed much more general than just these two examples and formation of clusters of galaxies or coagulation of blood can be seen as more complicated cases where cluster-cluster aggregation may be relevant.

To understand the new problems which arise in this field of research, it seems important to describe in details the standard model, insisting on the key points which can be relevant according to the experimental situations.

1) The standard Cluster-Cluster aggregation model

This model is defined as follows : in a square L^d box with periodic boundary conditions, disperse randomly N spheres of diameter δ, so that their concentration N/L^d is very small (we shall quantify more precisely this condition later). Two spheres can never overlap, and their centers are constrained to be situated on the vertices of a regular square lattice of step δ. Once the N spheres dispersed, one can begin the simulation. One chooses randomly one cluster in the box. At the beginning of this simulation there only exists clusters of size 1 (isolated particles). Then one chooses randomly a direction among the 2d possible directions on a d-dimensional square lattice. Now one translates the cluster of one lattice step in this direction. If after this movement, the cluster touches another one (a particle of the diffusive cluster is near-neighbour a particle of another cluster), they stick irreversibly in this relative position. Irreversibly means here that during all the rest of the simulation, the bond linking these two clusters cannot be broken.

Fractals' Physical Origin and Properties
Edited by L. Pietronero
Plenum Press, New York

Then this Monte-Carlo step is iterated : one chooses another (or the same cluster) and so on. The mean size of the clusters grows with time because of the successive sticking, and the simulation stops when there is just one cluster in the box.

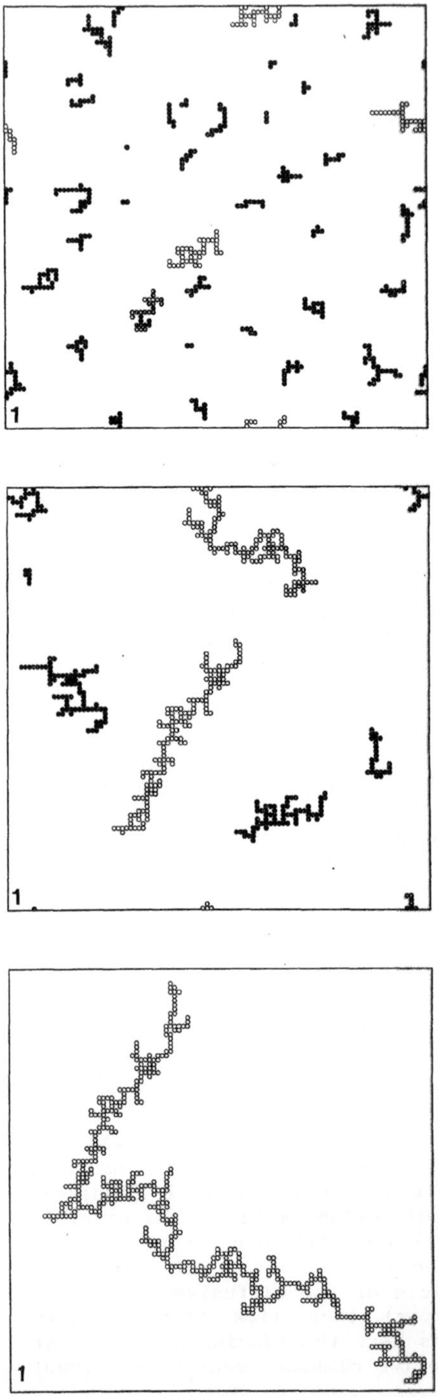

Fig. 1 Sketch of a 2 dimensional simulation of the Brownian cluster-cluster aggregation model. System of 500 particles in a 100 × 100 square box with periodic boundary conditions. Three different times are shown from up to down, with 40, 7 and 1 remaining cluster in the box respectively. Different grey tones correspond to different sizes. White is for the largest cluster.

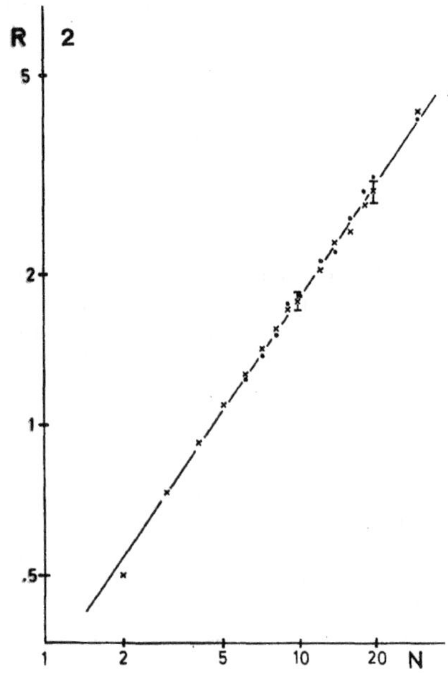

Fig. 2. Logarithm of the radius of gyration versus the number of particles for a typical 2-dimensional simulation like the one shown in figure 1. Crosses are the average of the square radius of gyration for given sizes N. Dots design the average of the square radius of gyration versus the average of the size N. Dots design the average of the square radius of gyration versus the average of the size N at different times. The two error bars show the statistical dispersion and the straight line is the slope D = 1.4.

A sketch of a bi-dimensional simulation is shown in Figure 1. An analysis of the logarithm of the radius of gyration of the clusters versus the logarithm of their size for all clusters appearing during the simulation, or the mean radius versus the mean size for regular times show (figure 2) that the clusters have a fractal structure with a fractal dimension $D \simeq 1.4$ for 2-dimension space. This result holds (with the same value for D) for every initial concentration in particles, if it is small enough.

2) The hierarchical Cluster-Cluster aggregation model

Since the scaling behaviour is found only in the low-concentration regime, it is interesting to study the limit of vanishing concentration in particles. In this limit, when, by chance, two clusters collide, they are so far from other clusters that this event occurs like these two clusters were alone in the world. To mimic this behaviour, one introduces the hierarchical model (Botet et al., 1984) where we use the sequence of the collisions instead of a real time. The model is defined as follows : take 2^n isolated particles. They are not situated in space. You choose two of them randomly. One (called the seed) is placed in the center of a square lattice (e. g.) and the other far away. This second particle begins a random walk on the lattice until it reaches a position neighbouring the seed. Then they stick irreversibly and form a cluster of 2 particles. This cluster is removed from the lattice and the scenario is played with two other particles, and so on. When you have obtained a collection of 2^{N-1} clusters of size 2, you do the same : you choose randomly two clusters of 2 particles, one is the seed, the other diffuses until they stick to form a cluster of 4 particles. And so on, you obtain at the end one cluster of 2^n particles. The hierarchy of the sizes during this simulation gives its name to the procedure. It is automatically in the 0-concentration limit, and clusters of same size are allowed to stick. This strong hypothesis has been checked on the standard model where the mobility of the clusters depend on their size (velocity of a cluster of size m is proportional to m^{α}, with $\alpha \lesssim 0$). In these cases, the size-distribution can be very different for various values of α, but the final cluster has the same fractal structure. The hierarchical model is just equivalent to impose a pecular size-distribution (strictly monodisperse) to a 0-concentration system. The values of the fractal dimension for different euclidean dimensions of space are collected on Table 1.

TABLE 1

Fractal dimension D of the standard clustering of clusters model aggregates as a function of the euclidean space dimension d. The value $D = \mathrm{Log}4/\mathrm{Log}\ 3/2$ for $d \geq 9$ is exact (Ball and Witten 1984). The error bars go from 0.04 for $d = 2$ to 0.1 for $d = 6$.

d	1	2	3	4	5	6	≥ 9
D	1	1.44	1.78	2.05	2.27	2.6	3.419

3. Long-range interactions (statement of the problem)

Many parameters of the model have been varied to know their relevance in the final geometric structure (see for example Botet and Jullien, 1988 for a review). In this paper we are only interested by the role of the interactions between the particles. The standard Cluster-Cluster model supposes that two particles do not interact until they are tangent. In this case they stick irreversibly and they cannot overlap. In other words the energy of interaction is 0 as long as the relative distance between the two particles is larger than δ, it is $-\infty$ when the distance equals δ, and is $+\infty$ for distances less than δ. This is of course a very pecular potential which is a rough approximation of the DLVO potential for colloids (Verwey and Overbeek, 1948). The realistic potential must be a mixing of the Van der Waals attractive interaction and the electrostatic (may be screened) repulsive interaction. The former is important for small distances, the latter for larger ones. Fickian molecular dynamics simulations of the standard Cluster-Cluster model have been performed by Ansell and Dickinson (1985) and their conclusions were that the fractal dimension of the aggregates remains unchanged, but they obtained an irrelevant local compactification of the geometric structure. Since simulations are done at finite temperatures, this is consistent with the idea that all models with short-range interactions belong to the same universality class.

But what happens for explicitely long-range interactions ? A typical realistic case appears when all colloidal particles have a magnetic moment. Long-range dipolar interactions are there present. Some experiments (Hurd and Schaeffer, 1985) have led to fractal dimensions smaller than those predicted by the standard model, and polarizability effects have been invoked to explain this discrepancy. A simple model (the tip-to-tip model, see Jullien 1985, 1986) has been introduced, able to explain quantitatively the fractal dimension in the experiments of Hurd and Schaefer as well as 3-dimensional experiments of aluminium hydroxide aggregation, as measured by low-angle X-ray scattering (Axelos et al. 1986).

A similar effect has been observed in experiments with magnetic (iron and cobalt) aerosols where it has been clearly observed that the fractal dimension of the aggregates decreases when the permanent magnetic moment of the individual particles increases (Kim and Brock, 1986, 1987, Niklasson et al. 1988). In this case all the particles carry a permanent momentum so that the problem is different from the tip-to-tip model.

Up to now it was difficult to have a clear idea of the behaviour of the clusters during aggregation so as the precise geometrical structure of the final aggregates. It is the reason why two of us (G. H. and A. T. S.) have imagined and realized a two-dimensional aggregation of magnetic microspheres which allows a clear visualisation of the whole aggregation in real time, and after the results of the experiment, we (P. N. M., R. B., R. J.) have imagined and simulated a simple numerical model reproducing the main features of the experimental aggregation.

4. Long range interactions (experiments)

The particles consisted of very uniformly sized sulfonated polystyrene spheres of diameter 3.6 μm produced using the Ugelstad (1980) swelling technique. By special methods (Ugelstad 1983) the spheres were made magnetic by introduction of 30 % (weight) magnetic iron oxides in the form of evenly distributed grains in a thin shell (of about 0.2 μm) near the surface. These spheres could be magnetized to various levels of remanent magnetization up to $M = 2.1$ emu.cm^{-3}. Measurements of the magnetization were done using a vibrating sample magnetometer. The spheres were dispersed in water and confined to a monolayer between two plane-parallel glass plates separated by about 5 µm. This separation could be adjusted evenly by using a small fraction of spheres of diameter 5 µm as spacers. The geometrical structures were observed directly in light microscopes. A video camera attachment and recorder allowed long term observations and digital analysis of the structures using a frame grabber with 512× 512 pixels resolution.

The aqueous dispersion was stabilized so that the electrostatic and Van der Waals interactions between the spheres were negligible compared to the magnetic forces.

For estimating the long-range interactions, the magnetized spheres may be considered as point dipoles of magnetic moment $\mu = M(\pi d^3/6)$. The magnetic interaction between two spheres labelled i and j, and separated by the distance $\vec{r}_{ij} = \vec{r}_i - \vec{r}_j$ is :

$$U_{ij} = \mu^2 \left[\vec{u}_i.\vec{u}_j - 3(\vec{u}_i\ \vec{r}_{ij})(\vec{u}_j\ \vec{r}_{ij})/r_{ij}^2\right]/r_{ij}^3$$

where $\vec{u}_i$ and $\vec{u}_j$ are unit vectors along the moments on spheres i and j. The dimensionless parameter which determines the effective strength of the dipole-dipole interaction relative to the disruptive thermal energy is :

$$K = \mu^2/d^3\ k_B T$$

In the experiments, the value of K could be adjusted from 0 to 1360 at room temperature.

The experiments were performed using low-concentration (less than 10 %) samples and a random initial distribution of spheres. To avoid the influence of the earth magnetic field and stray fields, the samples were enclosed in permalloy.

The typical aggregation time is about a few hours. During these experiments, it is clear that the clusters are rigid : there is no deformation nor restructuring of this geometrical structure. But reversibility is not rare : sometimes a cluster breaks into two smaller clusters. Nevertheless the number of such events is much smaller than the number of aggregations, so that one can suppose that reversibility is negligible within these experimental conditions.

Figure 3 shows a typical series of aggregated structures obtained after a few hours for various experimental conditions. From 3.a to 3.c, it is seen that there is an increasing tendency to form chains and open loops as M increases, reflecting the preference of alignment of the dipoles.

The fractal dimension of these aggregates were determined from an usual log-log plot of the radius of gyration versus the number of particles in each cluster. Figure 4 shows the variation of D versus the reduced magnetization K of the spheres. These results are based on approximately 70 measurements. Also included in Figure 4 is the earlier value $D = 1.49 \pm 0.06$ found for cluster aggregation of non magnetic spheres (Skjeltorp 1987). As may be seen, this result appears to be close to the limiting value for magnetized spheres as $K \to 0$.

The temporal evolution of the size-distribution of the clusters have also been studied in details and agrees with dynamical scaling relation of Vicsek and Family (1984). This point as well as the fractal features is developed in Helgesen et al. 1988.

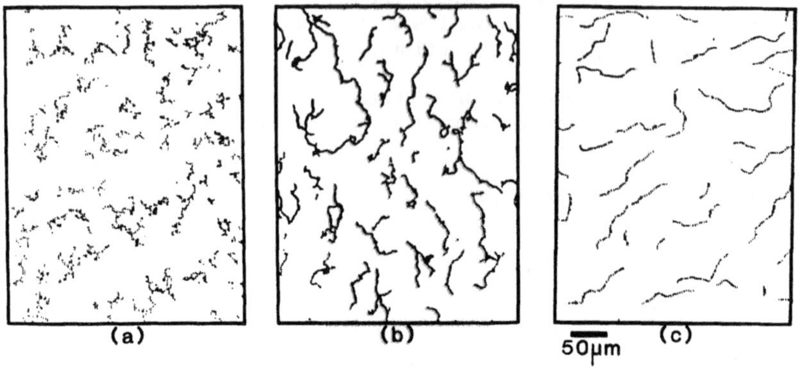

Fig. 3 Three 2-dimensional experimental aggregates of magnetic microspheres for different magnetizations ((a) K = 16, (b) K = 100, (c) K = 1360) in zero external field. As the magnetization increases, clusters tends to form chains.

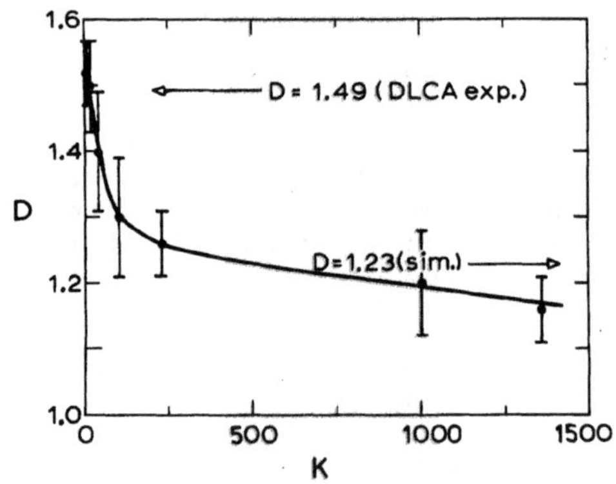

Fig. 4 Fractal dimension of the clusters in 2-dimensional experiments versus dipolar coupling constant K. The value $D = 1.49 \pm 0.06$ for $K \to 0$ was found in experiments with non magnetic spheres. Note the sudden drop of the value of D for small K.

5. <u>Long-range interactions</u> (simulations)

We have extended the cluster-cluster aggregation model to simulate these dipole-dipole magnetic interactions. We have kept the hypothesis of rigidity and irreversibility as discussed above. The first model is a variant of the hierarchical off-lattice, three-dimensional cluster-cluster aggregation model (see section 2.).

At each individual particle is attached a unitary vector $\vec{u}$ defining the direction of its momentum. It is randomly oriented at the beginning. When starting a collision process, two clusters are randomly rotated and placed apart in space with their centers of mass R_o apart. Since interactions are long-range, the choice of R_o is now important to avoid the influence of initial conditions. Systematic checks have shown that $R_0 = 2(R_1^M + R_2^M)$ was an optimum choice, where R^M_i is the maximum radius of cluster i.

Once placed, two types of Brownian movements are performed alternately : translation then rotation. The translation is of one unitary distance (diameter particle) in a random direction, except when an overlap occurs. In this case a partial movement is performed until a particle of cluster 1 comes in contact to a particle of cluster 2. They stick then irreversibly in this position.

The rotation is performed in one of the three planes (randomly chosen) defined by two of the three axes. The absolute value of the rotation angle is the one which allows for the most distant particle with respect to the center of mass of the cluster, a translation of one unitary distance. Here also the angle is chosen smaller if an overlap occurs. For numerical case, one of the clusters is the one which translates and the other one is the cluster which rotates. As usually, when the two centers of mass reach a distance apart greater than $2R_o$ (optimum value) the collision process is reinitialised. After the calculation of each movement, the quantity :

$$P = \exp(-K\Delta U)/(1 + \exp(-K\Delta U))$$

is computed. Here ΔU is the change in the dipolar energy of the whole system, resulting from the movement.

$$U = \sum_{(i,j)} U_{ij}$$

where U_{ij} is the dipolar energy between the two particles i and j which do not belong to the same cluster. After P is calculated, the movement is performed with probability P. This means that for large momentum, the movement is only performed if it lowers the total energy. On the other hand, for vanishing momenta, the movements are performed with a uniform probability $P = \frac{1}{2}$ independent of the change in the energy. This is a procedure quite similar to standard Monte-Carlo algorithms for these sorts of simulations. After each pair of movements (performed or not) a successive relaxation of the momenta may be done. We visit in a random order all the particles of the two clusters and, for each of them, we orientate its momentum in the direction of its local field. This procedure assumes a quite short relaxation time for dipole orientations. The fractal dimensions are estimated from the plot of the radius of gyration versus the number of particles after averaging over 15 independent samples. Since the computation of the total energy needs a sum over a large number (of order N^2) of couples of particles, we are limited to cluster sizes of 128 particles.

Without dipolar interactions, we recover a value $D = 1.75 \pm 0.08$ very close to the standard (more precise) value. But for very large moments ($K^{-1} = 0$) we find $D = 1.35 \pm 0.08$ which is a value significantly much smaller.

We have also modified the 2-dimensional standard off-lattice cluster-cluster aggregation model to take into account the dipolar interactions. There 100 particles were dispersed in a 50 × 50 box with periodic boundary conditions. The translation and rotation procedures were similar to the previous 3-dimensional ones : To compute the dipolar energy, particle separation $\vec{r}_{ij}$ is taken as the shortest distance in the extended zone under the periodic boundary conditions. The dipole momenta have of course three spatial components, and in the figures presented above, they are shown projected onto the plane. Figures 5 show typical aggregates obtained under different simulations : 5.a is without dipolar interactions and without Brownian rotation. The typical fractal dimension is $D = 1.41 \pm 0.02$. Figures 5 b includes rotational diffusion but is still without dipolar interactions ($D = 1.39 \pm 0.04$). At last, Figure 5 c, shows a typical cluster with dipolar interaction and rotational diffusion, and with very large momenta ($K^{-1} = 0$).

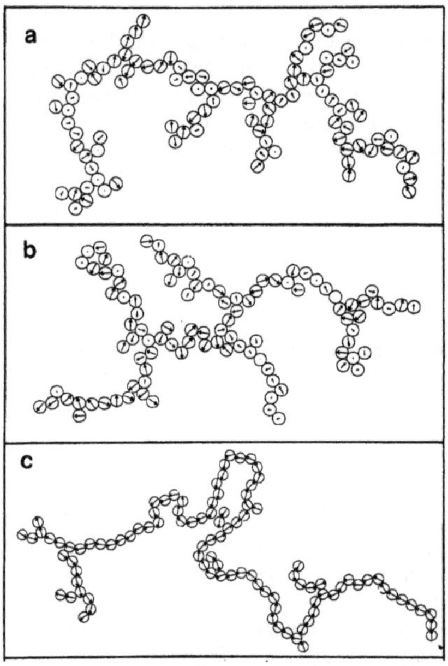

Fig. 5 Three typical simulated 2-dimensional clusters of 100 particles for different conditions : (a) without dipolar interaction and rotational diffusion ; (b) without dipolar interaction but including rotational diffusion ; (c) with strong dipolar interactions ($K^{-1} = 0$) and rotation diffusion. Concentration in particles is about 4 %.

The averaged fractal dimension is found to be $D = 1.23 \pm 0.12$. Although the statistical error is rather large because of the small samples, this value is significantly smaller than the preceding values. Moreover, the dipoles are well aligned and in the plane.

In the two cases (2- and 3-dimensional) we recover this feature that the fractal dimension of the aggregates decreases when the dipolar momentum increases.

6. Conclusion

Experiments of two-dimensional diffusion-limited cluster-cluster aggregation have been performed with magnetic microspheres which interact via long-range dipolar forces. The results show that the clusters are fractal and their fractal dimension decreases from 1.52 ± 0.05 to 1.16 ± 0.05 as the dipolar coupling increases. A simple numerical model is proposed, and the simulations show the same trend : the fractal dimension is found equal to 1.41 ± 0.02 for vanishing interaction and to 1.23 ± 0.12 for infinite coupling. Moreover, external magnetic fields produce very linear clusters with a fractal dimension close to 1 even for weak fields (Fig. 6).

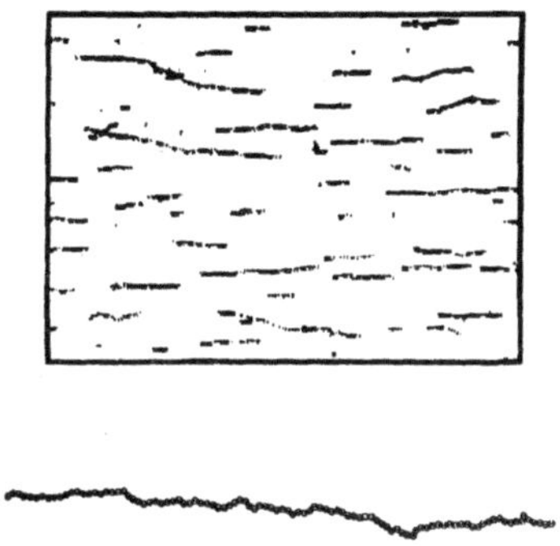

Fig. 6 Experimental (up) and simulated (down) clusters of magnetic spheres in presence of a weak external magnetic field ($H = 1$ Oe and $M = 21$ emu cm^{-3} for experiments ; $H = 0.2$ M for simulations).

REFERENCES

Axelos M. A. V., Tchoubar D. and Jullien R., 1986, J. Physique, 47, 1843
Ball R. C. and Witten T. A., 1984, J. Stat Phys. 36, 873
Botet R., Jullien R. and Kolb M., 1984, J. Phys. A, 17, L 75
Helgesen G., Skjeltorp A. T., Mors P. M., Botet R. and Jullien R., 1988, Phys. Rev. Lett. 61, 1736
Hurd A. and Schaefer D. W., 1985, Phys. Rev. Lett. 54, 1043
Jullien R., 1985, Phys. Rev. Lett., 55, 1697
Jullien R., 1986, J. Phys. A, 19, 2129
Kim S. G. and Brock J. R., 1986, J. Appl. Phys. 60, 509
Kim S. G. and Brock J. R., 1987, J. Colloid Interf. Sci., 116, 431
Kolb M., Botet R. and Jullien R., 1983, Phys. Rev. Lett., 51, 1123
Meakin P., 1983, Phys. Rev. Lett., 51, 1119
Niklasson G. A., Torebring A., Larsson C., Granqvist C. G. and Farestam T., 1988, Phys. Rev. Lett., 60, 1735
Skjeltorp A. T., 1987, Phys. Rev. Lett., 58, 1444
Ugelstad J. et al., 1980, Adv. Colloid Interface Sci. 13, 101
Ugelstad J., Soderberg L., Berge A. and Bergstrom J., 1983, Nature, 303, 95
Verwey E. J. W. and Overbeek J. T. G., 1948 : "The Theory of stability of lyophobin colloids", (Elsevier, Amsterdam).
Vicsek J. and Family F., 1984, Phys. Rev. Lett., 52, 1669

SHAPES OF DETERMINISTIC CRACKS OBTAINED UNDER SHEAR

H.J. Herrmann

SPhT, CEN Saclay, 91191 Gif sur Yvette, France

Abstract

Cracks are grown in a system submitted to external shear by solving the *full* Lamé equation on a two-dimensional lattice. One finds that deterministic fracture patterns are in general branched and can be fractal. This effect is due to the competition between the direction of global stress and the local growth direction imposed by the lattice anisotropy.

Introduction

The formation of cracks in an elastic medium and its subsequent failure is a question of widespread interest . The mechanisms leading to fracture are highly material dependent and have been studied quite extensively[1]. Despite the diversity of experimental situations one can hope to find generic features due to the underlying instabilities and their interplay with noise, anisotropy or memory effects. Recently two new approaches in this direction have been proposed[2] one inspired from random resistor networks[3,4] and another using DLA[5] as a guideline[6,7].

Here we will consider the growth of a single, connected crack. There have been numerical indications that cracks grown in central-force media with a probability proportional to the elongation of the springs are fractal[6,7]. The fractal dimension of these cracks seems to depend strongly on the type of external force that is applied (uniaxial tension, shear, uniform dilatation) but since only very small cracks can be grown, precise statements are difficult to make. We will investigate some of the origins of this fractal behaviour and obtain much better accuracy by considering deterministic models. In addition, in our studies we solve the full elastic equations which contain automatically angular forces and two elastic moduli, as compared to the central force model that has been studied before and which shows pathologies on most lattices.

Fractals' Physical Origin and Properties
Edited by L. Pietronero
Plenum Press, New York

The Model

The elastic medium is usually described by the field of displacement vectors $\mathbf{u}$ which obeys the Lamé equation[8]

$$(\lambda + \mu)\nabla(\nabla \mathbf{u}) + \mu \nabla^2 \mathbf{u} = 0 \tag{1}$$

where λ and μ are the Lamé coefficients. On the external boundary an imposed displacement is fixed. Suppose that in this medium one has already a crack and one wants to study how this crack grows. Then one will have on the surface of the crack a boundary condition $\partial_\perp \mathbf{u}_\perp = \partial_\perp \mathbf{u}_\parallel = 0$ and the crack will grow in the direction perpendicular to the surface at the point where the strain parallel to the surface is largest. The detailed growth law depends on the microscopic mechanism like how the elastic energy is transported away from the growing tip. We will use in this work a normal growth velocity $\mathbf{v}_n$ of the form

$$\mathbf{v}_n \propto ((\partial_\parallel \mathbf{u}_\parallel)^2 + q \cdot \partial_\parallel^2 \mathbf{u}_\perp)^\eta \tag{2}$$

where q and η are material dependent parameters. This growth law is inspired by the von Mises yielding criterion[1], but we cannot derive it from first principles. Physically q is the affinity of the breaking process to the bending mode (second term on rhs of Eq. 2) as compared to cleavage (first term on rhs of Eq. 2). In the above approach we have assumed that the relaxation of the local strain due to the growth of the crack is much faster than the velocity of the crack so that we do not consider viscoelastic effects. Also other possible time derivatives in Eq. 1, like inertia terms are neglected. Finally, we do not consider plasticity or non-linear elasticity.

We discretized these elastic equations on a square lattice by using the beam model[9]. This discretization introduces anisotropy and a cutoff at small length scales, two physical effects that are very often present in real materials.

A detailed description of the implementation of the beam model is given in Ref. 2. For each beam that is eligible for being broken one calculates the quantity p defined by

$$p = (f^2 + q \cdot max(|m_1|, |m_2|))^\eta \tag{3}$$

where f is the traction (and/or compression) force applied on the beam and m_1 and m_2 are the moments that are acting at the two ends of the beam; this p determines according to Eq. 2 if the beam will be broken. Each time a beam is broken the shape of the crack and consequently the boundary condition of the Lamé equation has changed and one has to solve the discretized equation again if one wants to know which beam to break next.

We consider a finite square lattice of linear size L, with periodic boundary conditions in the horizontal direction. On top and on bottom we impose an external displacement, usually a shear. We remove one beam in the center of the lattice which is the original microcrack. Next we consider the six nearest-neighbor beams of this broken beam. These include the two beams that are parallel to the broken beam and the four perpendicular beams that touch a common site with the broken beam. This choice of nearest-neighbors is due to the fact that the actual crack consists of the bonds that are dual to the set of broken beams[2]. Other connectivity conditions have also been used[7]. The Lamé equation is solved by a conjugate gradient method[10] to very high precision (10^{-20}) and the p's of Eq. 3 are calculated for each of the nearest-neighbor beams. We set $p = 0$ for a beam that is not a nearest-neighbor to the crack. Now various criteria for breaking are possible: I. One breaks the beam with the largest value of p; II. One breaks the beam for which $q_0 = p + f_0 \cdot p_{-1}$ is largest, where p_{-1} is the value of p that this beam had before the previous beam was broken; f_0 is a memory factor; III. On each beam of the lattice we put a counter c which is set to zero in the very beginning. Each time one has obtained the p's one calculates $\alpha = (1-c)/p$ and breaks the beam which has the smallest α, namely α_{min}. After the beam has been broken each counter c is set to $c = \alpha_{min} \cdot p + f \cdot c_{-1}$, where c_{-1} is the value the counter had before the breaking and f is another memory factor.

All three breaking criteria described above are deterministic. Criterion III corresponds for $f = 1$ to the limit of infinite noise reduction [11,12]. Noise reduction has been invented to reduce statistical noise in DLA simulations and has also been applied recently to central-force breaking[13]. What noise reduction certainly does is to introduce a memory effect with long range time correlations. Physically the three breaking criteria defined above correspond to three different situations. Criterion I describes ideally brittle and fast rupture. Criterion II contains a short time memory one would expect in cracks that propagate slower and produce strong local deformations at the tip of the crack as happens in many realistic situations. One could imagine applying this criterion to situations with very fast stress corrosion effects. Criterion III could be applied to situations of relatively slow stress corrosion, crazing of polymers or static fatigue. The memory factors f_0 and f measure the strength of these time correlations. In criterion III the limit $f \to 0$ gives criterion II with $f_0 = 1$, and in criterion II the limit $f_0 \to 0$ gives criterion I.

Results

In Figure 1 we see a crack broken according to criterion I under external shear for $L = 50$ and $q = 0.28$. Beams only break under tension and not under compression.

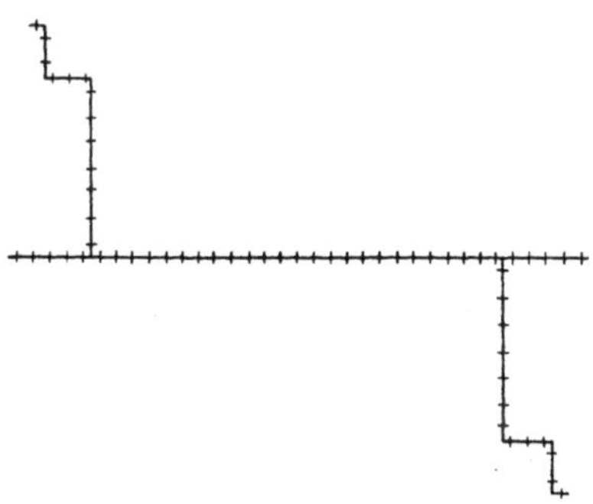

Fig. 1 Crack grown in a 50×50 system if an external shear is applied. Beams break under traction or with an affinity of $q = 0.28$ in the bending mode. Only the bond with the largest value of q breaks (criterion I). The first broken beam was vertical.

Cleavage tends to have the crack grow in the diagonal direction while the bending mode favours a horizontal rupture. The competition between these two effects can lead as seen in the figure to complex branched structures. The exact shape of these cracks depends strongly on q and the system size. For any finite q the horizontal rupture will eventually win if the system is large enough while for $q = 0$ one obtains diagonal cracks with eventual kinks. For this reason the cracks will not be fractal. However, we point out that in the analogous scalar model (i.e. DLA) only straight lines will be formed in criterion I; the different behaviour here is due to the fact that competing directions are possible in a vectorial model.

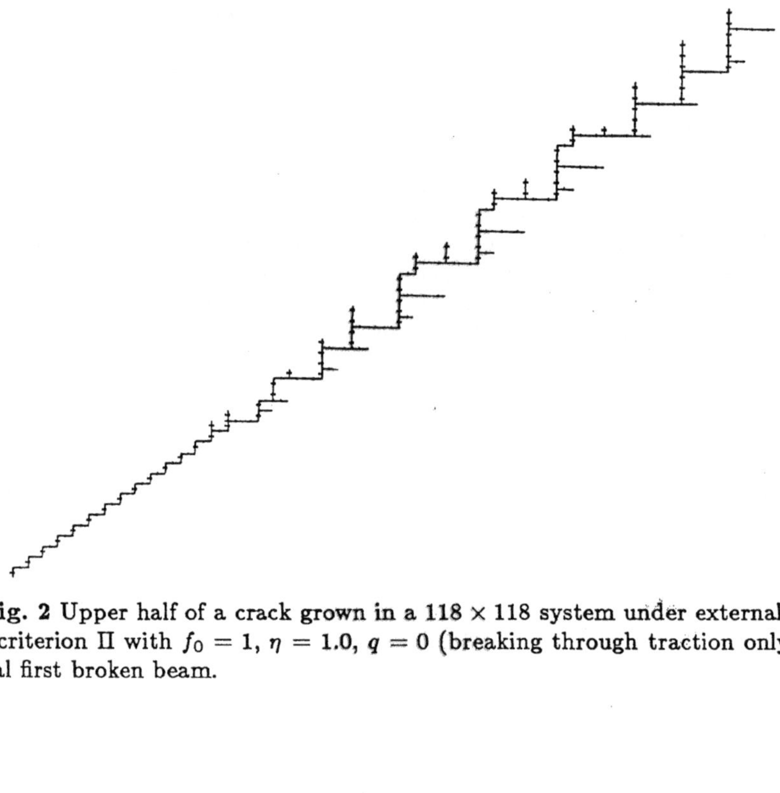

Fig. 2 Upper half of a crack grown in a 118×118 system under external shear using criterion II with $f_0 = 1$, $\eta = 1.0$, $q = 0$ (breaking through traction only) and vertical first broken beam.

Next we consider cracks grown using criterion II. We see in Fig. 2 and Fig. 3 cracks with $q = 0$ and $\eta = 1.0$ obtained in a system of size $L = 118$. Over four hours on one CrayXMP processor were needed to generate each of these structures. The crack in Fig. 2 is obtained by breaking only through tension while in Fig. 3 a beam can also break under compression. In Fig. 3 we show the whole crack which has a four-fold symmetry because it is grown deterministically, i.e. no random numbers are used and the result is independent on the roundoff errors of the computer. In Fig. 2 we only show the upper part of the crack the lower part being reflexion symmetric.

The very slight curvature of the crack is a finite size effect of the lattice but the fractality is not altered if the system size is changed.

If we count the number of broken beams inside a box of length l around the first broken beam and plot it as a function of l in a log-log plot ("sand box method") we find lines with slopes larger than unity which means that the cracks are fractals. In system sizes of $L = 118$ we find for the fractal dimensions d_f values that depend on η: $d_f = 1.3$ for $\eta = 1.0$, $d_f = 1.25$ for $\eta = 0.7$, $d_f = 1.15$ for $\eta = 0.5$ and $d_f = 1.1$ for $\eta = 0.2$. The structures are self-similar around the origin and probably directed fractals[14]. Changing the elastic constants (i.e. the Lamé coefficients) just changes the opening angle of the crack. If in Eq. 3 one uses an exponential instead of a power law, the structures seem to be dense[15].

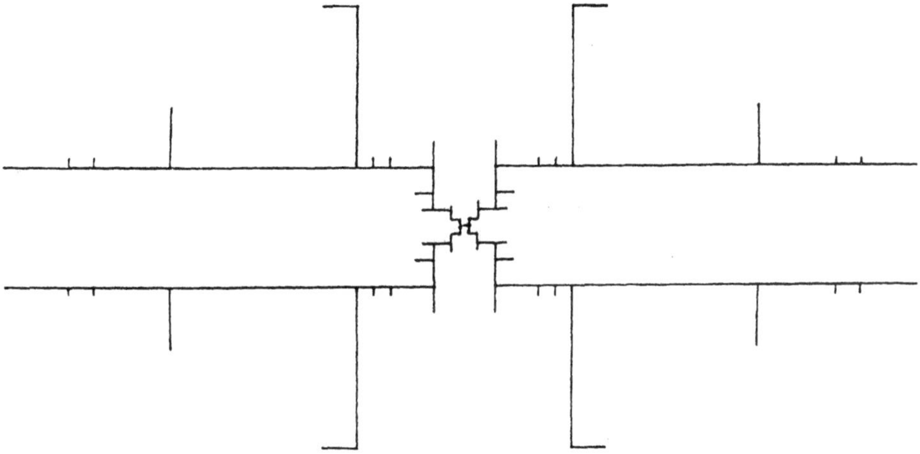

Fig. 3 Crack grown in a 118×118 system under external shear using criterion II with $f_0 = 1$, $\eta = 1.0$, $q = 0$ and vertical first broken beam. Here breaking occurs through traction and compression.

The effect that using criterion II gives fractal structures is novel and very distinct from what is seen in the scalar case of DLA. It shows that neither noise nor long range time correlations are necessary to obtain fractal breakdown. The origin of fractality is the competition between a global stress perpendicular to the diagonal and a local stress that tends to continue a given straight crack due to tip instability. Again we see the important role of the interplay of different directions which is only possible in a truly vectorial model. The relevance of a short memory in criterion II indicates that there might be a relation between this case and the models that have been put forward for snow flakes [16].

In Figs. 4 and 5 we show cracks grown using criterion III for $q = 0$, $f = 1$, $\eta = 1$ and $L = 118$. The physical situation is similar to that seen in criterion II, only the fractal dimensions are higher. This case can be directly compared to results obtained for DLA in the limit of infinite noise reduction[13,17] where needles, not fractals are predicted.

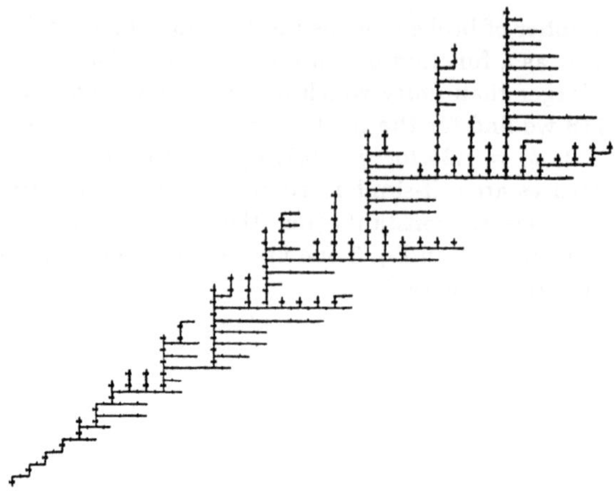

Fig. 4 Upper half of a crack grown in a 118 × 118 system using criterion III with $f = 1$, $\eta = 1$, $q = 0$ and vertical first broken beam when the beams break under traction only.

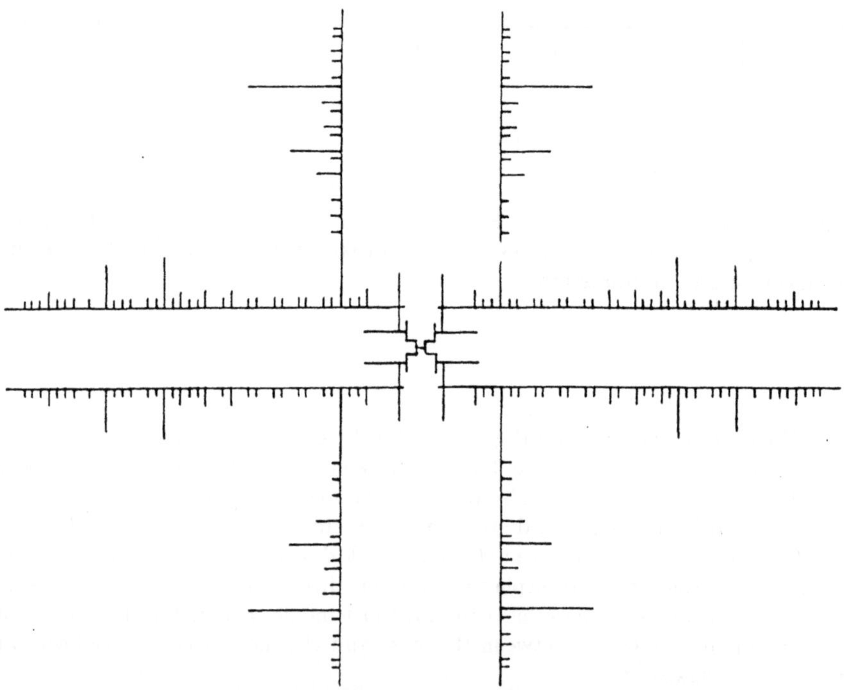

Fig. 5 Crack grown in a 118 × 118 system using criterion III with $f = 1$, $\eta = 1.0$, $q = 0$ and vertical first broken beam. Here breaking occurs through traction and compression.

In Fig. 6 we compare a deterministic crack with an experimental example of stress corrosion cracking in an alloy[18]. Due to the heuristic nature and simplicity of our model it makes no sense to compare numerical values of fractal dimensions. It seems also clear that the inhomogeneities of the medium in the experimental crack are important. The vague similarity that one can see between the patterns in Fig. 6 seems to indicate that the effects found in our model may explain to a certain degree the branching behaviour of experimental cracks.

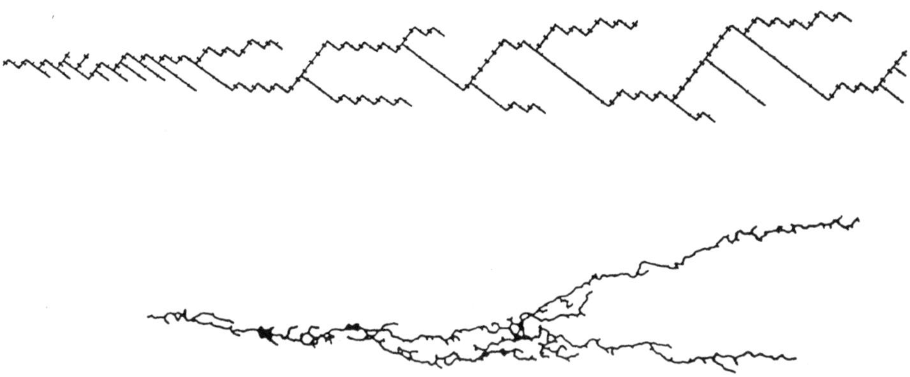

Fig. 6 Numerical and experimental cracks. The upper shape (rotated by 45°) is the upper halve of a crack grown in a 118×118 system under external shear with $q = 0$ and a vertical initially broken beam using criterion II with $f_0 = 1$ and $\eta = 0.2$. The lower picture shows the morphology of cracking in Ti - 11.5 Mo - 6 Zr - 4.5 Sn aged 100 hrs at $750°K$ and tested in 0.6M LiCl in methanol at -500mV under increasing stress intensity (taken from Ref. 18).

Conclusion

In conclusion, we have treated the problem of deterministic single crack propagation for finite square lattice samples. The patterns of cracks can become very complex and in particular they can be fractal with a fractal dimension that depends on the breaking criterion, i.e. the effect of memory. This phenomenon is due to the competition between the direction of global stress and the direction of local growth imposed by the lattice anisotropy. Therefore the *vectorial* nature of the elastic medium leads to crucially different results from what is known to occur in the *scalar* case of DLA. These differences must be taken into account also when randomness is introduced either quenched in the form of random elastic constants[19] or annealed in the form of breaking probabilities[6,7]. The dependence of shapes and fractal dimensions on the various parameters as well as the influence of noise, i.e. of a probabilistic growth rule, will be described elsewhere[15].

ACKNOWLEDGEMENTS

I thank my collaborators Lucilla de Arcangelis and Janos Kertész.

References

1. See e.g. H. Liebowitz (ed.), *Fracture*, Vols. I-VII, (Academic Press, New York, 1984)
2. H.J. Herrmann in *Random Fluctuations and Pattern Growth*, eds. H.E. Stanley and N. Ostrowsky (Kluwer, Dordrecht, 1988) , p.149
3. L. de Arcangelis, S. Redner and H.J. Herrmann, J. Physique Lett. **46**, L585 (1985); P.M. Duxbury, P.D. Beale and P.L. Leath, Phys. Rev. Lett. **57**, 1052 (1986); P.M. Duxbury and P.L. Leath, J. Phys. A **20**, L411 (1987) P.D. Beale and D.J. Srolovitz, Phys. Rev. B **37**, 5500 (1988) and references therein
4. B. Kahng, G.G. Batrouni, S. Redner, L. de Arcangelis and H.J. Herrmann, Phys. Rev. B **37**, 7625 (1988); H.J. Herrmann, A. Hansen and S. Roux, Phys. Rev. B **39**, 637 (1989) and references therein
5. T.A. Witten and L.M. Sander, Phys. Rev. Lett. **47**, 1400 (1981) ; L. Niemeyer, L. Pietronero and H.J. Wiesmann, Phys. Rev. Lett. **52**, 1033 (1984)
6. E. Louis, F. Guinea and F. Flores in *Fractals in Physics* eds. L. Pietronero and E. Tossatti (Elsevier, Amsterdam, 1986), p.117; E. Louis and F. Guinea, Europhys. Lett. **3**, 871 (1987)
7. E.L. Hinrichsen, A. Hansen and S. Roux, Europhys. Lett. **8**, 1 (1989); P. Meakin, G. Li, L.M. Sander, E. Louis and F. Guinea, J.Phys. A to be published
8. L.D. Landau and E.M. Lifshitz, *Theory of Elasticity* (Pergamon, Oxford, 1986)
9. S. Roux and E. Guyon, J. Physique Lett. **46**, L999 (1985)
10. G.G. Batrouni and A. Hansen, J. Stat. Phys. **52**, 747 (1988)
11. C. Tang, Phys. Rev. A, **31**, 1977 (1985); J. Szép, J. Cserti and J. Kertész, J. Phys. A **18**, L413 (1985); J. Nittmann and H.E. Stanley, Nature **321**, 661 (1986)
12. J. Kertész and T. Vicsek, J. Phys. A **19**, L257 (1986)
13. J. Fernandez, F. Guinea and E. Louis, J. Phys. A **21**, L301 (1988)
14. B.B. Mandelbrot and T. Vicsek, J. Phys. A to be published
15. H.J. Herrmann, J. Kertész and L. de Arcangelis, in preparation
16. F. Family, D.E. Platt and T. Vicsek, J. Phys. A **20**, L1177 (1987)
17. J.P. Eckmann, P. Meakin, I. Procaccia and R. Zeitak, Phys. Rev. A preprint
18. M.J. Blackburn, W.H. Smyrl and J.A. Feeney, in *Stress Corrosion in High Strength Steels and in Titanium and Aluminium Alloys*, ed. B.F. Brown (Naval Res. Lab., Washington, 1972), p.344
19. H. Takayasu in *Fractals in Physics*, eds. L. Pietronero and E. Tossatti (Elsevier, Amsterdam, 1986), p. 181; H. Takayasu, Phys. Rev. Lett. **54**, 1099 (1985)

Part 5

Diffusion and Vibrations on Fractals

SUPERLOCALIZATION, ANOMALOUS DIFFUSION AND SELF AVOIDING WALKS ON FRACTALS

Amnon Aharony

School of Physics and Astronomy
Raymond and Beverly Sackler Faculty of Exact Sciences
Tel Aviv University, Tel Aviv 69978, Israel

and

A. Brooks Harris

Department of Physics, University of Pennsylvania
Philadephia, Pennsylvania 19104, U.S.A.

1. INTRODUCTION

Many physical systems exhibit fractal geometry, at least over some range of length scales.[1] Much of the recent experimental and theoretical interest in such systems concentrated on alloys near the percolation threshold, p_c.[2,3] At p_c, such alloys are *self-similar*, and their properties exhibit an anomalous power law dependence on their linear size. Diferent physical properties turn out to depend on different subsets of sites (or bonds) on the percolating cluster, and hence require knowledge of a plenitude of fractal dimensionalities.[4] For example, the average total mass of the spanning cluster between two points a distance L apart scales as $M \sim L^D$, and the fractal dimensionality D equals $91/48, \sim 2.5, \sim 3.2$ and 4 for percolation clusters in dimensions d=2,3,4 and ≥ 6. The mass of the corresponding *backbone* (without the "dangling" bonds) has fractal dimensionalities $D_B \simeq$ 1.62, 1.83, 1.94 and 2, and that of the *minimal path*[5] (along bonds on the backbone) has $d_{min} \simeq$ 1.13, 1.36, 1.62 and 2. Similar fractal properties apply to other physical structures, e.g. *lattice animals*,[6] where $d_{min}=D_B \simeq$ 1.19, 1.33, 1.47 and 2 in d= 2,3,4 and ≥ 8.

Much of the recent study of physics on fractals has been devoted to *diffusion* and *conductivity* on fractals. In the *classical* regime, the diffusion of a random walker on a fractal is *anomalous*, and the mean square distance traveled after time t behaves as $\langle r^2 \rangle \sim t^{2/d_w}$, with[7] the fractal dimensionality of the random walk $d_w = D + \tilde{\zeta} = 2 + \theta$ where $\tilde{\zeta}$ describes the scaling of the two point resistance and θ describes the decay of the diffusion coefficient with distance. This result is related to an anomalous behavior of the *probability distribution of the random walker*, i.e. the probability P(r,t) that the walker reach a distance r after time t. Scaling arguments predict that

$$P(r,t) = t^{-\bar{\bar{d}}/2} \quad f(r^{d_w}/t) , \tag{1}$$

Fractals' Physical Origin and Properties
Edited by L. Pietronero
Plenum Press, New York

where $\bar{d} = 2D/d_w$ is the *fracton* dimensionality.[8-10] As we describe below, knowledge of the function P(r,t) yields results[11] concerning the decay of *localized wave functions*[12] on the fractal, the temperature dependence of thermally activated variable range *hopping conductivity*[13] and the fractal behavior of *self avoiding walks*[14,15] (or polymer chains) on the fractal.

As we discuss below, the scaling function f(x) is believed to decay exponentially. Whenever one encounters such exponential functions, one should be very careful with the *averaging procedures*, over the random distribution of clusters. There exist differences between results on *typical* clusters, which may be obtained theoretically by averaging over the log of the probability distribution, and those found by averaging the probability distribution itself. These differences are equivalent to those between *quenched* and *annealed* averages in random systems. One aim of the present paper is to emphasize the importance of the averaging procedure, and to study its consequences.

SUPERLOCALIZATION

In a very stimulating paper, Lévy and Souillard[12] considered the wave function of an electron near a single impurity on a fractal, and argued that it decays with distance as $|\psi(r)| \sim \exp(-cr^{a})$. Using path integrals between the origin and the point at distance r, they showed that $|\psi(r)| \leq \exp[t(E/J+2d)](1+\exp[t|V_0|/J])P(r,t)$, where J is the tight binding nearest neighbor hopping matrix element, $-|V_0|$ is the (delta function) bonding potential at the impurity and E is the eigen-energy, with $E < -2d\,J$ and $V_0 < -2d\,J$.

In a generalization of the Lévy-Souillard arguments, we assume[11] that P(r,t) is given by Eq. (1), with $f(x) \sim \exp(-x^{\alpha})$. Choosing also $t \sim r^{d_w\alpha/(\alpha+1)}$, the above inequality yields $|\psi(r)| \leq \exp(-c_1 r^{a})$, with

$$a = d_w\alpha/(\alpha+1) \ . \tag{2}$$

For the ground state, $\psi(r)$ may be chosen to be real and positive, and Lévy and Souillard found that $|\psi(r)| \geq \psi(0)\exp(tE/J)\,P(r,t)$, which yields $|\psi(r)| \geq \psi(0)\exp(-c_2 r^{a})$. Thus, we conclude that $\psi(r) \sim \exp(-cr^{a})$, with a given by Eq. (2).

Eq. (2) yields a relation between the "superlocalization" exponent a (previoulsy called d_ϕ by Entin-Wohlman *et al.*,[16]) and the new exponent α. The literature contains some confusion about α. If one takes[17] $\alpha=1$ then Eq. (2) yields the unreasonably high result[12] $a=d_w/2$. This led us[11] to start form the other end, obtain a and then deduce α.

Using a tight binding model on a d-dimensional dilute lattice, with $|V_0| > 2dJ$, so that the ground state energy obeys $|E| > 2dJ$, we found that

$$\psi_\ell = \sum_k G_{\ell k}(E)\, J_{ko}\psi_0 \ , \tag{3}$$

where $G(E) = ({}_0-E)^{-1}$, ${}_0$ being the Hamiltonian without the impurity site 0. Choosing all J's non-negative, and expanding G(E) in powers of J, we showed that $G_{\ell k}$ is positive and that $\partial G_{\ell k}(E)/\partial J_{ij} \geq 0$. This inequality reflects the intuitively clear expectation, that decreasing any J_{ij} to zero cannot cause an increase in $G_{\ell k}$, or in ψ_ℓ. The same expectation should hold for many two-point correlation functions.

Using this inequality, we have thus removed all bonds except those on the minimal path between 0 and k. Thus, $\psi_k/\psi_0 \geq G(L(k),E)$, where G(L,E) is the Green's function for two points at the ends of a chain of length L, and L(k) is the "mass" of the minimal path between 0 and k. For a long one dimensional chain, one has $G(L,E) \sim \exp(-L/\xi_1)$, with[11] $\xi_1^{-1} = \ln\{[|E|+(E^2-4J^2)^{1/2}]/2J\}$. Thus, for large L we have $\psi_k/\psi_0 \geq \exp[-L(k)/\xi_1]$, for *every* individual configuration.

The inequality $\partial G_{k\ell}/\partial J_{ij} \geq 0$ can also be used to obtain a lower bound on ψ_k: if we fill all the bonds on the lattice, we have an impurity on a regular lattice, and G decays exponentially. Thus, $\psi_k/\psi_0 \leq \exp(-r/\xi)$.

If we look at a *typical* cluster, then it is most probable that L(k) behaves (for large r) as the *average* minimal path, $L(k) \sim r^{d_{min}}$; (r is the Euclidean distance from 0 to k). On such a typical cluster we thus have $\psi(r) \sim \exp(-cr^{a})$, and

$$1 \leq a \leq d_{min} \qquad (4)$$

If we average ψ_k over *all* clusters, then the average will contain terms for which 0 and k are linked by a straight line, and $L(k) \sim r$. The weight of such clusters is of order p^r, hence for large r the average is dominated by $\exp(-\gamma r)$, and $a = 1$.

In real physical situations, one does not usually average over ψ, but rather over some measured physical property. For example, in a discussion of fracton wave functions, the relevant quantity is the strain, related to $\nabla\psi$. It has recently been argued[18] that the average strain scales like the conductance in a resistor network, i.e. like $r^{-\tilde{\zeta}}$. This might lead to the identification[18] of a (called d_ϕ in Ref. 16) with $\tilde{\zeta}$. Indeed, one always has[4] $\tilde{\zeta} \leq d_{min}$, in agreement with Eq. (4). However, the current value[3,4] of $\tilde{\zeta} \simeq 0.98$ in two dimensions may have problems with the left inequality in (4). This may imply a crossover of ψ_k, at large r, to a simple exponential.[19]

Using Eq. (2), we now find for *typical* clusters

$$1/(d_w-1) \leq \alpha \leq d_{min}/(d_w - d_{min}) , \qquad (5)$$

while averaging P(r,t) over *all* configurations yields $\alpha = 1/(d_w-1)$. Indeed, numerical simulations which average over many percolation clusters yield results[10] which are consistent with Eq. (5), and the measured α turns out to be quite close to the lower bound in (5).

Very recently, we found[19] a new lower bound on a, replacing Eq. (4) by

$$\max(1/\nu,1) \leq a \leq d_{min} , \qquad (6)$$

where ν is the percolation correlation length exponent ($1/\nu$ is the exponent for the number of the singly connected bonds between 0 and k, $L_{sc}(r) \sim r^{1/\nu}$). We also argued that in most typical cases, a is expected to be close to its upper bound, $a \simeq d_{min}$.

HOPPING CONDUCTIVITY

Following Ref. 12, Deutscher *et al*[13] argued that the quantum hopping conductivity between two impurities is given by[20]

$$\sigma_{ij} \sim \psi_{ij}\, e^{-\epsilon_{ij}/kT} , \qquad (7)$$

where ψ_{ij} is the overlap between the wave functions localized around i and j. Writing $\psi_{ij} \sim \exp(-cr^{a})$, replacing ϵ_{ij} by $[N(E_F)r^D]^{-1}$, and optimizing the exponential then yields

$$\sigma(T) \sim \exp[-(T_0/T)^{\beta}] , \qquad (8)$$

with $\beta = a/(D+a)$.

In order to identify what value of a to use here, we note that the distribution function of the σ_{ij}'s, which enters a more systematic derivation of the naive Mott arguement, is given by[21]

$$P(\sigma_{ij}, r_{ij}) = \int(-\ell n\, \sigma_{ij} + \ell n\, \psi_{ij})\, \theta\, (-\ell n\, \sigma_{ij} + \ell n\, \psi_{ij})\, P\, (\ell n\, \psi_{ij}, r_{ij})\, d\, (\ell n\, \psi_{ij}) , \qquad (9)$$

where $P(\ell n\psi_{ij}, r_{ij})$ is the distribution of $\ell n\psi_{ij}$ for fixed r_{ij}. Since (9) involves averaging over $\ell n\psi_{ij}$, and not over ψ_{ij}, we expect that $a \simeq d_{min}$, and this yields β of order 1/3 in both two and three dimensions.[11]

SELF AVOIDING WALKS

The function P(r,N) gives the number of configurations (or degeneracy) of chains with N "monomers" and end-to-end distance r. In order to study the partition function of self-avoiding-walks, one needs to supplement this *entropic* term by an *energetic* term, describing the potential self-replusion of the chain. Generalizing Flory's[22] argument, one may thus write the free energy as[14,23]

$$F = a(N^2/r^{D_B}) + b(r^{d_{w,B}}/N)^{\alpha} \quad . \tag{10}$$

In the entropic part, we use $\ell n\ P(r,N)$, but require that $d_{w,B} = D_B + \tilde{\zeta}$, since the self-avoiding-walks are restricted to move only on the *backbone.* similarly, we allow cross-intersections of monomers only within the backbone volume r^{D_B}.

Minimizing Eq. (10) yields $N \sim r^{D_{SAW}}$, with

$$D_{SAW} = \frac{D_B + \alpha\, d_{w,B}}{2 + \alpha} . \tag{11}$$

Rammal *et al*,[23] who first derived Eq. (11), used α=1 ("for simplicity") and obtained bad estimates. Havlin and Ben Avraham[10] recently used (11) with $\alpha = 1/(d_{w,B}^{min} - 1)$, where $d_{w,B}^{min} = d_{w,B}/d_{min}$, and found very good results. Their choice of this value of α was based on writing Eq. (10) in the "chemical" space, measuring distances by the corresponding minimal paths, and then following earlier arguments favoring $\alpha=1/(d_w-1)$. They also noted problems in using Eq. (11) with $\alpha=1/(d_{w,B}-1)$.

In the spirit of our earlier disucssion, it should be clear by now that α depends on the quantitiy which is averaged. As in quenched random systems, we believe[14] that one should average over the *free energy*, and not over the partition function. Since the free energy (10) involves $\ell n\ P(r,N)$, we expect the resulting α to be in the range (5). Accepting the conjecture[19] that $a \simeq d_{min}$, we have $\alpha = d_{min}/(d_{w,B} - d_{min})$. Substituting in Eq. (11) then yields

$$D_{SAW} = \frac{d_{min}\,\tilde{\zeta} + D_B^2 + D_B\tilde{\zeta}}{2D_B + 2\tilde{\zeta} - d_{min}} , \tag{12}$$

and the resulting numerical values are very close to all known simulations on percolation clusters, lattice animals, etc.[14] It is interesting that Eq. (12) was recently independently derived from completely different arguments.[15] It is also interesting that Havlin and Ben Avraham[10] obtained the correct answer (12) by working in the "chemical" space; it is only in that space that "typical" and "average" clusters have the same behavior!

In an earlier attempt to derive a Flory approximant for self-avoiding walks on fractals, Kremer[24] tried to substitute the fractal dimensionality D for the Euclidean dimensionality d in the usual Flory formula,[22] i.e. $D_{SAW} = (D + 2)/3$. Although we can argue that D_{SAW} depends only on properties of the backbone (rather than on D, a quantity which includes the effects of the dead ends), the Kremer formula gave excellent numerical estimates. This opens interesting directions for conjecturing approximate relations between D, D_B, $\tilde{\zeta}$ and d_{min}.[14]

CONCLUSIONS

A careful study of "superlocalized" wave functions on fractal has enabled us to produce non-trivial predictions concerning the probability distribution of random walks, the temperature dependence of hopping conductivity and the fractal dimensionalities of self-avoiding walks. We emphasize again that these results are sensitive to the averaging procedure used.

ACKNOWLEDGEMENTS

Work at Tel Aviv was supported by grants from the U.S.-Israel Binational Science Foundation and from the Israel Academy of Sciences and Humanities. Work at the University of Pennsylvania was supported by the NSF under grant DMR 85-20272.

REFERENCES

1. B. B. Mandelbrot, *"The Fractal Geometry of Nature,"* Freeman, San Francisco (1982).
2. D. Stauffer, *"Introduction to Percolation Theory,"* Taylor and Francis, London (1985).
3. A. Aharony, in *"Directions in Condensed Matter Physics,"* G. Grinstein and G. Mazenko, editors, World Scientific, Singapore (1986), p. 1.
4. A. Aharony, in *"Advances on Phase Transitions and Disorder Phenomena"*, G. Busiello, L. de Cesare, F. Mancini and M. Marinaro, editors, World Scientific, Singapore (1987), p. 185.
5. S. Havlin and R. Nossal, J. Phys. A*17*: L427 (1984).
6. S. Havlin, Z. V. Djordjevic, I. Majid, H. E. Stanley and G. H. Weiss, Phys. Rev. Lett. *53*: 178 (1984).
7. Y. Gefen, A. Aharony and S. Alexander, Phys. Rev. Lett. *50*: 77 (1983).
8. S. Alexander and R. Orbach, J. Phys. (Paris) Lett. *43*: 625 (1982).
9. R. Rammal and G. Toulouse, J. Phys. (Paris) Lett. *44*: 13 (1983).
10. For a recent review, see S. Havlin and D. Ben Avraham, Adv. Phys. *36*: 695 (1987).
11. A. B. Harris and A. Aharony, Europhys. Lett. *4*: 1355 (1987).
12. Y. E. Lévy and B. Souillard, Europhys. Lett. *4*: 233 (1987).
13. G. Deutscher, Y. E. Lévy and B. Souillard, Europhys. Lett. *4*: 577 (1987).
14. A. Aharony and B. Harris, J. Stat. Phys. *59*: 1091 (1989).
15. J. P. Bouchaud and A. Georges, Phys. Rev. B*39*: 2846 (1989).
16. O. Entin-Wohlman, S. Alexander and R. Orbach, Phys. Rev. B*32*: 8007 (1985).
17. J. R. Banavar and J. Willemsen, Phys. Rev. B*30*: 6778 (1984); B. O'Shanghnessy and I. Procaccia, Phys. Rev. A*32*: 3073 (1985).
18. A. Aharony, S. Alexander, O. Entin-Wohlman and R. Orbach, Phys. Rev. Lett. *58*: 132 (1987).
19. A. Aharony and A. B. Harris, Proceedings of STATPHYS 17, Physica A (in press).
20. N. F. Mott, J. Non-Cryst. Solids *1*: 1 (1968); Phil. Mag. *19*: 835 (1969).
21. U. Sivan, O. Entin-Wohlman and Y. Imry, Phys. Rev. Lett. *60*: 1566 (1988).
22. P. J. Flory, *"Statistical Mechanics of Chain Molecules"*, Interscience, New York (1969).
23. R. Rammal, G. Toulouse and J. Vannimenus, J. Physique *45*: 389 (1984).
24. K. Kremer, Z. Phys. B*45*: 149 (1981).

OBSERVATIONS OF FRACTONS

Eric Courtens

IBM Research Division
Zurich Research Laboratory
CH-8803 Rüschlikon, Switzerland

René Vacher and Jacques Pelous

Lab. de Science des Matériaux Vitreux*
Univ. des Sciences et Techn. du Languedoc
F-34060 Montpellier, France

ABSTRACT

The main theoretical predictions on vibrational excitations of fractal networks are first summarized. The application of the fracton theory to glasses and other amorphous materials is then critically discussed. The early experimental evidence for fractons obtained on demonstrated fractal systems is also surveyed. Finally, the extensive observations performed recently on silica aerogels are reviewed.

1. Vibrations of Fractal Media

Mathematicians have considered for quite some time the vibrations of systems with random boundary conditions.[1] Recently, they have been able to relate rigorously the vibrational density of states of objects with fractal boundaries to the Minkowski dimension of the boundary.[2] On the other hand, the vibrations of bulk fractal matter have been theoretically described by new collective excitations, which have been called fractons.[3] Fractons are highly localized modes[4] whose properties have recently been reviewed several times.[e.g. 5-7] In the present review, we summarize the main theoretical predictions on fractons, discuss the application of this concept to the vibrations of disordered solids, and show that fractons describe adequately the vibrational properties of silica aerogels.

Fractons are characterized by a length, ℓ, which is a measure of the spatial extent of the excitation. This length is essentially the size of a vibrating fractal "blob" loosely connected to other blobs.[7] The density of fracton states per unit frequency ω is given by $N(\omega) \propto \omega^{\bar{\bar{d}}-1}$. Here $\bar{\bar{d}}$ is the so-called spectral dimension, different from D, the Haussdorf dimension of the fractal, $\bar{\bar{d}} < D$. The fracton size ℓ is related to the fracton frequency ω by $\omega \propto \ell^{-D/\bar{\bar{d}}}$. This follows immediately from the counting of modes in fractal space. That relation replaces the usual phonon-dispersion relation of homogeneous media, associating ℓ with the inverse of a wave vector q. This is an unusual dispersion, as $D/\bar{\bar{d}} > 1$. Since fractons are eigenmodes, with

* Associated with the CNRS, Nr. 1119.

Fractals' Physical Origin and Properties
Edited by L. Pietronero
Plenum Press, New York

little overlapping with other fractons, their lifetime is expected to be very long.[8,9] This should not be confused with the lifetime of a plane-wave excitation of the same frequency, which is essentially equal to the frequency, since one expects to be in the Ioffe-Regel regime.[10]

A vibrational problem which continues to attract theoretical attention is that where the elastic waves are scalar waves. This assumes that scalar elasticity applies.[11] The vibrational problem then maps onto the problem of diffusion on the fractal.[12] The latter is characterized by an exponent θ related to $\bar{\bar{d}}$ by[3] $\bar{\bar{d}} = D/(1 + \frac{1}{2}\theta)$. In this case, the conjecture that $\bar{\bar{d}}$ assumes the value 4/3 for percolation networks in all Euclidean dimensions $d \geq 2$ was formulated.[3] On the basis of scaling arguments in the strong scattering regime, it was even made plausible that fractons could obey this conjecture irrespective of the detailed microscopic nature of the disordered materials.[10] More recently, it was recognized that the $\bar{\bar{d}}$ value, which is indeed 4/3 for percolation clusters, depends on the microstructure, and that it is for example different for a percolation backbone.[13]

In the real world, elasticity is mostly expected to be tensorial. Scalar elasticity can only be dominant in rubber-like materials, or when there is high internal pressure.[11] Simulations of percolation clusters, including bond bending elasticity, revealed $\bar{\bar{d}}$ values of 0.8 or 0.9, for $d = 2$ or 3, respectively.[14] Simulations on 3-d models of ruptured silica[15] have given $\bar{\bar{d}}$ values covering the range 0.5 to 2.5. Clearly, $\bar{\bar{d}}$ is a strong function of the microstructure of the fractal. Furthermore, real materials can at best be fractal over a restricted range of lengths,[16] ℓ, $a < \ell < \xi$, between typical particle dimensions a and correlation length ξ. Beyond ξ, the density ρ is well defined and the materials become homogeneous.[17] Corresponding to these boundaries, there are crossover frequencies between which fractons can be expected,[18] $\omega_{co2} > \omega > \omega_{co1}$. Well below ω_{co1}, one should observe usual long-wave phonons. Beyond ω_{co2}, particle modes should appear, starting at an ω_{min} which depends on the size of the particles and their elasticity rather than on properties of the fractal network.

The situation near the phonon-fracton crossover at frequency ω_{co1} and wave vector q_{co} has attracted considerable theoretical attention.[19-22, 10, 7] Scaling and mode counting arguments have been used to predict a hump in the density of states near crossover. Basically, the argument is as follows.[20,21] For a fractal of infinite extent, $\xi \rightarrow \infty$, the fracton density of states, $N_{fr}(\omega) = A\omega^{\bar{\bar{d}}-1}$, can be normalized to three modes per particle. This fixes the value of A. Isolating out of this fractal a blob of size ξ, the density of states of the blob is essentially unmodified for $\omega > \omega_{co1}$, where ω_{co1} is the fracton frequency at size ξ. The spectral weight of the missing lowest frequency modes is lumped into the remaining overall degrees of freedom of the blob. For sufficiently large blobs, the number of low-frequency modes is evidently very small compared to the total number of modes. Making up a material out of such blobs, these low-frequency modes give rise to long-wave phonons with a density of states $N_{ph}(\omega) \propto \omega_{co1}{}^{\bar{\bar{d}}-d}\omega^{d-1}$. With $d = 3$, $N_{ph}(\omega)$ decreases much faster with ω than $N_{fr}(\omega)$. In consequence, in order to keep the spectral weight, one anticipates that $N_{ph}(\omega)$ is higher than $N_{fr}(\omega)$ at ω_{co1}, *i.e.* that there should be a hump in the density of states. There is an indication for this effect in calculations of the specific heat for triangular lattices based on Sierpinski gaskets.[23] However, extensive simulations on infinite percolation clusters above threshold give no indication of a hump.[24,25] This needs to be explained.

The above argument ignores the modification of the modes that occurs at the junction of the blobs. This is illustrated in Fig. 1. From the Sierpinski gasket of Fig. 1(a), one can construct a large-scale homogeneous system following the procedure of Fig. 1(b) or (c). The former is the unit cell used by Southern and Douchant,[23] to which the arguments of the previous paragraph can apply, since the various blobs are held together just by their corners. The latter, however, is closer to a real situation where growing blobs eventually contact each other. One sees from Fig. 1(c) that along the boundary of the Sierpinski blobs the connectivity has been increased. It results that new high-frequency modes occur at all fractal scales. We propose that this is sufficient to distribute the "missing" spectral weight rather uniformly over the entire fracton regime, since the missing modes have such a small absolute weight and there is now no real discontinuity. The same should apply to all cases in which there is a fairly dense packing of blobs, including percolation clusters of finite ξ. Figs. 1(b) and (c) clearly present two extreme cases. In random fractals, an intermediate situation can be expected. Although these ideas still need to be supported by more calculations, it appears plausible that in real systems there should be no particular mode pile-up at the phonon-fracton crossover, but rather a very slight up-shift of the entire fracton density of states. This is particularly important as the presence of specific heat anomalies has often been interpreted as evidence for a crossover to fractons in amorphous materials.

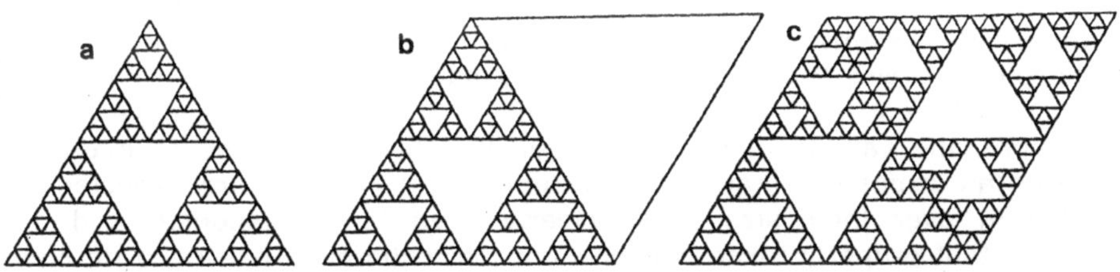

Fig. 1. Sierpinski-gasket models. The short segments between the nodes are identical springs. (a) is a section of the infinite gasket; (b) is the unit cell used by Southern and Douchant for their simulations;[23] (c) is a denser unit cell, possibly more representative of the steric hindrance that can occur during growth of a fractal and that leads to a homogeneous macroscopic object.

2. Applications to Glasses and Other Amorphous Materials

The thermal properties of glasses and other amorphous substances exhibit fairly universal features at low temperatures T.[26,27] At very low T ($\lesssim$ 1 K), one observes the specific heat $C \mathrel{\tilde{\propto}} T$, and the thermal conductivity $K \mathrel{\tilde{\propto}} T^2$. These dependences are now usually explained by the presence of two-level systems coupled to phonons.[28] Increasing the temperature beyond this regime, and plotting C/T^3 *vs.* T, one finds a more or less extended Debye plateau terminated by a hump which is followed by a decrease with some power law in T. Also, thermal conductivity changes over from T^2 to a plateau, $K \propto T^0$, approximately in the region of the hump in C/T^3, and it is followed by an approximately linear increase in T, $K \propto T$

It has been proposed[20] that the fracton model might explain the intermediate and upper T regions just described. In particular, the phonon-fracton crossover predicts C/T^3 going from T^0 to $T^{\bar{\bar{d}}-3}$ with increasing T. Also, if there were a hump in $N(\omega)$ near ω_{co1} this would lead to the hump in C/T^3 *vs.* T.[29] Since fractons are highly localized, the same crossover leads to a thermal conductivity plateau, and at higher T one should find $K \propto T$ owing to fracton hopping.[9]

Experiments on the density of states and thermal properties of epoxy resins cross-linked to various degrees have been presented as evidence for the applicability of the fracton model.[19,30-34] Although these experiments do show some power law behavior over restricted ranges of the relevant variables (ω or T), the basic question of the fractality of the medium has not really been answered. The same remark applies to glassy ionic conductors.[35,36] In the case of epoxies, the density of states crossover position implies a correlation length ξ as short as the molecules themselves (< 30 Å).[20] It is intuitively not clear how a material which is truly self-similar in its elasticity can be made at scales smaller than this small molecular size. Localization, and the resulting thermal conductivity plateau, are features which are not unique to fractals and fractons.[37] Furthermore, the use of the fracton model to interpret power-law exponents is only justified if self-similarity really applies either to the structure or to its connectivity.

In the case of Raman scattering experiments,[32,36,38-41] the observation of a power law for the Raman susceptibility does not establish fractality for the observed systems. If one investigates systems whose fractality was established otherwise,[39] one should still pay attention that fractons can only be seen between ω_{co1} and ω_{co2}, and in principle not above ω_{co2}. Furthermore, the validity of the expression that has been used to interpret the power-law exponent[39] has been challenged.[42,43] Fractons are expected to be coherent over their size ℓ, as clearly seen in simulations,[24] and an expression that properly takes into account this coherence has been derived in Ref. 18. As recently shown,[7] the exponent d_ϕ in the latter must be interpreted as an internal length scaling exponent σ.

In summary, there seems to be convincing evidence for features related to short range disorder in the thermal properties of these materials, in particular in the thermal conductivity plateau that should be associated with localization.[37] However, caution should be exerted in using strict fractal interpretations for the above experiments. Generally, density of states or thermal measurements alone are unlikely to be conclusive on this point. They must be combined with structural determinations of the fractality and, if possible, with measurements of the dynamical structure factor $S(q,\omega)$.

3. Early Experimental Measurements on Fractals

In view of their preparation method, it is intuitive that sintered metal powders could form experimental realizations of percolation structures. This is supported by elasticity and electrical conductivity measurements close to the onset of connectivity. The latter can be described as a percolation threshold.[44] It is also confirmed by scanning electron microscopy on porous copper-powder sinters.[45] Measurements of the variation with frequency of the ultrasonic attenuation in these sinters were compared quantitatively to the vibrational spectrum of a percolation system.[45] They revealed an anomalous power-law dependence of the attenuation on the ultrasonic frequency, and the onset of localization at a length which is within a factor of three of the percolation correlation length. This was interpreted as a phonon-fracton crossover. The experimentally observed crossover[45] is smoother than the one predicted by an effective medium approximation (EMA) theory.[46] To our knowledge, these measurements of phonon propagation have been the first conclusive observation of anomalous damping in a fractal medium near the phonon-fracton crossover. Such experiments, by their very nature, are unfortunately not able to observe real fractons which should be strongly localized excitations.

Another class of systems forming excellent realizations of percolation models are the diluted magnets. Among those, the randomly diluted antiferromagnet $Mn_xZn_{1-x}F_2$ has been extensively investigated, in particular by R.A. Cowley and collaborators. High-resolution inelastic-neutron scattering studies[47] of the spin dynamics in this material, with $x = 0.5$, has revealed spin waves, rather sharp at the zone center and broadening with increasing wave vector q. The signal was analyzed as the superposition of a spin-wave peak and a damped harmonic oscillator (DHO) function, the latter growing in intensity as q approaches the zone-boundary value q_{ZB}. The crossover from a dominant spin-wave to a dominant DHO response was found at $q \simeq 0.3q_{ZB}$. Remarkably, in energy space, this appears as a crossover from propagating waves to localized high-energy excitations. The crossover wave vector is in agreement with the percolation correlation length ξ determined from an independent elastic diffuse magnetic scattering measurement, $\xi^{-1} \simeq 0.3q_{BZ}$. These results provide strong evidence for a magnon-fracton crossover as expected theoretically.[48] The prediction is that the magnetic excitations are strongly spatially localized. An EMA calculation of $S(q,\omega)$ describes qualitatively the double peak structure observed experimentally. The broadening of the DHO should not be interpreted as the fracton lifetime, but as the lifetime of the plane-wave excitations observed in neutron scattering. These are clearly in the Ioffe-Regel regime.

Another magnetic system that has been experimentally investigated is a diluted amorphous ferromagnet, $(Co_xNi_{1-x})_{75}P_{16}B_6Al_3$. In that case, one has found a modification of the Bloch $T^{3/2}$ law for the dependence of the magnetization M(T) on temperature,[49] $M(T)/M(0) = 1-BT^{3/2}$. The system was investigated as a function of concentration, and the effects were interpreted in terms of a diffusion exponent in good agreement with percolation. This provides evidence that fracton excitations can be important in these magnets.

Finally, there is a broad class of systems which exhibit fractal structures, and are obtained by growth and aggregation.[50] Among these are the silica aerogels discussed in the following section. Fumed silica aggregates have also been found by various methods.[51] to be fractal over as much as two orders of magnitude in length scale. In compacted samples, a fractal dimension $D = 2.6$ was found.[52] More recently, the low frequency density of states of such samples has been measured by inelastic incoherent neutron scattering.[53] It shows $N(\omega) \propto \omega^p$, with $p = 0.8$ or 1.1 at two temperatures, T = 136 or 265 K, respectively. This yet unexplained temperature dependence may, we believe, be related to adsorbed water motion. Interpreting the low temperature value of p in terms of fractons, $\tilde{\tilde{d}}$ = p+1 = 1.8 is obtained, not inconsistent with present-day views[15] on the possible range of $\tilde{\tilde{d}}$.

As seen in this section, there are many different systems in which the fracton concept appears to be relevant. In some of these, in particular the diluted magnets, considerably more work could be performed. It is definitely of interest to study in sufficient detail the vibrations of systems that are well-identified fractals, as will now be shown.

4. Structure and Dynamics of Silica Aerogels

Silica aerogels are single-phase, highly porous, silica-based materials, obtained by hydrolysis of an alkoxysilane followed by polycondensation, gelation, and subsequent hypercritical drying.[54] The properties of these materials are very dependent on the preparation conditions, in particular on the dilution of the reactants which adjust the final density ρ of the dried solids. The addition of catalysts during preparation can also strongly modify the microstructure of the materials. Base catalyzed aerogels with $\rho \approx 100$ kg/m^3 are known to be fractal over restricted length scales.[55] Ultrasonic measurements[56] have also shown a rapid variation of the sound velocity with ρ. In the lightest samples, sound velocities as small as that in air had in fact been reported.

In view of the above, it appeared that silica aerogels could be excellent candidates for a systematic study of the phonon-fracton crossover and of the density of states in the fracton regime. The results of our investigations, which have been documented and also reviewed[57,58] elsewhere, will now be summarized.

Small-angle neutron scattering experiments have been performed to determine the fractal structure of various series of aerogels.[16,59] It is generally possible to extract three parameters from such measurements: 1) the mean particle size a; 2) the correlation length ξ; 3) the fractal dimension D. One important result[16] is that series of materials can be prepared for which: 1) ξ is progressively changed; 2) D is constant; and 3) ξ is related to the macroscopic density ρ by $\xi \propto \rho^{1/(D-3)}$, with the same value of D and a constant proportionality factor across the series. Such materials can be called *mutually self-similar*. They allow scaling as a function of length in the fractal regime ($a < \ell < \xi$) to be investigated, without actually performing microscopic experiments at these lengths.[58] It is such a series of neutrally reacted aerogels with D $\simeq$ 2.4 that was used to obtain most of the following dynamical results.[60-62, 18]

The phonon-fracton crossover frequency and wave vector are accessible to Brillouin scattering experiments.[60,61] Spectra can be measured for various sample densities ρ, and for each ρ for various momentum exchanges q. Each spectrum is determined by three fitting parameters, namely ω_{co1}, q_{co}, and the absolute intensity. Using the former two, and assuming that mutual self-similarity also extends to dynamical properties, one obtains the fracton "dispersion curve",[61,57] $\omega \propto q^{D/\tilde{\tilde{d}}}$. A plot of ω_{co1} *vs.* q_{co}

obtained from a number of Brillouin spectra on a series of mutually self-similar samples is shown in Fig. 2. The line is a fit to the experimental points, with $D/\bar{\bar{d}} = 1.9$. From q_{co} alone, one also derives an acoustical correlation length, $\xi_{ac} \propto 1/q_{co}$. Using $\xi_{ac} \propto \rho^{1/(D-3)}$, one finds a value for D in agreement with the direct structural information.[61,58] From $D/\bar{\bar{d}}$ and D, one finds $\bar{\bar{d}} = 1.3 \pm 0.1$.[61] Such a value can either be caused by scalar elasticity in the infinite percolation cluster, or by tensorial elasticity in structures that are more connected than percolation clusters. The latter appears much more likely.[58]

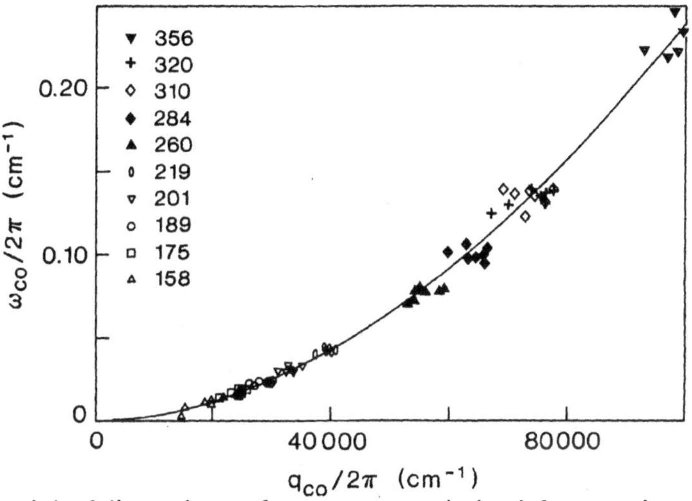

Fig. 2. A plot of the values of ω_{co1} *vs.* q_{co} derived from various Brillouin scattering measurements performed on a series of mutually self-similar aerogels. Different symbols correspond to different sample densities, as indicated in kg/m^3. The points for each individual sample have been obtained at various scattering angles. (From Ref. 57, © 1988 Kluwer Academic Publishers.)

In addition to coherent contributions, there are incoherent contributions to light scattering in which fractons of characteristic size smaller than the optical wavelength scatter independently from each other. In that case, the scattered intensity is the sum of individual scattering intensities, while for coherent contributions it is the scattered amplitude which is the sum of amplitudes. The incoherent (Raman) spectrum of fractons falls typically in the range of 1 to 300 GHz.[18] Beyond this frequency, particle modes are observed. In the fracton range, the dependence of the Raman susceptibility χ on frequency ω is given by $\chi \propto \omega^{-2+2\sigma\bar{\bar{d}}/D}$.[18, 7] Here, σ is an internal length exponent, $s_\ell \propto \ell^\sigma$, where s_ℓ is the internal length of an element of Euclidean size ℓ.[7] The measurement yields $\sigma \simeq 1.5$.

Of considerable interest is to obtain a measurement of $N(\omega)$ for *one* single sample. This should allow $\bar{\bar{d}}$ to be determined independently of scaling and mutual self-similarity. A power law in $N(\omega)$ has already been derived from specific heat measurements by Calemczuk *et al.*[62] in the fracton regime, they found $C \propto T^{1.1}$, for an aerogel of density $\rho = 0.21$ g/cm^3. This was interpreted as indicating $\bar{\bar{d}} = 1.1$.

Incoherent neutron scattering allows a spectral determination of $N(\omega)$. Among the various approaches, we used a difference technique that allows us to extract a contribution mostly due to incoherent scattering from protons.[63] The first results covered the region of particle modes, and probably the upper frequency fractons. The particle density of states can also be calculated and compared to experiment, affording an approximate absolute calibration of $N(\omega)$. Combined with the Brillouin results, the overall behavior of $N(\omega)$ was obtained.[63] This result was recently confirmed by a different neutron-scattering approach.[64] The thermal properties which are calculated from this agree remarkably well with the absolute values of Calemczuk *et al.*[62]

More recently, new measurements[65] with higher resolution, on a sample prepared in a *different* manner, have confirmed an extended fracton region. The power law now observed in the fracton domain over more than one order of magnitude has a slope $\bar{\bar{d}} - 1 \simeq 0.85$. We propose that this increased value of $\bar{\bar{d}}$ is due to a different microstructure of the materials. In contrast to the aerogels studied in our previous experiments, which were allowed to age 15 days before being hypercritically dried, this sample was dried soon after gelation. In the latter case, the small clusters floating in the solution are transported by the moving fluid, and clutter on the infinite cluster. This modification in the cluster-cluster aggregation regime can be expected to produce a more compact structure at small scales.[66] Hence, one anticipates a greater relative density of small clusters, and thus of modes at high frequency, leading to a larger effective $\bar{\bar{d}}$. This experiment confirms that $\bar{\bar{d}}$ is not a universal dimension, but rather an additional one sensitive to the microstructure of the fractal.

The experimental work on which this review is based has been performed in collaboration with G. Coddens, J. Phalippou, Y. Tsujimi, and T. Woignier. The neutron results were obtained at the Laboratoire Léon Brillouin, a Laboratoire mixte Centre National de la Recherche Scientifique (CNRS) - Commissariat à l'Energie Atomique, Saclay, France. The authors thank Profs. Aharony, Alexander, Entin-Wohlman, Orbach, and Teixeira for many discussions.

References

1. H.P. McKean and I.M. Singer, J. Differential Geometry **1,** 43 (1967).
2. M.L. Lapidus and J. Fleckinger-Pellé, C. R. Acad. Sci. Paris **306,** Série I, 171 (1988).
3. S. Alexander and R. Orbach, J. Phys. (Paris) Lett. **43,** L625 (1982).
4. R. Rammal and G. Toulouse, J. Phys. (Paris) Lett. **44,** L13 (1983).
5. R. Orbach, in *Scaling Phenomena in Disordered Systems*, R. Pynn and A. Skjeltorp, Eds. (Plenum, New York, 1985) p. 335.
6. S. Alexander, Physica **140A,** 397 (1986).
7. S. Alexander, presented at this workshop and to be published.
8. S. Alexander, O. Entin-Wohlman, and R. Orbach, Phys. Rev. B **34,** 2726 (1986).

9. A. Jagannathan, R. Orbach, and O. Entin-Wohlman, Phys. Rev. B (to be published).
10. A. Aharony, S. Alexander, O. Entin-Wohlman, and R. Orbach, Phys. Rev. Lett. **58,** 132 (1987).
11. S. Alexander, J. Phys. (Paris), **45,** 1939 (1984).
12. Y. Gefen, A. Aharony, and S. Alexander, Phys. Rev. Lett. **50,** 77 (1983).
13. O. Entin-Wohlman, Y. Kantor, and R. Orbach, private communication.
14. I. Webman and G. Grest, Phys. Rev. B **31,** 1689 (1985).
15. J. Kieffer and C. A. Angell, J. Non-Cryst. Solids **106,** 336 (1988).
16. R. Vacher, T. Woignier, J. Pelous, and E. Courtens, Phys. Rev. B **37,** 6500 (1988).
17. E. Courtens and R. Vacher, Z. Phys. B **68,** 355 (1987).
18. Y. Tsujimi, E. Courtens, J. Pelous, and R. Vacher, Phys. Rev. Lett. **60,** 2757 (1988).
19. P.F. Tua, S.J. Putterman, and R. Orbach, Phys. Lett. **98A,** 357 (1983).
20. S. Alexander, C. Laermans, R. Orbach, and H.M. Rosenberg, Phys. Rev. B **28,** 4615 (1983).
21. A. Aharony, S. Alexander, O. Entin-Wohlman, and R. Orbach, Phys. Rev. B **31,** 2565 (1985).
22. A. Aharony, O. Entin-Wohlman, and R. Orbach, in *Time-dependent Effects in Disordered Materials*, R. Pynn and T. Riste, Eds. (Plenum, New York, 1987) p. 233.
23. B.W. Southern and A.R. Douchant, Phys. Rev. Lett. **55,** 966 (1985).
24. K. Yakubo and T. Nakayama, Phys. Rev. B **36,** 8933 (1987).
25. T. Nakayama, K. Yakubo, and R. Orbach, Phys. Rev. B (to be published).
26. R.C. Zeller and R.O. Pohl, Phys. Rev. B **4,** 2029 (1971).
27. See, e.g., *Amorphous Solids: Low-Temperature Properties*, W.A. Phillips, Ed. (Springer, Berlin, 1981).
28. P.W. Anderson, B.I. Halperin, and C.M. Varma, Philos. Mag. **25,** 1 (1972); W.A. Phillips, J. Low Temp. Phys. **7,** 351 (1972).
29. As discussed above, such a hump is not an intrinsic feature of the fracton model. It is also not a specific feature of glasses, since good single crystals often show such a hump, e.g. W.N. Lawless, Phys. Rev. B **14,** 134 (1976). In fact, humps of comparable size are found in fused silica and in crystalline quartz.[26]
30. H.M. Rosenberg, Phys. Rev. Lett. **54,** 704 (1985).
31. A.J. Dianoux, J.N. Page, and H.M. Rosenberg, Phys. Rev. Lett. **58,** 886 (1987).
32. A. Boukenter, E. Duval, and H.M. Rosenberg, J. Phys. C **21,** L541 (1988).
33. M. Arai and J.E. Jörgensen, Phys. Lett. A **133,** 70 (1988).
34. J.E. de Oliveira, J.N. Page, and H.M. Rosenberg, Phys. Rev. Lett. **62,** 780 (1989).
35. A. Avogadro, S. Aldrovandi, and F. Borsa, Phys. Rev. B **33,** 5637 (1986).
36. A. Fontana, F. Rocca, and M.P. Fontana, Phys. Rev. Lett. **58,** 503 (1987).
37. J.E. Graebner, B. Golding, and L.C. Allen, Phys. Rev. B **34,** 5696 (1986); J.E. Graebner and B. Golding, Phys. Rev. B **34,** 5788 (1986).
38. E. Duval, G. Mariotto, M. Montagna, O. Pilla, G. Viliani, and M. Barland, Europhys. Lett. **3,** 333 (1987).
39. A. Boukenter, B. Champagnon, E. Duval, J. Dumas, J.F. Quinson, and J. Serughetti, Phys. Rev. Lett. **57,** 2391 (1986).
40. G. Mariotto, M. Montagna, G. Viliani, R. Campostrini, and G. Carturan, J. Phys. C **21,** L797 (1988).
41. A. Boukenter, B. Champagnon, E. Duval, J.L. Rousset, J. Dumas, and J. Serughetti, J. Phys. C **21,** L1097 (1988); J.L. Rousset, E. Duval, A. Boukenter, B. Champagnon, A. Monteil, J. Serughetti, and J. Dumas, J. Non-Cryst. Solids **107,** 27 (1988).
42. T. Keyes and T. Ohtsuki, Phys. Rev. Lett. **59,** 603 (1987).
43. A. Boukenter, B. Champagnon, E. Duval, and J. Serughetti, Phys. Rev. Lett. **59,** 604 (1987).

44. D. Deptuck, J.P. Harrison, and P. Zawadski, Phys. Rev. Lett. **54**, 913 (1985).
45. J.H. Page and R.D. McCulloch, Phys. Rev. Lett. **57**, 1324 (1986).
46. O. Entin-Wohlman, S. Alexander, R. Orbach, and K.-W. Yu, Phys. Rev. B **29**, 4588 (1984).
47. Y.J. Uemura and R.J. Birgeneau, Phys. Rev. Lett. **57**, 1947 (1986) and Phys. Rev. B **36**, 7024 (1987).
48. R. Orbach and K.-W. Yu, J. Appl. Phys. **61**, 3689 (1987).
49. M.B. Salamon and Y. Yeshurun, Phys. Rev. B **36**, 5643 (1987).
50. These phenomena have recently been reviewed in *Random Fluctuations and Pattern Growth: Experiments and Models* H.E. Stanley and N. Ostrowsky, Eds. (Kluwer Academic Publishers, Dordrecht, 1988).
51. J.H. Page, W.J.L. Buyers, G. Dolling, P. Gerlach, and J.P. Harrison, Phys. Rev. B (15 March 1989).
52. T. Freltoft, J. Kjems, and S.K. Sinha, Phys. Rev. B **33**, 269 (1986).
53. T. Freltoft, J. Kjems, and D. Richter, Phys. Rev. Lett. **59**, 1212 (1987).
54. See, e.g., the Proceedings of the two Int'l Conferences on Aerogels: (a) *Aerogels*, J. Fricke, Ed., (Springer, Berlin, 1985); and (b) R. Vacher, J. Phalippou, J. Pelous, and T. Woignier, Rev. Phys. Appl. **24**, C4 (1989).
55. D.W. Schaefer and K.D. Keefer, Phys. Rev. Lett. **56**, 2199 (1986).
56. B. Nouailhas, F. Michard, R. Gohier, and A. Zarembowitch, in *11th I.C.A.* (Paris, 1983) p. 179.
57. E. Courtens and R. Vacher, in *Random Fluctuations and Pattern Growth: Experiments and Models* H.E. Stanley and N. Ostrowsky, Eds. (Kluwer Academic Publishers, Dordrecht, 1988) p. 21.
58. E. Courtens and R. Vacher, Phil. Trans. Roy. Soc. (London), Series A (to be published).
59. R. Vacher, T. Woignier, J. Phalippou, J. Pelous, and E. Courtens, J. Non-Cryst. Solids **106**, 161 (1988). p. 145.
60. E. Courtens, J. Pelous, J. Phalippou, R. Vacher, and T. Woignier, Phys. Rev. Lett. **58**, 128 (1987).
61. E. Courtens, R. Vacher, J. Pelous, and T. Woignier, Europhys. Lett. **6**, 245 (1988).
62. R. Calemczuk, A.M. de Goër, B. Salce, R. Maynard, and A. Zarembowitch, Europhys. Lett. **3**, 1205 (1987).
63. R. Vacher, T. Woignier, J. Pelous, G. Coddens, and E. Courtens, Europhys. Lett. **8**, 161 (1989).
64. G. Reichenauer, J. Fricke, and U. Buchenau, Europhys. Lett. **8**, 415 (1989).
65. R. Vacher, E. Courtens, G. Coddens, J. Pelous, and T. Woignier, Phys. Rev. B (1st April 1989).
66. P. Meakin, in *On Growth and Form*, H.E. Stanley and N. Ostrowsky, Eds. (Nijhoff, Dordrecht, 1986) p. 111.

Part 6

Diffusion Fronts and Invasion Percolation

DIFFUSION, INTERCALATION AND INVASION NOISE

B. Sapoval, M. Rosso and J.F. Gouyet

Laboratoire de Physique de la Matière Condensée
Ecole Polytechnique, 91128 Palaiseau, France

Y. Boughaleb

Département de Physique, Faculté des Sciences
Hassan II , Ben M'Sick, Casablanca, Maroc

ABSTRACT

Whenever fractal interfaces are obtained by diffusion, they may present, besides the anomalous electrical properties due to their static geometry, an anomalous noise related to the fluctuation in time of this geometry. These fluctuations occur at very high frequencies as compared to the atomic jump rate. They may then be a source of noise in heterogeneous systems or diffused contacts which can be otherwise considered as quenched. This "geometrical" noise is calculated in the framework of gradient percolation Monte Carlo simulations in d=2. Scaling arguments based on fluctuations of cutting bonds are given to account for the results. We predict a high-frequency power noise spectrum in $1/f^2$ and a low-frequency power spectrum in $1/f$. The cross-over between the two regimes occurs at a frequency which has a power law dependence as a function of the gradient of concentration at the interface. The scaling behaviour of these phenomena agrees with simple predictions from percolation theory.

INTRODUCTION TO DIFFUSION FRONTS AND RELATION TO PERCOLATION

Objects generated by diffusion naturally have a fractal geometry[1,2] This geometry is closely related to the geometry of percolation clusters and may show up in invasion and corrosion patterns[3,4]. The most general concept which permits a unique discussion of these structures is the concept of percolation in a gradient[2-8]. The fractal interfaces should present anomalous noise which is related to their anomalous impedance through the Nyquist theorem[9-11].

Besides, a striking characteristic of these interfaces is their instability. They fluctuate at frequencies much higher than the average probability per unit time for atomic jump. Therefore fluctuations of diffused interfaces may be a source of noise in heterogeneous systems which can be otherwise considered as quenched[12-14]. The purpose of this work is to propose a quantitative analysis of this "geometrical" noise of a diffused interface.

A diffusion geometry, such as that in Fig.1, is obtained by Monte Carlo simulation of particles jumps from a source of particles kept at a

Fractals' Physical Origin and Properties
Edited by L. Pietronero
Plenum Press, New York

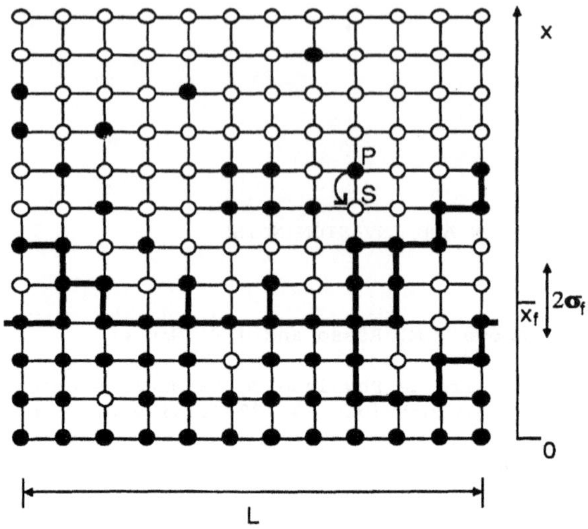

Fig.1. Diffusion front in the square lattice. The diffusion source is at the bottom of the figure. The diffusion front is the thick line. It is situated at a distance x_f and has a finite width σ_f. A sample has a lateral width L, but the correlation has only the range σ_f. If the particle P jumps into the site S, it connects a "large" cluster (island) which becomes a peninsula.

constant concentration $p = 1$ (at the bottom of the figure). The sites which are occupied by the diffusing particles ("A-sites") are represented by solid circles. The empty sites ("B-sites") are shown as empty circles.

In such a system we have defined a diffusion front[2]. Suppose that A atoms are metallic atoms. Metallic atoms are considered to be electrically connected if they are first-nearest neighbours. If an electric potential is applied at the bottom of the A region, all A atoms which are first-nearest neighbours to the potential source will be at the same potential. The limit of this equipotential region is the diffusion front, shown in Fig.1 as a thick line. The geometry of this line is the true geometry of the electrical contact. It is fractal[2]. The diffusion front may also be defined as the external frontier of the largest cluster of particles. Hence, the study of the diffusion front reduces mainly to the study of cluster external boundary. Our problem becomes similar to a percolation problem, except that there exists here a gradient of the occupation probability ∇p. This is gradient percolation[2-8]. The percolating cluster must be limited to a certain distance from the source because the concentration tends to zero. The concentration of particles at the mean position x_f of the frontier is very close to the percolation concentration p_c[5,15] : $p(x_f) \equiv p_c$ and the front is asymptotically identical to the external boundary or "hull" of the usual percolation cluster[16] in the limit where the local gradient tends to 0 around x_f. It then has a fractal dimension[2,17,18].

$$D_f = (1+\nu)/\nu \qquad (1)$$

where ν is the correlation length exponent, equal to 4/3 in d=2 [19]. Hence

$D_f = 7/4$. The front may be described by three macroscopic quantities (see Fig.1) : its position x_f, its width σ_f, and the total number N_f of atoms of the front. It can be easily deduced that the following power laws are obeyed[2] :

$$\sigma_f \propto (\nabla p)^{-\alpha_\sigma} \quad \text{with } \alpha_\sigma = \nu/(1+\nu) = 4/7 \tag{2}$$

$$N_f \propto L\,(\nabla p)^{-\alpha_N} \quad \text{with } \alpha_N = \alpha_\sigma(D_f-d+1) = 3/7 \tag{3}$$

for d=2. Here ∇p is the local gradient at the position x_f. L is the lateral width of the sample.

FLUCTUATIONS OF THE FRONT FOR d=2

The dynamical behaviour of the diffusion front was revealed by simulation calculations. The most striking result of these simulations is that the behavior of the system is "erratic". By this we mean that the geometry may remain unmodified for a period of time, then suddenly it may undergo a "catastrophic" change, i.e. a change on a semi-macroscopic scale. The reason for this phenomena is that the jump of a single particle can dis connect or connect a large group of particles (for example a large isolated cluster near the front which may contain $\sigma_f^{D_f}$ particles). This would occur for instance, if the particle P in Fig.1 jumps to the S position.

The most remarkable feature about front fluctuations is their very high frequency, much higher than the hopping frequency. For a fluctuation to appear, it is not necessary to wait the jump time θ; the jump time θ/N_f is enough for something to happen on the front[13]. For a macroscopic system N_f can be a very large number. Thus a system, which may be considered as quenched because θ is very long, can still show interfaces fluctuations at measurable time intervals θ/N_f. We define $\Delta N_f(t)$ to be the absolute change of the number of points on the frontier in the time interval t

$$\Delta N_f(t) = |\,N_f(t) - N_f(0)\,| \tag{4}$$

The results of the Monte Carlo simulation of this process are shown in Fig.2. The average value $<(\Delta N_f(t))^2>$ is given as a function of time. The calculation was carried out by taking a finite sample of width L=524 which contains the front and the neighboring region. The front is recognized after each 2^n steps. For one value of the gradient the data reported in Fig.2 is obtained in a time of the order of one hour on a main frame computer (NAS 9080). We studied various values of the local gradient in order to understand the scaling behavior of the fluctuations.

We concentrate here on the study of the fluctuations of the geometry of the frontier. A second step would be to calculate the "electrical" noise due to "geometrical" noise. The general behavior of the fluctuations as a function of time shows that for small time intervals the average square fluctuations increase; they saturate for a cross-over time interval t_c. The fluctuations follow the law

$$<(\Delta N_f(t))^2> \sim t^{2H} \tag{5}$$

where H is the Hurst exponent[20]. For short times, the value of H is 0.5 corresponding to a $1/f^2$ noise at high frequency. For longer times the mean fluctuations $<(\Delta N_f(t))^2>$ stabilize. This corresponds to H = 0 and to a 1/f noise at low frequency.

We first study the long time behavior ($t>\theta$) where $H = 0$. To understand this behavior we treat our system as a collection of a number L/σ_f of independent percolating "boxes". Each box of lateral size σ_f is considered to have a constant concentration $p = p_c$. This is allowed in first approximation because the presence of the concentration gradient has the effect of reducing the correlation from infinity to σ_f. The fact that there is a saturation of the fluctuations is related to the finite width of the front due to the existence of a finite gradient. For short time intervals the probability of a catastrophic event is very small. For long time intervals, on the contrary, all the possible large events have appeared. In a frontier of lateral extent L, the number of uncorrelated (independent) zones is L/σ_f. The maximum fluctuation of one part of the frontier of lateral width σ_f is due, for example, to the connection or disconnection of one large cluster of size σ_f which contains $\sigma_f^{D_f}$ points on its hull. Thus, for large time intervals the variance of the resulting fluctuation is of the order of

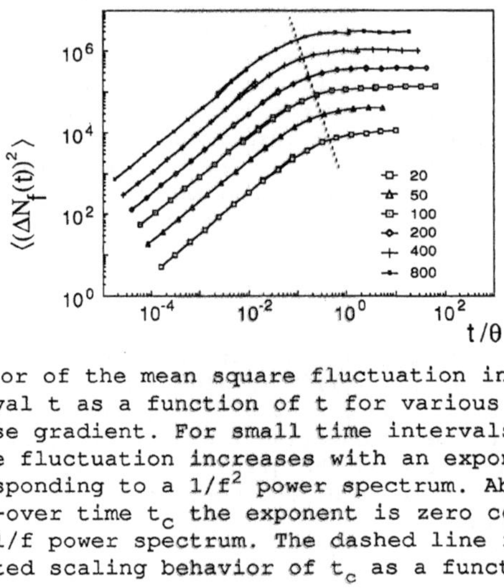

Fig.2. Behavior of the mean square fluctuation in a time interval t as a function of t for various values of the inverse gradient. For small time intervals the mean square fluctuation increases with an exponent one corresponding to a $1/f^2$ power spectrum. Above a cross-over time t_c the exponent is zero corresponding to a 1/f power spectrum. The dashed line represents the expected scaling behavior of t_c as a function of ∇p.

$$<(\Delta N_f(t))^2> \approx (L/\sigma_f) \, . \, \sigma_f^{2D_f} \approx L.(\nabla p)^{-10/7} \qquad (6)$$

and is independent of the time interval. In Fig.3 this predicted power law is compared to the numerical data. We determine an exponent 1.50 ± 0.05 instead of the predicted value $(10/7)=1.428...$ .Note that relation (6) is not only a proportionality relation, it gives also the correct order of magnitude. For example, for $(\nabla p)^{-1}=800$ and $L=524$ we predict a value $7.35.10^6$ for $<(\Delta N_f(t))^2>$ and we observe a value of the order of 4.10^6. The numerical prefactor in relation (6) is, therefore, of order 2.

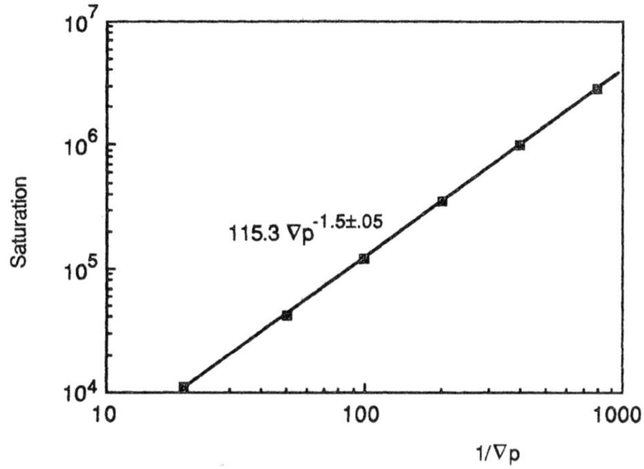

Fig.3. Saturation (long term fluctuations) as a function of the gradient. The observed slope is 1.50±0.05 (estimated error); the theoretical value is 1.428.

HIGH FREQUENCY NOISE

For short times (high frequency) one can explain the observed behavior by considering the simplest possible mechanism[14]. Fluctuations are created by connection (or disconnection) of isolated clusters through a single jump of a particle. Of course there are other types of events. For instance, the opening of a lake (a cluster of empty sites) near the front so that the lake becomes a bay; but this is basically the same kind of event if one considers the symmetry of occupied and empty sites. Notice that the probability that a single atomic jump creates no front fluctuation at all is of order one. This is because most particles in the system of N particles are not generally found near or on the front because the front is very diluted (its fractal dimension is 7/4). However, due to the hyperbolic behavior of the distribution of events, the variance Σ^2 for the probability distribution of an elementary event of size h is dominated in a rough estimate[14] by the very few "catastrophic" events of size $\sigma_f^{D_f}$. In an ordinary percolation situation, large fluctuations of the percolating cluster may be created by connections or disconnections of "cutting" or "red" bonds[21]. We suppose that the fluctuations of the gradient percolation frontier are due to the same type of bonds. We recall that when one considers standard, uniform, percolation it is clear that all the "cutting" bonds sit on the "hull" of the percolation cluster. Here the "hull" is the front. We have to calculate the probability that one point of the frontier is a "cutting" bond. This can be done from the following: In a square of side σ_f, the mass of frontier is $\sigma_f^{D_f} = \sigma_f^{1+(1/\nu)}$. The number of cutting bonds[21] is $\sigma_f^{1/\nu}$. The probability for a point of the frontier to be a cutting bond is then $\sigma_f^{1/\nu} / \sigma_f^{1+(1/\nu)} = \sigma_f^{-1}$. Neglecting the events of small size we can write the variance Σ^2 for a single simulation step as

$$\Sigma^2 \propto (1/\sigma_f) \, . \, (\sigma_f^{D_f})^2 \, . \, (N_f/N) \qquad (7)$$

The factor (N_f/N) takes into account that only this proportion of atoms are active in connecting or disconnecting isolated clusters. Considering a system of lateral width L as a collection of independent percolating systems of size σ_f, the total number of points on the frontier is[2] $N_f \approx (L/\sigma_f)\sigma_f^{D_f}$. The variance of the elementary event is

$$\Sigma^2 \approx L.N^{-1}.\sigma_f^{(3D_f-2)} \approx L.N^{-1}.(\nabla p)^{-13/7} \tag{8}$$

The mean square fluctuation $<(\Delta N_f(t))^2>$ over a time interval t corresponds to the fluctuation of the sum of $\mathcal{N}$ quasi identical random variables, where $\mathcal{N}$ is proportional to t. This explains why the exponent $H \approx 0.5$ is observed in simulations for short times. The correspondance between $\mathcal{N}$ and the real time t is

$$\mathcal{N} = N.(t/\theta) \tag{9}$$

because the physical jump time θ is the time for which all the particles have jumped (or tried to jump) once. The variance of the sum of the $\mathcal{N}$ random variables corresponding to the time t is $<(\Delta N_f(t))^2>$, where

$$<(\Delta N_f(t))^2> = N.(t/\theta).\Sigma^2 = C.L.(t/\theta).(\nabla p)^{-13/7} \tag{10}$$

C is a constant of order unity. The scaling behavior of the short time fluctuations as a function of the gradient is shown in Fig.4. We have plotted the quantity $\mathcal{A} = <(\Delta N_f(t))^2>.(\theta/t) = C.L.(\nabla p)^{-13/7}$. The value of the exponent in the simulation is found to be 1.83±0.05. The predicted value is 13/7=1.857. Here again the agreement which the simple prediction is good. The order of magnitude predicted by relation (10) is also good. The predicted value of $\mathcal{A} = C.L.(\nabla p)^{-13/7}$ for L=524 and ∇p=100 is equal to 2.7 10^6C and one measures a value of approximately 10^6. This shows that C is approximately 3.

The cross-over time t_c between the H=0 regime and the H=0.5 regime is found by equating (6) and (10). The result is : $t_c \approx C^{-1}.\theta.\sigma_f^{1-D_f}$. This last exponent is equal to $-1/\nu$. The expected scaling behavior of t_c as a function of ∇p ($t_c \propto \nabla p^{3/7}$) is shown as the dashed line in Fig.2. The cross-over frequency $f_c = t_c^{-1}$ is independent of the size of the sample. Its value is

$$f_c \approx C.\theta^{-1}\cdot\sigma_f^{1/\nu} = C.\theta^{-1}.(\nabla p)^{-1/(1+\nu)} \tag{11}$$

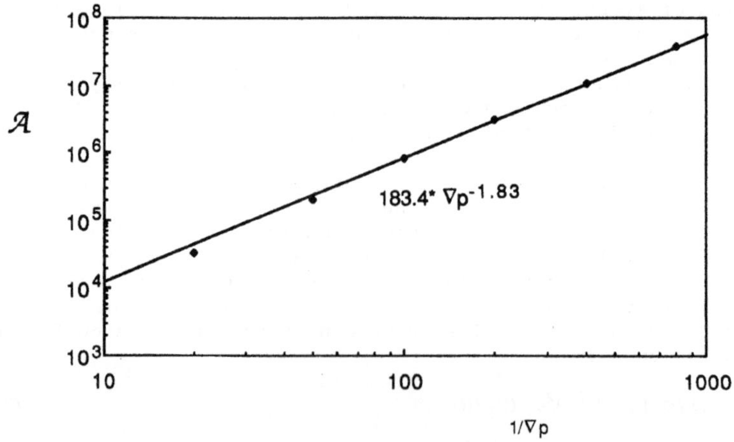

Fig.4. Short time fluctuations as a function of the gradient. The observed slope is 1.83±0.05 (estimated error); the theoretical value is 1.857.

It is interesting to note that this cross-over frequency is equal to the atomic jump rate θ^{-1} multiplied by the number of cutting bonds in a domain of size σ_f. These results could be slightly modified by correcting for finite size effects[22]. The value of the exponent $1/(1+\nu)$ is $3/7 = 0.428571....$ We recall that such a "geometric" noise has a very high cut-off frequency which is of the order of $\theta^{-1}.N_f$. This is because only one atom of the frontier or near the frontier need to jump to create a fluctuation. The number N_f in a macroscopic sample is enormous. This can reduce the order of the frequency θ^{-1} from frequencies corresponding to (millions of years)$^{-1}$ to hertz [12-14]. The geometrical noise will exhibit a $1/f^2$ power spectrum for frequencies superior to the cross-over frequency, $f_c < f < \theta^{-1}.N_f$. It will exhibit a $1/f$ power spectrum for low frequencies, $f < f_c$. Even the cross-over frequency is increased as compared to θ^{-1}; f_c is proportional to the factor $(\nabla p)^{-1/(1+\nu)}$ which can be a large number.

STATISTICS OF THE EVENTS

We now explain the statistics of the events. We call Nev(h) the number of events of size h. An event of size h is the connection or disconnection of a cluster of perimeter h and diameter $d=h^{1/D_f}$. The diffusion front is made of a number L/σ_f of fractal lines of diameter σ_f. Each of these lines, due to its fractal structure, is made of $(\sigma_f/d)^{D_f}$ parts of size d. Each of these parts countains $d^{1/\nu}$ cutting bonds which are effective in creating fluctuations of size of order h. Since h is the number of points in each of these clusters, the probability that such a bond will be cut is $(d^{1/\nu})/h$. Therefore the number Nev(h) of events of size h after all the particles of the front have jumped (or tried to jump) is approximately

$$\begin{aligned} Nev(h) &\approx (L/\sigma_f)(\sigma_f/d)^{D_f}\, d^{1/\nu}\, h^{-1} \\ &\approx N_f\, h^{-2+(1/\nu D_f)} \approx L.(\nabla p)^{-\alpha_N} .\, h^{-2+1/\nu D_f} \qquad (12) \\ &\approx L.(\nabla p)^{-3/7}.h^{-11/7} \end{aligned}$$

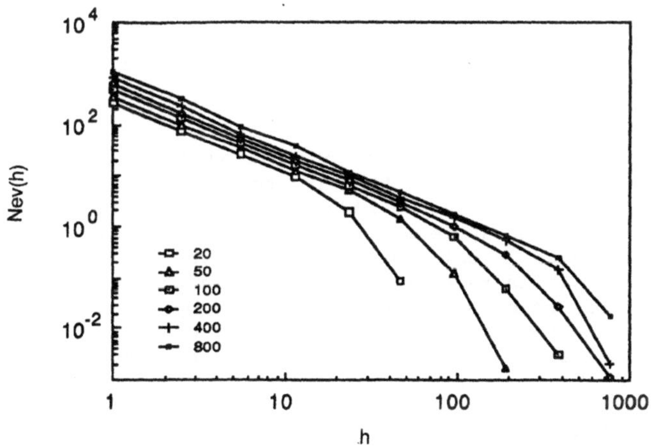

Fig.5. Statistics of the events : Number of events of size h as a function of h for various values of the inverse gradient. The observed slope is 1.42±0.05 (estimated error) whereas the theoretical value is 1.57.

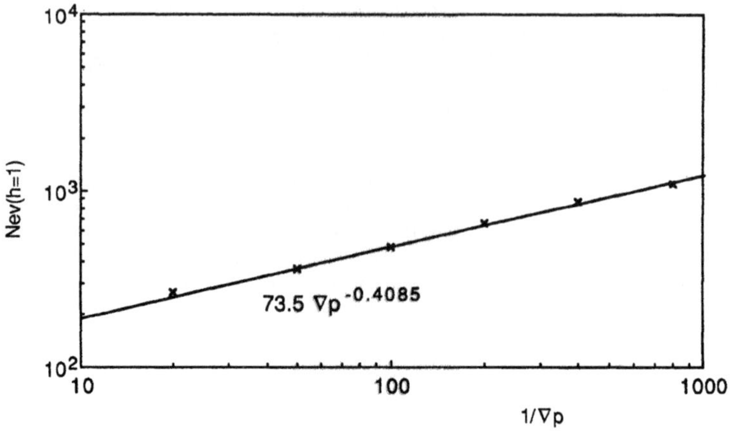

Fig.6 Number of events of size 1 as a function of the gradient. The observed slope is 0.408±0.02 (estimated error); the theoretical value is 0.428.

A plot of the result of the simulation is given in Fig.5 for various values of the inverse gradient. We observe a power law followed by an abrupt decrease at the value corresponding to the maximum size of an event, approximately $\sigma_f^{D_f} \sim \nabla p^{-1}$. The average slope of this line is -1.42±0.05 whereas the predicted value is -11/7 = -1.57. This discrepancy may indicate that noise cannot be strictly identified with the fluctuations of the "cutting" bonds. This point is under current investigation. For h=1, Nev(1) $\approx L(\nabla p)^{-\alpha_N}$. A plot of Nev (1) as a function of $(\nabla p)^{-1}$ is shown in Fig.6. The measured value for the exponent is 0.408±0.02 whereas the predicted value is 3/7 = 0.428.

The numerical values of Nev(h) also show that the numerical prefactors in equation (12) are of order unity. For example, for $(\nabla p)^{-1}$=800, L=524 and h=10, one predicts Nev(10) = 247; one measures, in Fig.5, a numerical value of the order of 300.

CONCLUSION

Although a macroscopic object obtained by diffusion can be considered as quenched at room temperature, the time scale for semi-macroscopic fluctuations of the system can be reduced by enormous factors so that in strongly non-homogeneous systems, 1/f noise due to atomic diffusion could be observed. The lines of calculation followed above should apply equally well to the d = 3 case. It is remarkable that whithin the range of gradients considered here the problem can be approximated by considering standard percolation in afinite box of size σ_f. A more detailed calculation taking into account the existence of a gradient is proposed by Gouyet and Boughaleb in ref.(22) and confirms the simple predictions given above. The existence of interactions between the particles [23,24] should modify our results because the number of cutting bonds should be strongly dependent on the strength of the interaction.

The same approach should apply to the calculation of "invasion noise". Experimental data on slow invasion of a random medium by a non wetting fluid indeed exhibit large fluctuations[25]. The calculation of the electrical noise of a contact possessing this fractal geometry is still to be made.

REFERENCES

1. B. Mandelbrot, The fractal geometry of Nature, W.H. Freeman and Company, San Francisco (1982)
2. B. Sapoval, M. Rosso and J.-F.Gouyet, J. Phys. Lett. (Paris) 46 : 149 (1985). J.Feder, Fractals, Plenum press, New York (1988)
3. J.-P. Hulin, E. Clement, C. Baudet, J.-F. Gouyet and M. Rosso, Phys. Rev. Lett. 61: 333 (1988)
4. B. Sapoval, M. Rosso, J.-F. Gouyet, Fractal interfaces in diffusion, invasion and corrosion in "The fractal approach to the chemistry of disordered systems, polymers, colloids and surfaces". Edited by D. Avnir. To be published by John Wiley and sons (1989)
5. M. Rosso, J.-F. Gouyet and B. Sapoval, Phys. Rev. B32: 6053 (1985)
6. M. Rosso, B. Sapoval and J.-F. Gouyet, Phys. Rev. Lett. 52: 3195 (1986)
7. J.-F. Gouyet, M. Rosso and B. Sapoval, Phys. Rev. B37: 1832 (1988)
8. J.-F. Gouyet, M. Rosso and B. Sapoval, in Fractals in Physics, ed. by Pietronero L. and Tosatti E., Elsevier, Amsterdam (1986) p.137
9. A. Le Méhauté and G. Crépy, Solid State Ionics, 9&10,17 (1983)
10. S.H. Liu, Phys. Rev. Lett. 55,529 (1985)
11. B. Sapoval, J-N. Chazalviel and J. Peyrière, Phys. Rev.A, 38,5867 (1988)
12. B. Sapoval, M. Rosso, and J.-F. Gouyet, Materials Research Society Fall Meeting, Boston (1985), Symposium on Fractals in Materials
13. B. Sapoval, M. Rosso, J.-F. Gouyet and J.F. Colonna, Solid State Ionics, 18&19: 21 (1986)
14. B. Sapoval, Philosophical Magazine B, Jan.1989
15. R. Ziff and B. Sapoval, J.Phys.A:Math. Gen.19: 1169 (1986)
16. R.F. Voss, J. Phys. A. Math. Gen. 17: L373 (1984)
17. A. Bunde and J.-F. Gouyet, J. Phys. A 18: L285 (1985)
18. H. Saleur and B. Duplantier, Phys. Rev. Lett. 58: 2325 (1987)
19. D. Stauffer, Introduction to percolation theory,Taylor & Francis, London (1985)
20. B. Mandelbrot and J.W. Van Ness, SIAM Review 10: p.422 (1968)
21. H.E. Stanley, J. Phys. A 10: L211(1977),A. Coniglio, J. Phys. A 15, 3829 (1982)
22. J.-F. Gouyet, B. Sapoval, Y. Boughaleb and M. Rosso, ETOPIM 2 Conference, Paris, Sept. 88, to be published by Plenum Publishing Corporation, New-York. J.F. Gouyet and Y. Boughaleb, to be published
23. M. Kolb, J.F. Gouyet and B. Sapoval, Europhys. Lett. 3: 33 (1987)
24. J.F. Gouyet, Solid State Ionics, 28-30: 72 (1988)
25. A.J. Katz and A.H. Thompson,Phys. Rev. Lett. 58: 29 (1987)

DYNAMICS OF INVASION AND DISPERSION FRONTS

Jens Feder[1], Torstein Jøssang[1], Liv Furuberg[1], Knut Jørgen Måløy[1]
Finn Boger[1] and Amnon Aharony[1,2]

(1)Department of Physics, University of Oslo
Box 1048 Blindern, 0316 Oslo 3, Norway

(2)School of Physics and Astronomy,
Beverly and Raymond Sackler Faculty of Exact Science
Tel Aviv University, Tel Aviv 69978, Israel

INTRODUCTION

The displacement of one fluid by a another fluid in a porous medium is a process of both scientific and practical importance. Depending on the displacement rates, viscosity ratios, miscibility, interfacial tensions and pore geometry a bewildering variety of displacement front behaviors arises. Lenormand[1–4] has studied many of the regimes observed under various conditions during two-fluid displacement processes in micromodels of porous media.

At high displacement rates the front structure is now relatively well understood and is best best characterized as a *fractal* fingering structure. Chen and Wilkinson[5] and Måløy et al.[6] demonstrated that viscous fingering in a random porous medium at high capillary numbers, $Ca >> 10^{-4}$, generates structures with a fractal[7,8] geometry. This fractal structure closely resembles that obtained from the diffusion limited aggregation (DLA) model of Witten and Sander.[9,7] Similar structures have also been obtained by fluid-fluid displacement in radial Hele-Shaw cells using non-Newtonian viscous fluids.[10] The relationship between fluid-fluid displacement in porous media and DLA was first discussed by Paterson.[11] The original DLA model of Witten and Sander specifies a time ordered sequence of events but is not explicitly time dependent. While the time dependent aspects of DLA and closely related processes have been explored theoretically[12,13] and by means of computer simulations,[14,15] this aspect of DLA has only recently been explored experimentally.[6,16] The dynamics of the viscous fingering structures have also been discussed in terms of multifractal measures.[16–18] A crossover function has recently been shown to describe the structure of DLA and viscous fingers, whis is not self-similar.[19]

Fractal structures are also observed for the *invasion percolation*[20,21] process at very low displacement rates. The *dynamics* of the processes that arise at low dis-

Fractals' Physical Origin and Properties
Edited by L. Pietronero
Plenum Press, New York

placement rates has been much less studied experimentally and theoretically. We have recently shown[22] that the growth of planar invasion percolation clusters exhibits a novel dynamic scaling which we describe here in the first part of the paper. Tis dynamical scaling structure has so far not been observed experimentally in a quanitative fashion. However, we are preparing experiments in order to test if the dynamics found in simulations is also valid for fluid invasion process in porous media.

In the last part we discuss the movement of tracers in a fluid flowing through the two-dimensional porous model. In this case there is *no* hydrodynamic instability in the fluid flow. However, we find that the *dispersion* of tracers, which map the fluid flow through the porous medium, move in such a way that equal concentration contours in fact are self-affine fractal curves.[7,23,24] The dispersion of tracers is in fact the simplest flow problem in porous media (apart from the flow of a single component fluid) and the front dynamics (motion and spreading) is well understood in terms of the diffusion-convection equation. Our observation of a fractal front structure was surprising and it remains a theoretical challenge to explain these results.

INVASION PERCOLATION

Introduction to invasion percolation

Invasion percolation[20,21] is a *dynamic* percolation process introduced by Wilkinson and Willemsen[21] motivated by the study of the displacement of one fluid by another fluid in a porous medium.[25,26] Both standard percolation processes[27–29] and invasion percolation generate self-similar *fractal*[7] structures. A review of fractals and of experimental results[2,30–32] obtained in fluid displacement processes is given in a recent book.[8]

Dynamics of displacement fronts is essential for understanding displacement processes in oil production, and invasion percolation is the simplest model with nontrivial front structure and dynamics.

When water is injected very slowly into a porous medium filled with oil, the capillary forces dominate the viscous forces, and the dynamics is determined by the local pore radius r. Capillary forces are strongest at the narrowest pore necks. It is consistent with both a simple theoretical model and experimental observations to represent the displacement as a series of discrete jumps in which at each time step the water displaces oil from the smallest available pore. The experimental result shown in figure 1a illustrates the results of an invasion percolation process where air (the non-wetting fluid) displaces glycerol (the wetting fluid). The figure also shows the result of a simulation of the invasion percolation process.

The algorithm

Wilkinson and Willemsen[21] simulated the model on a regular lattice. Sites and bonds represented pores and throats and were assigned random 'radii'. For convenience, one assumes that the easily invaded throats are invaded instantaneously, and one assigns random numbers r in the range $[0,1]$, representing the pore sizes, to the sites.

Growth sites are identified as the sites that belong to the defending fluid and are neighbors to the invading fluid. The growth sites represent the *external perimeter*.[33] At every time step the invading fluid is advanced to the growth site that has the lowest random number r.

The invading fluid may *trap* regions of the defending fluid. As the invader advances

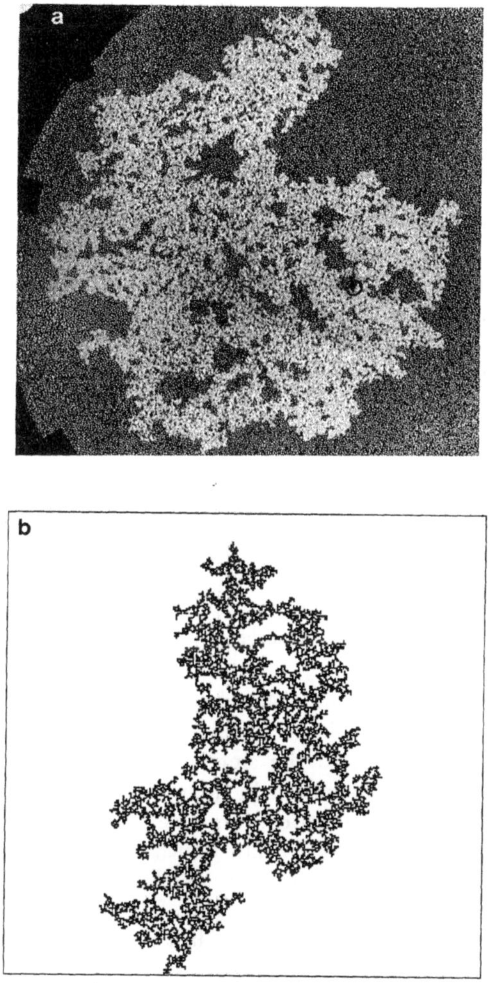

Figure 1. (a) Invasion percolation of air (white) displacing glycerol (black) in a two-dimensional model[30] (see the experimental section). (b) Invasion percolation with trapping on a 500 × 500 lattice. The invader (black) enters from the center and the defender (white) escapes through the square rim indicated. right-hand edge. At break-through the invader reaches the edge and has invaded 20 368 sites.

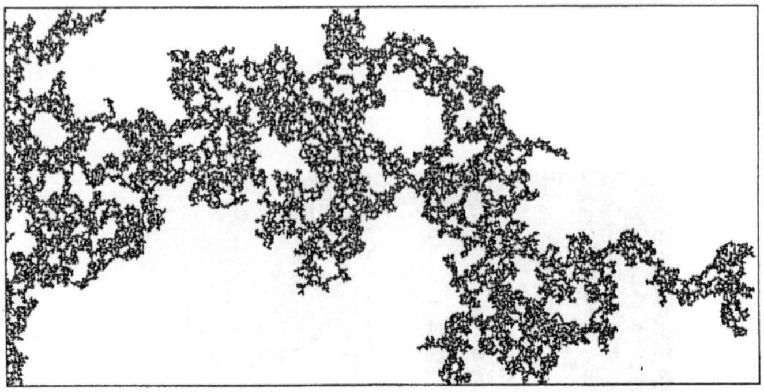

Figure 2. Invasion percolation with trapping on a 300 × 600 lattice. The invader (black) enters from sites on the left-hand edge and the defender (white) escapes through the right-hand edge. At breakthrough the invader first reaches the right-hand edge and has invaded 31802 sites. A color version of this figure which shows sites added within successive time intervals in different colors may be found in reference [22].

it is possible for it to completely surround regions of the defending fluid, i.e., completely disconnect finite clusters of the defending fluid from the exit sites of the sample. This is one origin of the phenomenon of 'residual oil,' a great economic problem in the oil industry. Since oil is incompressible, Wilkinson and Willemsen[21] introduced the rule that water cannot invade trapped regions of oil. This rule is implemented by removing growth sites in regions completely surrounded by the invading fluid from the list of growth sites.

In our simulations we used the algorithm described above on lattices of size $L \times 2L$ with L in the range 50–400. We used impermeable horizontal walls, injected the invader at the left hand side and terminated the simulation when the invader reached the right hand edge (see figure 2). As shown in figure 1b we also made simulations on $L \times L$ lattices with injection at the center site. The trapping rule is implemented as follows. The cluster of uninvaded sites in contact with the sink is found by the Hoshen-Kopelman[34] algorithm. If a growth site does *not* belong to this cluster, then it is trapped and removed from the list of growth sites. This global search for trapping is time consuming and is performed only when the last pore invaded is in a position that *may* trap a region of the defender.

Invasion percolation structures

Figures 1a and 2 shows the results of simulations of the invasion process. The number of sites, $M(L)$, that belong to the central $L \times L$ part of an $L \times 2L$ lattice, with injection from one side, scales with the size of the lattice,[21]

$$M(L) = AL^D \,, \quad \text{with} \quad D \simeq 1.82 \,. \tag{1}$$

This result is consistent with the experiments of Lenormand and Zarcone,[2] of air invading slowly into a network of ducts filled with glycerol. These results should

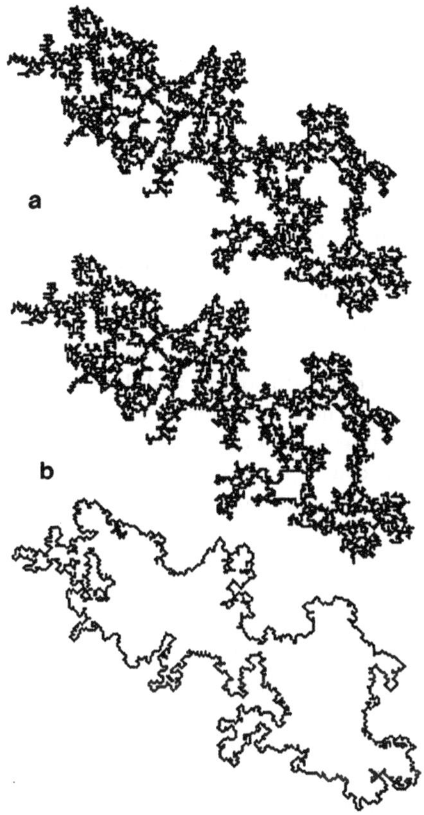

Figure 3. (a) The hull and (b) external perimeter of the invasion percolation cluster shown in figure 1b.

be contrasted with the ordinary percolation process for which the cluster is found by occupying all available sites with random numbers $r \leq p$ that are connected to the seed, and p is a pre-chosen occupation probability. At the percolation threshold $p = p_c$, the incipient percolation cluster also obeys equation (1), but with the higher fractal dimensionality[27–29] $D = 91/48 \simeq 1.895...$ There are two main differences between ordinary and invasion percolation. First, invasion percolation will *always* span the region between the injection and extraction sites. There is no analog to the occupation probability p, and there are no finite clusters of 'invaders.' Second, invasion percolation is a *dynamic* process, with a well defined sequence of invaded sites. Previous studies measured only the *static* fractal dimension D of the final aggregate.

Hull and External perimeter

The front of the invading fluid is of particular interest. Fractal fronts have been studied by means of computer simulation.[15,33,35–37] The fractal fronts of percolation clusters include the *hull*,[15] i.e., the edge of the cluster, with a fractal dimension of $D = {}^7\!/_4$

and the *external perimeter*,[33] i.e., the contour of the cluster seen when tested from the outside by a finite probe, which has a fractal dimension $D_e = 1.37$. The difference between the fractal dimensions of the hull and the external perimeter emphasizes that the details in the definition of the front may be important.

In figure 3 we show the hull and the external perimeter of the invasion percolation cluster shown in figure 1b. It is clear from the figure that the hull includes most of the occupied sites of the cluster itself. We find that the fractal dimension of the hull is $D_h = 1.80 \pm 0.07$, which is indistinguishable from the fractal dimension of the hull and of the cluster itself to the resolution of our simulations.

Numerical simulations[38] show that the growth sites form a fractal curve — the external perimeter. The number of growth sites in a circle of radius r is $M_g(r) \sim r^{D_g}$, where we find[38] $D_g \simeq 1.37$. In the simulations on strips of width L, we find that the number of growth sites becomes stationary and fluctuates around an average value $M_g(L) \sim L^{D_g}$. It is interesting to note that this new value is consistent with the fractal dimension of the external perimeter for ordinary percolation[33] given by $D_e = 1.37$. In the simulations on strips of width L, we find that the number of growth sites becomes stationary and fluctuates around an average value $M_g(L) \sim L^{D_g}$.

INVASION DYNAMICS

The first hints to the nature of the dynamics came from experiments on drying[31,32] and on slow fluid displacements.[39] In both cases, the front moved by invading local areas in *bursts*. Figure 4 shows a similar behavior: once a new site was invaded, the front tended to stay in that vicinity. The growth within a time interval t tends to occur within a *connected* region, and the different colored regions have similar linear extensions, of order $r_t \sim t^{1/D}$. Qualitatively, this can be understood: The invading front exhausts all easily invaded pores, then by forcing the invader through a difficult pore a new region which may have new easily invaded areas is made available to the front. The front then moves into this area until it gets stuck again having exhausted the new easily invaded pores.

To obtain a *quantitative* measurement of these time correlations, we considered the pair correlation function $N(r,t)$, giving the probability that a site a distance r from a reference site is invaded a time t later than the reference site. Thus $N(r,t)drdt$ is the conditional probability that if a site at the position $\mathbf{r}_0$ was invaded at time t_0, another site at a distance between r and $r + dr$ away from $\mathbf{r}_0$ is invaded in a time interval dt around $t_0 + t$. During the simulations the reference site is successively chosen to be the last invaded site. After some initial transient effects, the function $N(r,t)$ is found to be independent of t_0. This is expected since the invasion process is governed by local rules, and the surroundings of every new invaded site are statistically similar to the surroundings of any other invaded site independent of how far the process has developed.

We find that the correlation function obeys the *dynamic scaling* form

$$N(r,t) = r^{-1} f(r^z/t) , \qquad (2)$$

with the new dynamic exponent

$$z = D . \qquad (3)$$

We also find that the scaling function $f(u)$ is peaked at $u \sim 1$, and has an unusual limiting power law behavior at both limits,

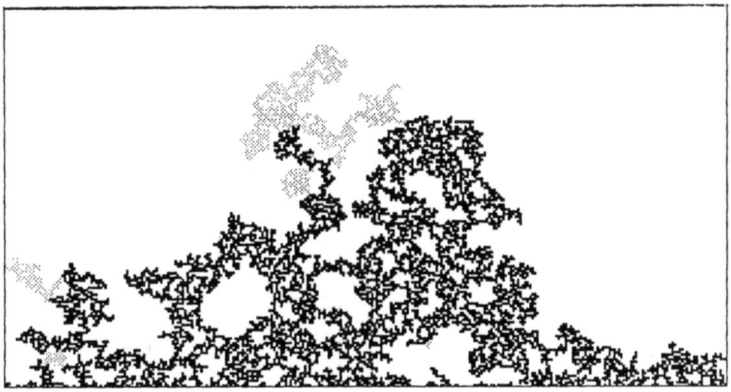

Figure 4. The growth dynamics of invasion percolation is characterized by regional invasion. The black sites represent the first 7 000 sites invaded on from the line at the bottom (300 sites wide). Around the last site invaded we have drawn a circle of radius $r = 25$. The next 1 000 invaded sites gray are clustered at a few locations.

$$f(u) \sim \begin{cases} u^a , & u \ll 1 \\ u^{-b} , & u \gg 1 \end{cases} \qquad \text{with} \quad a \simeq 1.4 \,, \quad b \simeq 0.6 \,. \tag{4}$$

This implies that the most probable growth occurs at $r_t \sim t^{1/D}$. At time t, most of the region within distance r_t has already been invaded, the rest of the region contains trapped defender fluid, and new growth there is rare. On the other hand, the probability to select a new growth site at $r \gg r_t$ decays rapidly with r.

We find that the initial effects due to the line source of the invading fluid decay rapidly and may be ignored for times that roughly correspond to the time when the invader first reaches a distance of $1/2 \cdot L$ from the source line. Beyond that time we find that $N(r,t)$ does not depend on t_0 (that is how far from the source it is evaluated). We thus average over t_0 to obtain an estimate for $N(r,t)$.

In figure 5 we show the correlation function $N(r,t)$ obtained in extensive simulations. First we note that for $t = 1$ growth is most probable close to the previously invaded site, and that the growth decreases as a power law r^{-2} as r increases. For $t > 1$, we find that after a time t has passed, growth is most probable at some distance r_t away. We find that $r_t \sim t^{1/z}$ with $z \simeq 1.8$. These results suggest the scaling form given in (2), which leads to the very satisfying data collapse shown in figure 6 with $z = 1.82$.

The straight segments in figure 6 give rise to the limiting behaviors in equation (4), implying that

$$N(r,t) \sim \begin{cases} r^{aD-1} t^{-a} , & r \ll r_t \\ r^{-bD-1} t^{b} , & r \gg r_t \end{cases} \tag{5}$$

The r^{-1} factor in the scaling expression (2) is a result of the normalization of the correlation function: Using r^{-x} instead gives

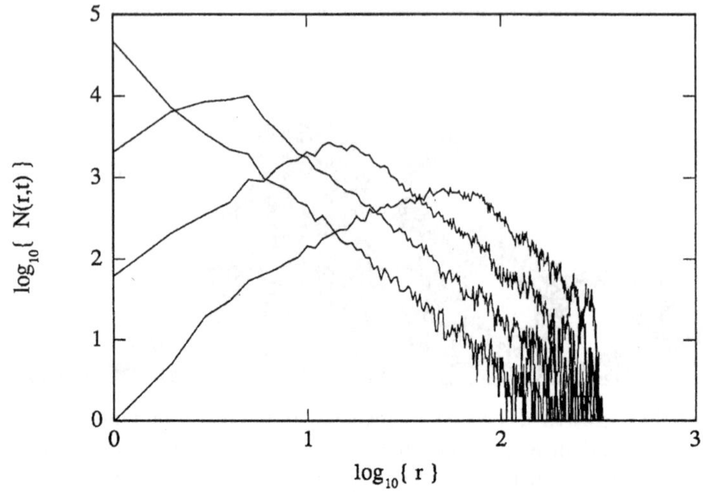

Figure 5. The correlation function $N(r,t)$ as a function of the separation r between sites invaded with a time separation t on a log–log plot, for time separations $t = 1$, 10, 100 and 1000. The data in the figure were generated in 8 simulations of the invasion percolation process on a lattice of size 300×600. The slope of the rising part of the curves is about 1.4, and that of the falling part is about -2.

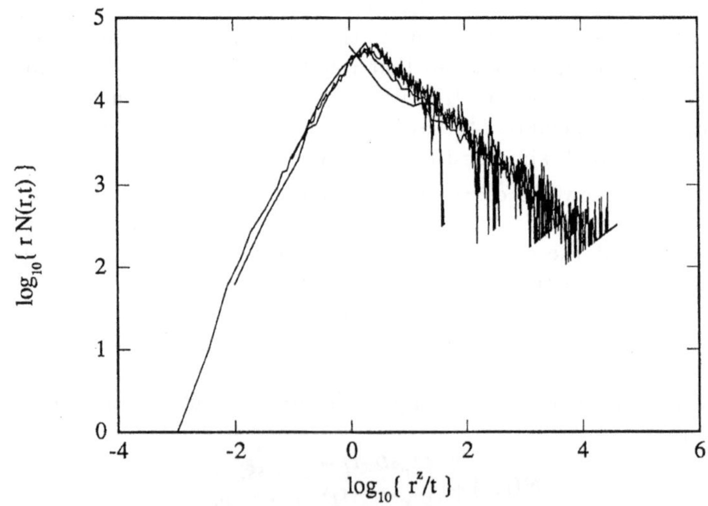

Figure 6. Log-log plot of the scaling function $f(u) = r \cdot N(r,t)$ as a function of $u = r^z/t$ and with $z = 1.82$ obtained by replotting the results shown in figure 5. Finite size effects result in a violation of the data collapse for $r \sim L$.

$$1 = \int_0^\infty r^{-x} f(r^z/t)\, dr = \frac{1}{z} t^{(1-x)/z} \int_0^\infty u^{(1-x-z)/z} f(u)\, du\,, \tag{6}$$

which is independent of time only for $x = 1$.

Equation (3) follows from the *pair connectedness* function $G(r)$, which is the probability that a site at a distance r from an occupied site is also occupied. We may express $G(r)$ in terms of $N(r,t)$ noting that (in d Euclidean dimensions) the number of sites a distance r away is $\sim r^{d-1}$

$$G(r) \sim \int_0^\infty N(r,t)/r^{d-1}\, dt \sim r^{z-d} \int_0^\infty u^{-2} f(u)\, du\,. \tag{7}$$

Here the integral converges. The pair connectedness function scales[27–29] as $G(r) \sim r^{D-d}$ and it follows that $z = D$ as given in equation (3). This result can be easily intuited: t is equal to the mass of an invasion percolation cluster grown around the reference site, as represented by different colors in figure 2.

DISPERSION IN POROUS MODELS

When a tracer is added to a fluid flowing in a porous medium it disperses because of molecular diffusion and convection. Dispersion plays an important role in oil production, hydrology, chemical processing and chromatography. Here we show that the dispersion front of miscible displacement has a fractal structure not previously described or analyzed.

The macroscopic description of dispersion[40–50] has the following form

$$\frac{\partial C}{\partial t} = \nabla \cdot (\mathbf{D} \cdot \nabla C - \mathbf{U} C) \tag{8}$$

Here $C(\mathbf{r},t)$ is the tracer concentration as a function of position $\mathbf{r}$ and time t. The dispersion tensor $\mathbf{D}(\mathbf{U})$ depends in general on the imposed hydrodynamic (average) flow velocity $\mathbf{U}$. For homogeneous porous media this dispersion tensor is characterized by only two independent components: the longitudinal, $D_{\|}$, and the transverse, $D_{\perp}$, dispersivities. For poorly connected porous media one observes *anomalous* dispersion and diffusion.[51,52]

Dispersion of tracers in a stationary fluid ($\mathbf{U} = \mathbf{0}$) is due to ordinary molecular diffusion and $D_{\|} = D_{\perp} = D_m$, where D_m is the diffusion constant of tracers in the fluid. Tracers are carried along the flow for finite velocities, $U > 0$, and the dispersion depends on U, i.e., the magnitude of $\mathbf{U}$. The relative importance of convective to diffusive transport is characterized by the *Péclet* number $\mathrm{Pe} = Ud/D_m$, where d is a typical pore size. The question of the dependence of $D_{\|}$ on Pe is a delicate problem. Any given stream-line meanders through the porous medium. It is important to realize that streamlines through one pore may separate into different pores and also meet again in a later pore. Therefore tracers that follow streamlines from one pore to another in effect perform independent random walks through the medium. Also, the velocity along the streamline fluctuates being slow through large pores and in stagnant regions, and faster than the average flow in narrow pore necks oriented parallel to the average flow. For large Péclet numbers the position of a tracer (relative to the position expected from the average flow) is described by a random walk process with an effective diffusion constant given by the Einstein relation: $D_{\|} = \frac{1}{2}d^2/\tau$, where the average time between 'steps' of length d is $\tau \sim d/U$. Therefore one finds[40,41] $D_{\|} \sim Ud$, i.e., the longitudinal dispersion

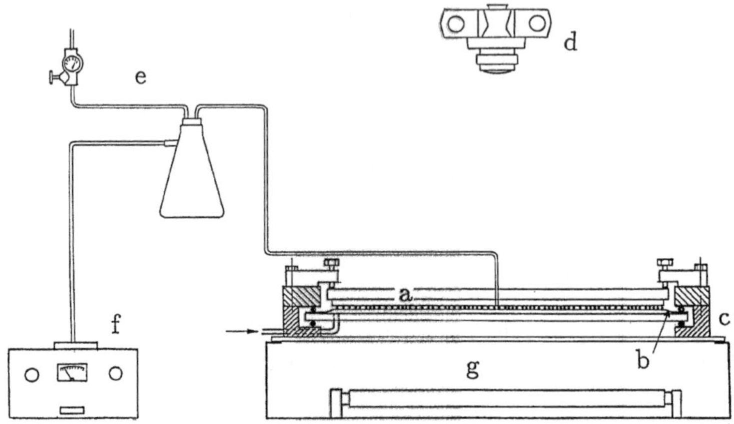

Figure 7. Experimental setup. a: porous model with glass spheres, b: plastic film, c: external aluminum ring, d: camera, f: pressure gauge, e: pressure reduction system, g: light board.

is proportional to the flow velocity U for $Ud \gg D_m$. When stagnation effects are included the expression is modified by logarithmic terms $D_{\|} \sim Ud\ln(U\ell/D_m)$, where ℓ is a length scale for diffusion out of stagnant regions.[40–50] We will use the form $D_{\|} = Ud_{\|}$, where $d_{\|}$ is the effective hydrodynamic correlation length.

At lower Péclet numbers molecular diffusion across stream lines leads to *Taylor dispersion*[53] with a longitudinal dispersion given by $D_{\|} = D_m + a^2U^2/48D_m$. This result was derived for flow in capillaries of radius a. Taylor dispersion dominates if the transverse mixing is large enough, i.e., if the time needed for diffusion across the capillary a^2/D_m is short enough compared with the convective time d/U.

The *new feature* presented here appears when we analyze the dispersion front itself: Contours of constant tracer concentration are *self-affine fractal curves*[7,8,23,24] confined by the width of the dispersion front. This fractal structure does *not* arise in dispersion of fluid flow in Hele-Shaw cells or capillaries, it is characteristic of dispersion in porous media. We also stress that our results have been obtained in homogeneous models. The fractal dimension is different for dispersion fronts in fractally porous media, such as dispersion in models that are near the percolation threshold.[51,52]

Sapoval et al.[35] discussed the diffusion of particles from a source, a process that is controlled by the diffusion equation, which is equation (8) *without* the convection term. They found that the front of the region of diffusers *connected* to the source was a fractal curve corresponding to the hull of a percolation cluster. The experiments of Shaw[31,32] on drying appear to be well described by a percolation front.

Experimental Methods

The experimental setup is shown in figure 7. The porous model consisted of 1 mm diameter glass spheres sandwitched between a stiff plexiglass disk (40 cm in diameter) and a thin plastic sheet held in contact with the spheres by compressed air. This assembly was supported from above and below by 10 mm thick glass discs, and clamped in an aluminum ring as illustrated in figure 7. We connected the space between the plastic film and the lower glass plate to a compressed air supply in order to force the film into contact with all of the glass spheres. This air pressure was higher than the pressure of the fluid injected into the porous model, and was held constant during the experiment. Fluids are injected at the center and leave the model at the rim. The model, which (porosity $\phi \simeq 0.7$) was filled by injecting a glycerol–water mixture through a hole in the center. Filling the model before increasing the pressure on the plastic film, makes it easier to fill pores with high viscosity fluids without trapping air bubbles.

In a typical experiment air injected at the center displaces glycerol filling the pore space of the model. The displaced glycerol was accumulated at the ambient pressure, p_0, in a channel at the rim of the circular model. Air at a constant pressure p_i, was introduced into the porous layer through a 1 mm hole at the center of the plexiglass disc. A stable pressure of the air displacing the glycerol was obtained using a Mortanair B11-M3 pressure regulator and a Norgren low pressure regulator connected with an external reservoir of about 5 l. The pressure of the air during the injection process was measured with a Texas Instrument Fused Quartz Pressure Gauge, and the pressure fluctuations at the center were typically less than 0.5%.

The resulting front structure was photographed with a Nikon F3 camera controlled from an IBM PC. Uniform lighting of the transparent model was provided from below. The pictures were enlarged using an Agfa Gevaert reprodoline 716 transparent film. figure 1a shows a typical invasion percolation pattern obtained in this way.

The dispersion experiments consisted of injecting a black glycerol-water-Negrosine solution, having the same viscosity and density as the clear mixture ($\mu = 49.9 \pm 0.4$ cP, $\rho = 1.21 \pm 0.03$ g/cm^3; $T = 25$ °C) at a rate of $Q = 0.173$ cm^3/s through the central hole. The resulting dispersion front was photographed and the negatives digitized with a resolution of 4000×4000, using a Data Copy scanning digitizing camera interfaced to an Apollo DN3000 workstation. The resolution used corresponds to 0.2 mm per pixel. In the digitizing process we selected a logarithmic response curve so that the resulting gray levels (0–255) are roughly proportional to the concentration of Negrosine in the volume imaged onto a pixel.

Observation of Fractal Dispersion

Our experiments on dispersion in miscible flow show that the dispersion front *on the average* is accurately described by equation (8) at high Péclet numbers. However, the front has a fractal structure that extends over the width of the front. The structure of the front is quite different from the fractal diffusion front discovered by Sapoval et al.[35,36]

An examples of a digitized picture is shown in figure 8. The figure illustrates the strong fluctuations of the fractal dispersion front caused by geometrical dispersion, which generates concentration 'spikes' in the radial direction.

The simplest geometry for solving equation (8) is the case where the tracers are added as a step-function in a linear geometry at $x = 0$. The concentration profile is then given by

$$C(x,t) = \frac{1}{2}(1 - \mathrm{erf}[(x - R_0)/\lambda]) \ , \qquad (9)$$

Here erf(x) is the error function, $R_0 = Ut$ is the position of the front and the width of the dispersion front is $\lambda = 2\sqrt{D_{\|}t}$. The solution of equation (8) for the radial geometry used here is more complicated. However, for the present purposes sufficient accuracy

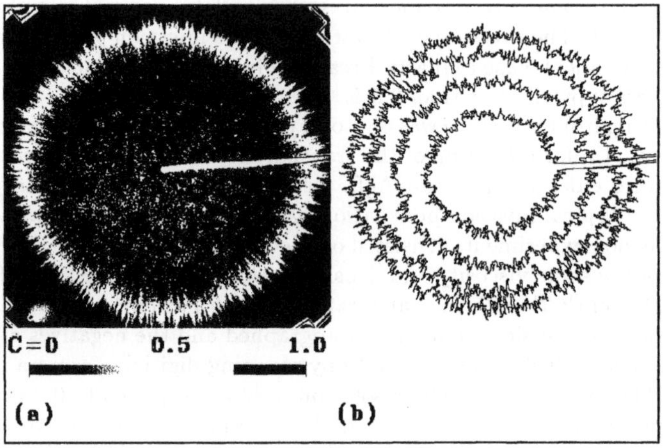

Figure 8. The dispersion obtained by injecting glycerol colored by Negrosine into glycerol of the same viscosity and density in a two-dimensional porous model. (a) The logarithm of the transmitted light intensity is color coded as shown in the insert. Time $t = 160$ s. (b) The time development of the fractal contour where the concentration is $1/2$ the injected tracer concentration. The four contours correspond to increasing times: $t = 36$ s; $t = 77$ s; $t = 122$ s; $t = 160$ s.

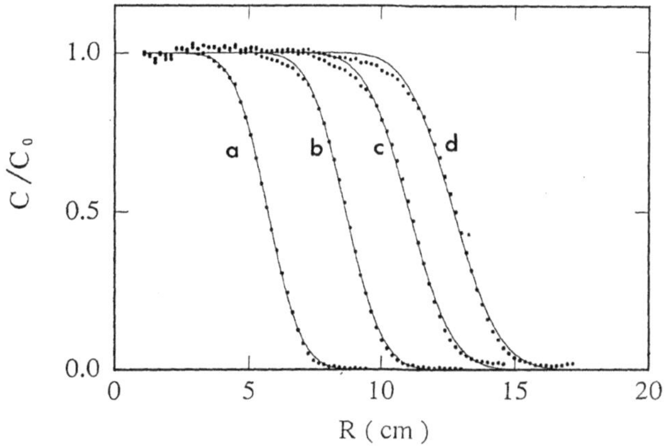

Figure 9. The average concentration $C(r,t)/C_0$ as a function of r for different times. The fitted functions $C/C_0 = \frac{1}{2}(1-\text{erf}\,[(r-R_0)/\lambda])$ are shown as solid lines in the figure. (a): $t = 36$ s, $R_0 = 5.71 \pm 0.01$ cm, $\lambda = 1.44 \pm 0.02$ cm. (b): $t = 77$ s, $R_0 = 8.67 \pm 0.01$ cm, $\lambda = 1.55 \pm 0.02$ cm. (c): $t = 122$ s, $R_0 = 12.72 \pm 0.02$ cm, $\lambda = 1.95 \pm 0.03$ cm. (d): $t = 160$ s, $R_0 = 11.06 \pm 0.02$ cm, $\lambda = 1.83 \pm 0.04$ cm.

is obtained by estimating the average concentration as $C(r,t) = \sum c(r_i,t)/2\pi r_i$, where the sum extends over the observed concentrations, $c(r_i)$, in the pixels labeled by i. Of course, the position of the front R_0 is no longer given by Ut but by $R_0 = \sqrt{qt/\pi}$, where $q = Q/b\phi$ is the injection rate per unit area given in terms of the volumetric injection rate Q the sample porosity ϕ and the sample thickness b. Figure 9 shows that equation (9) (full curves) approximates the observed average concentration profile well.

The values of $R_0(t)$ obtained from the fits of equation (9) to the observations are in good agreement with the measured injection rate Q. The width of the front λ obtained from the fits, increases with time. For the linear displacement we have $\lambda^2 = 4D_{||}t = 4d_{||}Ut = 4d_{||}R_0$. We find that, for the results shown in figure 9, this relation gives $d_{||} = 0.78 \pm 0.05$ mm, which is somewhat below the particle diameter $d = 1$ mm and consistent with the values of $d_{||} = 0.5d$ to $1.5d$ observed in porous media.[50] In the radial geometry used here the dispersion coefficient $D_{||}$ depends on the distance from the center of injection and the estimates made for $d_{||}$ are only approximate. At the leading edge of the average fronts shown in figure 9 we have a small discrepancy between the observations and the theoretical curve which is due to nonlinearities in the detection system. The deviation between equation (9) and the observed points at the trailing end of the front increases as the front moves is due to anomalous dispersion.

The structure of the dispersion front was studied in terms of the fractal dimension of the contour of the interface where the local concentration $C \in [0.500, 0.504]$. The fractal coastlines for four time stages are shown in figure 8b. Any practical fractal structure will have a lower and an upper length scale cut-off. In the present case the particle dimension $d = 1$ mm which corresponds to a five pixels is the lower cut-off. The upper cut-off is given by the width λ of the dispersion front. In figure 10 we show

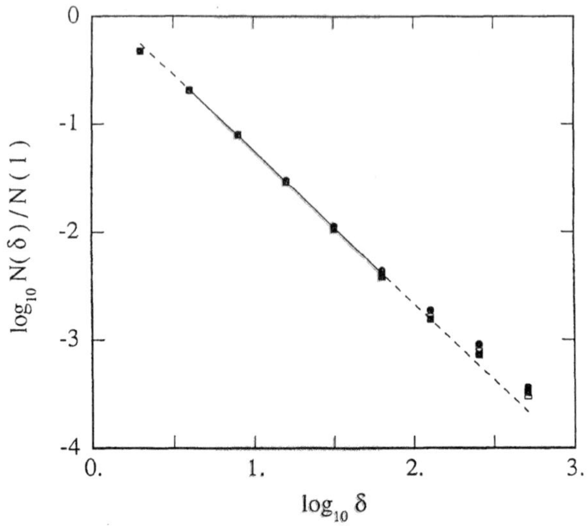

Figure 10. The number of 'boxes' $N(\delta)$ needed to cover the contours where the tracer concentration equals 1/2 the injected concentration as a function of the box size δ given in pixels. $N(1)$ is the total number of pixels in the contour. The fractal dimension is $D = 1.42 \pm 0.01$ estimated from the fit in the region drawn with a full curve.

the result of using the 'box-counting' method to estimate the fractal dimension of the front. The number of boxes $N(\delta)$ needed to cover the front with a box size δ (in pixels) is[7,8] $N(\delta) \sim \delta^{-D}$. We find that the dispersion front is fractal with $D = 1.42$. The uncertainty in the fractal dimension as estimated from the fit in figure 10 is ± 0.01. However, this uncertainty reflects only how well the points fall onto the straight line. Including the points for smaller and or larger δ changes the estimate and it is more realistic to conclude that $D = 1.42 \pm 0.05$. In order to obtain better estimates of the fractal dimension of the dispersion front much larger models must be constructed so that very wide dispersion fronts may be obtained.

In figure 10 we see that for $\delta > \lambda$ there is a crossover to a lower fractal dimension. In fact this is to be expected since the front on a scale $\delta \gg \lambda$ is a circle (with $D = 1$) and therefore is a self-affine[7,8,23,24] curve for which one must distinguish between *local* and *global* fractal dimensions.

Discussion of Fractal Dispersion

The concentration profiles of the dispersion front in a two dimensional porous medium have been measured. The results are described quite well by the solution of the convective diffusion equation (8) in a linear geometry which is given in equation (9). We find that the hydrodynamic dispersion coefficient $D_{\parallel} = Ud_{\parallel}$ with the parallel velocity correlation length is equal to $d_{\parallel} = 0.78d$, where $d = 1$ mm is the particle diameter. The width λ of the dispersion front is $\lambda = 2\sqrt{D_{\parallel}t} = 2\sqrt{d_{\parallel}R_0}$ and increases with the radius of the dispersion front.

We have shown that the detailed structure of a dispersion front in a two dimensional porous medium is fractal and that the contour of the concentration where

$C = 0.5$ has a fractal dimension of $D = 1.42 \pm 0.05$. It is tempting to relate the fractal contours we observe to the fractal diffusion front discovered by Sapoval et al.[35] which has a fractal dimension of $D = 1.75$ for the hull and $D = 4/3$ for the external perimeter. However, the diffusion front is defined in terms of the *connectivity* between diffusing particles whereas the fractal structure of the dispersion front reflects the probability distribution of where diffusing tracers end after time t. This probability distribution is the result of the combined diffusion and random convection in the porous medium. The physics of the two fronts is therefore different. The the diffusion front has been successfully mapped onto the percolaton problem which is also a problem of connectivity, and one may say that this front is theoretically well understood but not well established experimentally. The dispersion front contains different physics and we know of no model of fractal physics onto which the dispersion front may be directly related. Simulations of dispersion in porous media[47,49,50,54] have been restricted to very small systems due to limitations in computer resources and the structure of the front has not been studied. Comparing the contours shown in figure 9b to the self-similar diffusion fronts[36] obtained in simulations one finds that the dispersion contours look quite different. We therefore suggest that dispersion contours in fact belong to a universality class that is distinct from that of the diffusion front.

CONCLUSIONS

We have shown that the front of the invader in invasion percolation is characterized by a dynamic correlation function with the scaling form $N(r,t) = r^{-1} f(r^z/t)$ where the new dynamic exponent z is equal to the fractal dimension $D \simeq 1.82$ of the invaded region. The scaling function $f(u)$ behaves as u^a for $u \ll 1$ and as u^{-b} for $u \gg 1$. Such a power law behavior for both large and small arguments is rather surprising and remains a challenge for future theories.[55] We expect the exponents a and b to be related to D and D_g and possibly to other exponents characterizing the growth process. However, such relations remain to be derived.

Hopefully, the present study will stimulate similar studies on other growth and fluid displacement phenomena. For example, fluid displacement at high capillary numbers leads to *viscous fingering*[30] having a fractal structure[5,6] with a fractal dimension[6] $D = 1.64$. However, the scaling structure of this growth dynamics has not been investigated.

Why is the dispersion front fractal? Since the dispersion on the average is well described by Eq. (1) we know that the front is characterized by only two length scales: the average position of the front, and the width of the dispersion front, that both depend on time. This leads to the conclusion that dispersion has no intrinsic length scale independent of time in the range between the pore size and the width of the front. It is by now well established both from the study of phase transitions and from the applications of fractals that for problems which have no intrinsic length scale we expect *scaling* behavior, and that the geometry of the system is *fractal*. Unfortunately, we can say little in general about the expected fractal dimension for the dispersion process. A proper understanding of the fractal structure of the dispersion front remains a challenge for future theories.

ACKNOWLEDGEMENTS

Many interesting discussions with Einar Hinrichsen, Unni Oxaal and Paul Meakin have been very helpful. This work has been supported by VISTA, a research cooperation between the Norwegian Academy of Science and Letters and Den norske stats oljeselskap a.s. (STATOIL), and by NAVF. Work at Tel Aviv University was supported by the Israel Academy of Sciences and by the U.S. – Israel Binational Science Foundation.

REFERENCES

[1] Lenormand R. and Zarcone C. *Physico-Chemical Hydrodynamics*, **6**, 497, (1985).

[2] Lenormand R. and Zarcone C. *Phys. Rev. Lett.*, **54**, 2226–2229, (1985).

[3] Lenormand R. *C. R. Acad. Sci. Paris Ser. II*, **301**, 247–250, (1985).

[4] Lenormand R. *J. Fluid Mech.*, **189**, 165, (1988).

[5] Chen J. D. and Wilkinson D. *Phys. Rev. Lett.*, **55**, 1892–1895, (1985).

[6] Måløy K. J., Feder J., and Jøssang T. *Phys. Rev. Lett.*, **55**, 2688–2691, (1985).

[7] Mandelbrot B. B. *The Fractal Geometry of Nature*. W. H. Freeman, New York, 1982.

[8] Feder J. *Fractals*. Plenum, New York, 1988.

[9] Witten T. A. and Sander L. M. *Phys. Rev. Lett*, **47**, (1981).

[10] Vicsek T. *Fractal Growth Phenomena*. World Scientific, Singapore, 1988.

[11] Nittmann J., Daccord G., and Stanley H. E. *Nature*, **314**, 141–144, (1985).

[12] Paterson L. *Phys. Rev. Lett.*, **52**, 1621–1624, (1984).

[13] Deutch J. M. and Meakin P. *J. Chem. Phys.*, **78**, 2093, (1983).

[14] Hentschel H. G. E., Deutch J. M., and Meakin P. *J. Chem. Phys.*, **81**, 2496, (1984).

[15] Meakin P. and Deutch J. M. *J. Chem. Phys.*, **80**, 2115, (1984).

[16] Voss R. F. *J. Phys. A*, **17**, L373–L377, (1984).

[17] Måløy K. J., Boger F., Feder J., and Jøssang T. In Pynn R. and Riste T., editors, *Time-Dependent Effects in Disordered Materials*, pages 111–138, Plenum Press, New York, 1987.

[18] Meakin P. Fractal aggregates and their fractal measures. In Domb C. and Lebowitz J. L., editors, *Phase Transitions and Critical Phenomena*, pages 336–489, Academic Press, New York, 1987.

[19] Lee J. and Stanley H. E. *Phys. Rev. Lett.*, **61**, 2945–2948, (1985).

[20] Hinrichsen E. L., Måløy K. J., Feder J., and Jøssang T. *J. Phys. A: Math. Gen.*, (1989), in press.

[21] Chandler R., Koplik J., Lerman K., and Willemsen J. F. *J. Fluid Mech.*, **119**, 249–267, (1982).

[22] Wilkinson D. and Willemsen J. F. *J. Phys. A*, **16**, 3365–3376, (1983).

[23] Furuberg L., Feder J., Aharony A., and Jøssang T. *Phys. Rev. Lett*, **61**, 2117–2120, (1988).

[24] Mandelbrot B. B. *Phys. Scr.*, **32**, 257–260, (1985).

[25] Mandelbrot B. B. In Pietronero L. and Tosatti E., editors, *Fractals in Physics*, pages 3–28, North-Holland, Amsterdam, 1986.

[26] de Gennes P. G. and Guyon E. *J. Mec.*, **17**, 403–432, (1978).

[27] Lenormand R. *C. R. Acad. Sci. Paris B*, **291**, 279, (1980).

[28] Essam J. W. *Rep. Prog. Phys.*, **43**, 833–912, (1980).

[29] Stauffer D. *Introduction to Percolation Theory.* Taylor, Francis, London, 1985.

[30] Aharony A. Percolation. In Grinstein G. and Mazenko G., editors, *Directions in Condensed Matter Physics*, pages 1–50, World Scientific, Singapore, 1986.

[31] Feder J., Jøssang T., Måløy K. J., and Oxaal U. In Englman R. and Jaeger Z., editors, *Fragmentation Form and Flow in Fractured Media*, pages 531–548, 1986. Ann. Isr. Phys. Soc. **8**.

[32] Shaw T. M. *Better Ceramics Trough Chemistry II, Materials Research Society Symposia Proceedings*, **73**, 1671, (1986).

[33] Shaw T. M. *Phys. Rev. Lett.*, **59**, 1671–1674, (1987).

[34] Grossman T. and Aharony A. *J. Phys. A*, **19**, L745–L751, (1986).

[35] Hoshen J. and Kopelman R. *Phys. Rev. B*, **14**, 3428, (1976).

[36] Sapoval B., Rosso M., and Gouyet J. F. *J. Phys. Lett.*, **46**, L149–L156, (1985).

[37] Sapoval B., Rosso M., Gouyet J. F., and Colonna J. F. *Solid State Ionics*, **18**, 21–30, (1986).

[38] Meakin P. Fractal aggregates and their fractal measures. In Domb C. and Lebowitz J. L., editors, *Phase Transitions and Critical Phenomena*, pages 336–489, Academic Press, New York, 1987.

[39] Furuberg L. *Computer Simulations of Percolation Phenomena.* Master's thesis, University of Oslo, 1988.

[40] Måløy K. J., Feder J., and Jøssang T. 1985. Unpublished observations made during the preparation of reference[30].

[41] Saffman P. G. *J. Fluid Mech.*, **6**, 321, (1959).

[42] Saffman P. G. *J. Fluid Mech.*, **7**, 194, (1960).

[43] Bear J. *Dynamics of fluids in porous media.* American Elsevier, New York, 1972.

[44] Scheidegger A. E. *The physics of flow through porous media.* University of Toronto Press, Toronto, 1974.

[45] Dullien A. L. *Fluid Transport and Pore Structure.* Academic Press, New York, 1979.

[46] Sahimi M., Davis H. T., and Scriven L. E. *Chem. Eng. Com.*, **23**, 329, (1983).

[47] Sahimi M. *J. Phys. A*, **20**, L1293, (1987).

[48] Koch D. F. and Brady J. F. *J. Fluid Mech.*, **154**, 399, (1985).

[49] Baudet C., Charlaix E., Clement E., Guyon E., Hulin F. P., and Leroy C. In Pynn R. and Riste T., editors, *Scaling Phenomena In Disordered Systems*, pages 399–422, Plenum, 1985.

[50] de Arcangelis L., Koplik J., Redner S., and Wilkinson D. *Phys. Rev. Lett.*, **57**, 996, (1986).

[51] Charlaix E., Hulin J. P., and Plona T. J. *Phys. Fluids*, **30**, 1690, (1987).

[52] de Gennes P. G. *J. Fluid Mech.*, **136**, 189, (1983).

[53] Gefen Y., Aharony A., and Alexander S. *Phys. Rev. Lett.*, **50**, 77–80, (1983).

[54] Taylor G. I. *Pros. Roy. Soc. A*, **219**, 186, (1953).

[55] Koplik J., Redner S., and Wilkinson D. *Phys. Rev. A*, **37**, 2619, (1988).

[56] Scaling functions which vanish both at small and large arguments were seen before [Kolb M., and Herrmann H. J., J. Phys. A **18**, L435 (1985)] in other problems, but they have not been analyzed for power law behavior.

Part 7

Random Surfaces

FRACTAL BEHAVIOR OF TETHERED NETWORKS

Mehran Kardar

Department of Physics
Massachusetts Institute of Technology
Cambridge, Massachusetts 02139, USA

Abstract

Tethered networks are large macromolecules with regular (D-dimensional) connectivity, embedded in a d-dimensional space. Such networks may exhibit a variety of non-trivial fractal behaviors. A "Landau-Ginzburg" field theory is proposed to describe statistical mechanics of such structures. Effective elasticity and rigidity terms emerge naturally as a consequence of connectivity, while longer-range interactions are also included. A combined Mean-Field/Flory treatment reveals crumpled, rigid, and compact phases. Fluctuations (as explored by various renormalization-group schemes) play a crucial role in determining the fractal exponents in each of these phases, as well as at the phase transitions.

1. MODEL

1.1 Motivation

Recently much attention has been devoted to understanding the statistical mechanics of surfaces.[1] The interest spans particle physics (string and gauge theories), condensed matter physics (microemulsions, lamellar phases), and biology (membranes). However, the statistical mechanics of two-dimensional manifolds has turned out to be considerably more complex than that of one-dimensional objects[2] (polymers). Indeed a variety of different macroscopic behaviors can emerge from the choice of different starting microscopic surface models. In view of this complication, the microscopic model under consideration has to be carefully defined. Recently we introduced[3] a surface model composed of permanently connected particles. This can be regarded as the simplest generalization of polymers. Indeed, one can further generalize by considering D-dimensionally connected structures.[4] Such "macromolecules" will be referred to as "tethered networks".

The constraint of fixed connectivity is easily implemented by assigning a d-dimensional coordinate $\vec{r}_i$ to each particle, and an energy cost $V(|\vec{r}_i - \vec{r}_j|)$ which diverges for large separations. (Note that d = 3 for any real problem, but it is convenient to consider the general case.) Such a description clearly applies to covalently bonded atoms at low temperatures. (There can, in addition, be many body interactions.) For a statistical description of a large network the positions $\vec{r}_i$ of individual particles are no longer appropriate. Instead, we consider a coarse-grained average $\vec{r}(\mathbf{x})$; where a <u>continuous</u> coordinate $\mathbf{x}$ replaces the discrete index i for the <u>internal</u> position of the particle in the network, and the external coordinate $\vec{r}$ is the average of the positions of particles in the vicinity of $\mathbf{x}$ on the network.

All information about connectivity now resides in the topology of the domain Ω, which is the collection of all possible coordinates $\mathbf{x}$. Here, to proceed further, we make the assumption that Ω is a regular D-dimensional space of typical linear size L. (The volume L^D is proportional to N, the total number of atoms in the molecule.) For example, D = 1 corresponds to a linear macromolecule, while D = 2 refers to a planar structure such as a fisherman's net. Gels can be regarded as D = 3 networks, while non-integer D may approximate fractal structures.

The interparticle interactions can be separated into two groups[4]: (i) Corresponding to strong bonds between neighboring particles on the network (these are responsible for the primary conformations of biological molecules); and (ii) Weaker hydrogen bonds, van der Waals, and hard-core interactions between particles that are far away along the internal coordinate $\mathbf{x}$, but are actually close in real space (responsible for secondary and tertiary conformations). The role and consequences of each type in a statistical description is now described separately.

1.2. Internal Connectivity

First consider the strong bonds holding the network together, and ignore interactions between particles not close in internal space. In the terminology of polymers[2], these are "phantom networks". The probability of a particular configuration $\{\vec{r}(\mathbf{x})\}$ is given by the Boltzmann weight $P(\{\vec{r}(\mathbf{x})\} \propto \exp[-\beta H\{\vec{r}(\mathbf{x})\}]$. Rather than calculating the energy function βH from first principles, we deduce its form from symmetry considerations. This is similar in spirit to the Landau-Ginzburg approach to superconductivity, and phase transitions[5]. The basic symmetries in external space are invariance under translations and rotations. The former implies that βH can depend only on derivatives such as $\partial_\alpha \vec{r} \equiv \partial \vec{r}(\mathbf{x})/\partial x_\alpha$ and $\partial_\alpha \partial_\beta \vec{r}$; while the latter allows only scalar products such as $\partial_\alpha \vec{r} \cdot \partial_\beta \vec{r}$. For a uniform <u>and isotropic</u> network we can then expand βH in powers of $\partial_\alpha \vec{r}$

$$\beta H_1 = \int d^D x \left[\frac{t}{2}(\partial_\alpha r_i)^2 + u(\partial_\alpha r_i \partial_\beta r_i)^2 + v(\partial_\alpha r_i \partial_\alpha r_i)^2 + \frac{K}{2}(\partial_\alpha^2 r_i)^2 + \ldots\right], \tag{1}$$

where $\alpha = 1, 2, \ldots, D$; $i = 1, 2, \ldots, d$; and summation convention is used.[4]

The terms in Eq.(1) have simple physical interpretations: t represents a Hookian elasticity, while u and v are anharmonic elastic terms; κ corresponds to a rigidity that arises from bond-bending forces. Thus elasticity and rigidity emerge naturally as macroscopic manifestations of internal connectivity. For polymers, entropy-generated elasticity is well known and easily proved by the central limit theorem.[2] Its presence for $D = 2$ has been shown from simulations, and can be seen in all D from an approximate Migdal-Kadanoff rescaling.[3] In fact Eq.(1) describes a variety of macroscopic behaviors,[4] in the same way that Landau theories of magnetism describe ordered and disordered phases.[5] A detailed description of these phases will be given after inclusion of long-range interactions. It is clear, for example, that for $t < 0$ and $(u, v) > 0$, the tangents $\partial_\alpha \vec{r}$ obtain a non-zero expectation value. This broken symmetry state is, in fact, a rigid phase.[6]

1.3. Long-Range Interactions

The entropy generated elastic energy is minimized when the network has a small size R in external space.[3] Consequently particles that are far apart along the backbone of the manifold are brought to close physical proximity and their interactions can no longer be ignored. A general two body term is described by $\int d^D x\, d^D y\, U(|\vec{r}(\mathbf{x}) - \vec{r}(\mathbf{y})|)$. At temperatures higher than typical van der Waals energies, particles feel only the hard-core repulsion which can be described by $U \equiv b(T)\, \delta^d[\vec{r}(\mathbf{x}) - \vec{r}(\mathbf{y})]$. As in polymers, the "excluded volume" b(T) is related to the second virial coefficient in a solution of such networks, and may change sign as temperature is reduced, or the quality of the solvent is changed.[2] When this happens, higher order terms are necessary to prevent collapse to very high densities. With this in mind we approximate the effects of these remote interactions by an energy,

$$\beta H_2 = b \int d^D x_1\, d^D x_2\, \delta^d[\vec{r}(\mathbf{x}_1) - \vec{r}(\mathbf{x}_2)] +$$
$$c \int d^D x_1\, d^D x_2\, d^D x_3\, \delta^d[\vec{r}(\mathbf{x}_1) - \vec{r}(\mathbf{x}_2)]\; \delta^d[\vec{r}(\mathbf{x}_2) - \vec{r}(\mathbf{x}_3)] \;. \qquad (2)$$

The probability for a configuration $\{\vec{r}(x)\}$ is now controlled by a Hamiltonian $\beta H = \beta H_1 + \beta H_2$, which includes both neighboring and remote interactions. The terms in the Hamiltonian have been written down on the basis of symmetry, and hence the parameters t, u, v, κ, b, and c are all expected to be functions of temperature, microscopic parameters, solution pH, and so on. As in usual Landau theories, the signs of these effective parameters determine the macroscopic phase of the network.[5] Such analogies are formally correct only for $L, N \to \infty$, but for large N similar behavior is expected up to some "finite-size rounding" effects which are discussed in the next section.

2. MEAN-FIELD/FLORY TREATMENT

Consider a network of internal linear size L (or mass L^D), embedded in d-dimensions. The scaling of the actual network size R in external space with L characterizes the macroscopic "phase" of the system. This dependence can be estimated by comparing typical values for the various terms in βH_1 and βH_2. These estimates[6] are summarized by a free energy,

$$2\beta F/D \approx \kappa R^2 L^{D-4} + t R^2 L^{D-2} + w R^4 L^{D-4} + b L^{2D}/DR^d + c L^{3D}/DR^{2d}, \qquad (3)$$

where the βH_1 terms are evaluated approximately by replacing $\partial_\alpha r_i$ with R/L, and $w = u + Dv$. The terms in βH_2 are calculated in the usual Flory approximation.[2] As R/L is typically small, the expansion in Eq.(3) is justified, and only the most important terms need to be kept. For example the rigidity term is always smaller than the elastic terms and can be neglected. Since b and t can change sign with temperature[2,6], the other terms with $c, w > 0$ are necessary to ensure stability.

The optimal radius is obtained by minimizing Eq.(3) with respect to R for fixed L. At sufficiently high temperatures both t and b are positive, and these two terms asymptotically dominate the rest. Minimization leads to the generalized Flory expression[6,7]

$$R \sim \left(\frac{b}{t}\right)^{\frac{1}{d+2}} L^{\frac{D+2}{d+2}}, \qquad (4)$$

i.e. balancing the self-avoiding repulsion with the elastic attraction leads to a crumpled network with a non-trivial fractal dimension. The Flory exponent $\nu_F = (D + 2)/(d + 2)$, although not exact, is quite accurate for polymers (D = 1);[2] and $\nu_F = 4/5$ is quite close to the result obtained numerically[3] for surfaces (D = 2) in d = 3.

Eq.(4) indicates a divergence in R as $t \to 0$; and indeed for $t < 0$ the anharmonic term wR^4L^{D-4} is needed for stability. The competition between the elastic terms leads[6] to $R \sim L\,|t|^{1/2}$. This clearly describes an expanded rigid phase with stretched bonds between particles on the network. The average bond length plays the role of an order parameter, and vanishes with the mean-field exponent $\beta = 1/2$ close to the transition ($|t| \to 0$).

At $t = 0$, the anharmonic elasticity competes with self-avoidance, leading to[6] $R \sim L^{\nu_c}$ with $\nu_c = (D + 4)/(d + 4)$. The distinct scaling forms in the vicinity of $t \sim 0$ can be combined into a single homogeneous function $R \sim L^{\nu_c}\,\psi(t\,L^y)$, where $\psi(0) = \text{constant}$, $\psi(x) \to |x|^{\phi_\pm}$ for $x \to \infty$, $y = 2\,(d - D)/(d + 4)$, $\phi_- = 1/2$, and $\phi_+ = -1/(d + 2)$. Similar homogeneous functions, with the same crossover exponent, y, can be constructed for other variables such as the free energy and heat capacity.[6] For example, approaching the transition from the crumpled side, the specific heat per particle scales anomalously, $C \sim t^{-\alpha} L^{-k}$ with $\alpha = (d + 4)/(d + 2)$ and $k = 2\,(d - D)/(d + 2)$. These results only hold for $t > t_x \sim L^{-y}$; and may be experimentally observable.

Again Eq.(4) predicts $R \to 0$ as $b \to 0$; and for $b < 0$ the three body interaction with $c > 0$ is necessary for stability. Consequently $R \sim \left(\frac{c}{b}\right)^{1/d} L^{D/d}$ which describes a compact structure with a density that vanishes linearly with b. The point $b = 0$ is referred to as a θ-point in polymer terminology[2], and is similar to a tricritical point[5]. At this point,

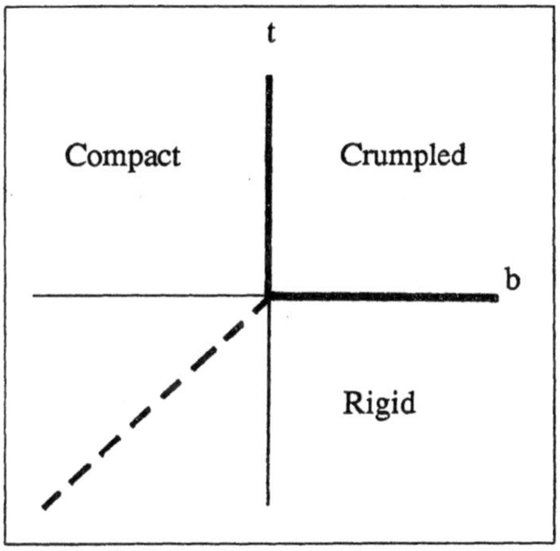

FIGURE 1

Schematic phase diagram obtained from Eq.(3).

balancing the three-body and elastic energies leads to $R \sim L^{\nu_\theta}$ with $\nu_\theta = (D + 1)/(d + 1)$. In the vicinity of $b \sim 0$, again, a scaling form $R \sim L^{\nu_\theta} \Phi(bL^{y_\theta})$ tcan be matched to the forms given for $b > 0$ and $b < 0$. There is again a specific heat anomaly approaching the θ point from the crumpled side.[2] One should note however that for $b < 0$, a solution of such networks phase separates,[3] and the results from considering just a single network are no longer meaningful.

For $b, t < 0$ there is a first order transition between the rigid and compact phases for $b^2/c \sim t^2/w$. The resulting phase diagram in indicated in Fig.(1). The three phase boundaries come together in a special multicritical point at $b = t = 0$. At this point scaling is determined by the competition of anharmonic and three body terms, leading to $R \sim L^{\nu^*}$ with $\nu^* = (D + 2)/(d + 2)$ which coincides with the Flory exponent ν_F.

3. FLUCTUATIONS

3.1. Crumpled Networks

The crumpled phase is "critical" in the sense that it has no characteristic length scale. (Tangent-tangent correlations, for example, decay algebraically.) It can be shown that[4,8] for $d > d^*(D) = 4D/(2 - D)$ self-avoidance is irrelevant and ν takes the free-field value $\nu_0 = (2 - D)/2$. For $d < d^*(D)$, upon including fluctuations, R behaves as $R \sim b^{\omega'} t^{-\omega} L^{\nu}$. The exponent ν can be calculated systematically by an $\varepsilon = 4D - d(2 - D)$ expansion[4,8]. Furthermore, since there is a general scaling form

$$R^2 \sim K L^{2-D} f(b K^{-d/2} L^{\varepsilon/2}), \tag{5}$$

with $f(x) \sim x^{2(2\nu + D - 2)/\varepsilon}$ for large x; where the effective elastic constant K diverges as $t^{-\gamma}$. Relaxation of these surfaces is by diffusive modes, and their critical dynamics have been described in detail elsewhere.[3]

3.2. The Rigid Phase

In the rigid phase, there is a spontaneously broken symmetry as the network orients itself along a particular direction in space. We should therefore consider fluctuations in the form of Goldstone modes that tend to restore the symmetry. The lowest energy modes are undulations h_β ($\beta = D + 1, ..., d$) in directions perpendicular to the chosen orientation of the network. These modes are, however, coupled to phonons u_α ($\alpha = 1, ..., D$), along the stretched network backbone. Substituting $\vec{r}(\mathbf{x}) = \zeta [(x_\alpha + u_\alpha)\hat{e}_\alpha + h_\beta \hat{e}_\beta]$ in βH_1 and using $\zeta \sim R/L \sim |t|^{1/2}/w$ leads to[6]

$$\beta H_f = \int d^D x \left[\frac{\kappa}{2}(\nabla^2 h_\beta)^2 + \mu\, u_{ij}{}^2 + \frac{\lambda}{2} u_{kk}{}^2\right], \tag{6}$$

where the strain tensor is $u_{ij} = \frac{1}{2}[\partial_i u_j + \partial_j u_i + \partial_i h_\beta \partial_j h_\beta]$, and the elastic constants are

$\mu = 4u\zeta^4$ and $\lambda = 8v\zeta^4$. Eq.(6) generalizes the expression for the bending of plates.[9] Note that the elastic constants μ and λ vanish at the transition.

Naively, one expects that the undulation modes will restore the full symmetry for $D \leq 2$, and that the rigid phase is unstable for $D = 2$. (Indeed this mechanism is responsible for absence of rigid-rod polymers). However, the non-linear coupling of undulation and phonon modes tends to stiffen the flat surface at large distances. This is seen both in a mode-coupling approximation[10], and in a rigorous $\varepsilon = 4 - D$ expansion.[11] A flat tethered surface has also been observed upon inclusion of bending rigidity in the numerical simulations.[12]

3.3. The Compact Phase

Minimizing the free energy in Eq.(3) for $b < 0$ led to a compact phase. This phase can also be obtained by exerting an external pressure p on the network. However, the compact equilibrium configuration may not be easily accessible dynamically, and the system may get trapped into metastable configurations. Indeed, although it is easy to compactify a string, attempts to compactify aluminum foil[4], or to crush paper[13] lead to fractal objects with $\nu \sim 4/5$ rather than 2/3, i.e. with a fractal dimension of 2.5. These results, although quite reproducible, have not been satisfactorily explained.

3.4. The Rigid to Crumpled Transition

The mean-field approach described in Sec.2 ignores critical fluctuations. As the crumpling transition is approached from the flat phase, a Ginzburg criterion[6] shows that mean-field theory breaks down for $t^2 (\kappa/-t)^{D/2} \lesssim 1$. If the transition remains continuous, we expect $R \sim L|t|^\beta$ with $\beta \neq 1/2$ due to fluctuations. Since self-avoidance is irrelevant in the flat phase, the exponent β can in fact be probed systematically by $\varepsilon = 4 - D$ expansions.[5] To the lowest order in $\varepsilon = 4 - D$, the transition is in fact driven first order by fluctuations[6] for $d < d_c \approx 219$. It is however possible that a continuous transition is recovered for $\varepsilon = 0(1)$ as suggested by Monte-Carlo simulations[12] in $D = 2$ and $d = 3$.

Another approach that includes fluctuations at the rigid to crumpled transition is a 1/d expansion (analogous to the 1/n expansion for O(n) models[5]). Indeed this approach at $D = 2$ has suggested a continuous transition[14], and its extension to general D is quite natural.[15,16] The resulting field theory has the remarkable property of having lower critical dimension $D_l = 2 - 2/d + O(1/d^2)$, which is less than two. This theory can thus be used to systematically probe, for the first time, the approach to a nontrivial lower critical dimension.[16]

4. CONCLUSIONS

Guided by considerations of symmetry, we have constructed a field theory describing embeddings of a regular isotropic network in d-dimensional space. Elasticity and rigidity terms naturally appear as a result of internal connectivity, and interactions between particles remote on the network are also included. This theory is capable of describing various phases of the network: crumpled, rigid, compact, etc. The behavior of these phases and the transitions between them is described both in a mean-field/Flory approach, and upon including fluctuations. This model represents a unified approach to regular networks (D = 1 for polymers, D = 2 for tethered membranes, and D = 3 for gels). Including fluctuations has led us to consider some remarkable field theories. The crumpled phase is described by a theory of fractional manifolds, and perturbation theory requires calculation of manifold diagrams with similarities to string-theory diagrams. Consideration of the rigid phase indicates unusual couplings between Goldstone modes, yielding anomalously scaling elastic constants. Consequently the Mermin-Wagner theorem no longer holds, and a spontaneous symmetry breaking is allowed in lower than two dimensions.

ACKNOWLEDGEMENTS

The work described here has resulted from collaborations with Y. Kantor, D.R. Nelson, and M. Paczuski. The research was supported by NSF through grant No. DMR86-20386.

REFERENCES

1. *Statistical Mechanics of Membranes and Surfaces*, Proceedings of the Fifth Jerusalem Winter School, edited by D.R. Nelson, T. Piran, and S. Weinberg (World Scientific, Singapore, 1989).
2. P.G. De Gennes, *Scaling Concepts in Polymer Physics* (Cornell University Press, Ithaca, NY, 1979).
3. Y. Kantor, M. Kardar, and D.R. Nelson, Phys. Rev. A 35, 3056 (1987).
4. M. Kardar and D.R. Nelson, Phys. Rev. A 38, 966 (1988).
5. K.G. Wilson and J. Kogut, Phys. Reports 12C, 75 (1974).
6. M. Paczuski, M. Kardar, and D.R. Nelson, Phys. Rev. Lett. 60, 2638 (1988).
7. M.E. Cates, Phys. Lett. 161B, 363 (1985); Phys. Rev. Lett. 53, 926 (1984).
8. J.A. Aronovitz and T.C. Lubensky, Europhys. Lett. 4, 395 (1987).
9. L.D. Landau and E.M. Lifshitz, *Theory of Elasticity*, (Pergamon Press, 1986).
10. D.R. Nelson and L. Peliti, J. Physique 48, 1085 (1987).
11. J.A. Aronovitz and T.C. Lubensky, Phys. Rev. Lett. 60, 2634 (1988).
12. Y. Kantor and D.R. Nelson, Phys. Rev. A 36, 4020 (1987).

13. M.A.F. Gomez and G.L. Vasconcelas, Phys. Rev. Lett. 60, 237 (1988); Y. Kantor, M. Kardar, and D.R. Nelson, Phys. Rev. Lett. 60, 238 (1988).

14. F. David and E. Guitter, EuroPhys. Lett. 5, 709 (1988).

15. J.A. Aronovitz, L. Golubovic, and T.C. Lubensky, J. Phys. (Paris) 50, 609 (1989).

16. M. Paczuski and M. Kardar, Phys. Rev. A 39, 6086 (1989).

SURFACE GROWTH, DIRECTED POLYMERS, AND 1/f NOISE

YI-CHENG ZHANG

INFN, Dipartimento di Fisica,
Università di Roma, 00185 Roma, Italy

ABSTRACT

Three seemingly unrelated topics are discussed: surface growth, directed polymers, and $1/f$ noise. From the discussion of surface growth, a nonlinear differential equation is motivated. It is shown to be related to the problem of Directed Polymers in a random medium. The partition function of these Directed Polymers can be regarded as a hybrid of sums and products of random numbers, we show its distribution is a natural generalization of the log-normal distribution. We use this knowledge to explain why is $1/f$ noise in nature so robust.

Growth Problem

Recently there has been progress in understanding interfaces which are not at equilibrium. Such interfaces are often seen in *nature*: forest fire spreading, tumor growth—this inspired Eden to propose his well-known model[1], crystal growth, ballistic deposition, etc. If a growth mechanism is local—various segments of an advancing interface do not interact at long distances (DLA is thus excluded), homogeneously and stochastically, the above growing interfaces are believed to fall in the same universality class[2].

One of the first attempts to model an advancing interface with an average constant velocity was made by Edwards and Wilkinson[3], who proposed the following equation:

$$dh(\vec{x},t)/dt = \Delta h(\vec{x},t) + v + \eta(\vec{x},t), \tag{1}$$

Fractals' Physical Origin and Properties
Edited by L. Pietronero
Plenum Press, New York

where $\eta(\vec{x},t)$ is short-range correlated noise, v is the constant velocity and $h(\vec{x},t)$ is the interface height, as shown in the figure below.

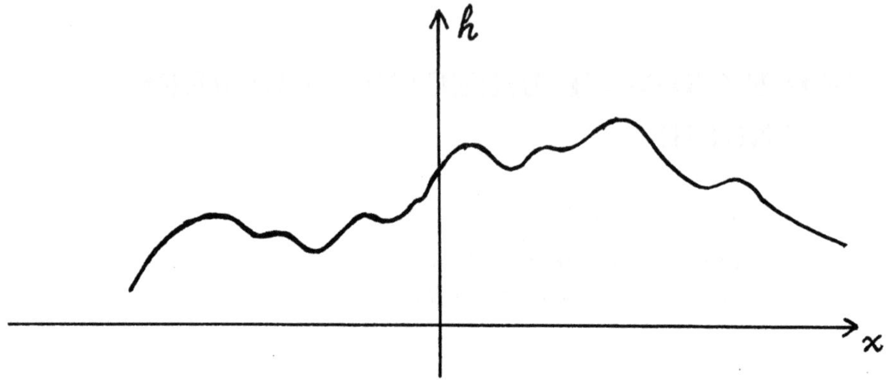

Figure 1.

The above equation would be the stochastic equation of a free interface at equilibrium, except for the constant velocity added.

An interface advances because the phase on one side of the interface is growing into the other. Let us check if eq.(1) is enough to describe the growth phenomena discussed above. In Fig.2 we show a segment of the interface in Fig.1, and it has been shifted a constant distance in the growth direction. Apart from stochastic noise, this is implied by eq.(1) .

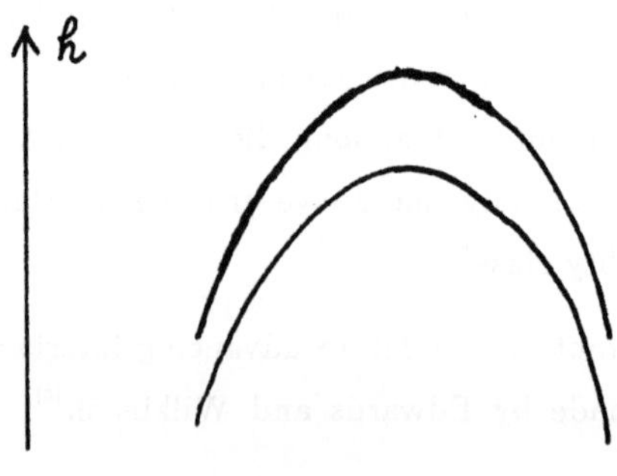

Figure 2.

It is clear that there is bias—the lateral growth has been under-estimated. From common knowledge it is clear that, if a fire or infection is spreading, it should have equal chance to affect the surrounding regions; the growth should take place towards the local normal direction of the interface. It is not hard to show how to correct this bias in eq.(1)—a term $\sqrt{1+(\vec{\nabla}h)^2}$ has to be included to compensate lateral growth. For $(\vec{\nabla}h)^2$ not very large, it can be expanded $1+1/2(\vec{\nabla}h)^2+\cdots$. Since we are interested only in the large scale and long time limits, according to commom folklore of scaling concepts, higher order terms can be neglected. The equation now becomes (apart from a constant):

$$\partial h/\partial t = \Delta h + \frac{1}{2}(\vec{\nabla}h)^2 + \eta(x,t), \tag{2}$$

Note that the above equation has many desirable ingredients for describing a growing interface: it is translationally invariant; it does not has the symmetry $h \to -h$: the interface differentiates the two sides as it should ($-\lambda$ would describe corrosion rather than growth); another point is somewhat hidden—it enjoys a Galilean invariance[4], which can be seen by mixing the spatial and temporal variables, or in other words by tilting the reference frame-work in Fig.1 by a small angle. Note also that this equation *cannot* be treated as a Lagevin equation of the form $\partial h/\partial t = -\delta H/\delta h + \eta$. Such a Hamiltonian H does not exist. This shows that we are dealing with a genuine dynamical phenomenon—equilibrium à *la* Boltzmann does not exist.

If one is in the moving frame, one should see effective dynamical equilibrium. We are interested the scaling behavior,

$$< |h(\vec{x},t) - h(\vec{x}',t')|^2 > \sim |\vec{x}-\vec{x}'|^{2\chi} f(|t-t'|/|\vec{x}-\vec{x}'|^z), \tag{3}$$

where χ and z are the two scaling exponents, $f(u)$ is a scaling function. Due to the Galilean invariance[4], we have the relation $\chi + z = 2$. Thus there is only one scaling exponent to be found. The equation (2) can be readily analysed by the dynamical renormalization group (RG) technique[2], which leads us to $z = 3/2$ for $d = 2$. For $d > 2$ cases, the RG analysis shows that physical fixed points cannot be probed perturbatively, one has to rely on direct or indirect numerical simulations.

The equation (2) can be rewritten in other forms. Defining $\vec{v} = \vec{\nabla}h$, we have

$$\partial\vec{v}/\partial t = \Delta\vec{v} + \vec{v}\cdot\vec{\nabla}\vec{v} + \vec{f}(x,t), \tag{4}$$

where $\vec{f} = \vec{\nabla}\eta$. This equation is called the noise-driven Burgers' equation, $\vec{v}$ is the vortex-free fluid velocity. It has applications in describing shock waves in fluid transport, and has been studied extensively.[5]

If we define $W = \exp[\frac{1}{2}h]$, W satisfies

$$\partial W/\partial t = \Delta W + \eta(x,t)W, \tag{5}$$

which describes diffusion in a time-dependent random medium.

Directed Polymers

The above equation (5) has the Feynman path integral solution

$$W(\vec{x},t) = \int_{(\vec{0},0)}^{(\vec{x},t)} D[\vec{x}] \exp - \int_0^t d\tau \{\frac{1}{2}\dot{\vec{x}}^2(\tau) + \eta(\vec{x}(\tau),\tau)\}. \tag{6}$$

It is a sum of all the oriented paths that connect $(\vec{0},0)$ to $(\vec{x},t)$, hence called directed polymers.[6] On a space-time lattice, the above expression becomes

$$W = \sum_{path} \prod_{i \in path}^{t} a_i, \tag{7}$$

where a_i is the random quenched variable on lattice bond, which assumes positive values. The following figure shows an example of the square lattice, on which a few paths are drawn.

For each random sample, $W(\vec{x},t)$ in general is not symmetric with respect to the geometrical center $(\vec{0},t)$. We are interested in its deviation, defined by $x_c(t) = \overline{|<\vec{x}>|}$ where the overbar denotes the sample average, $<\cdot>$ is the average using the normalized probability density function $P(\vec{x},t) = W(\vec{x},t)/\int d\vec{y}W(\vec{y},t)$. We

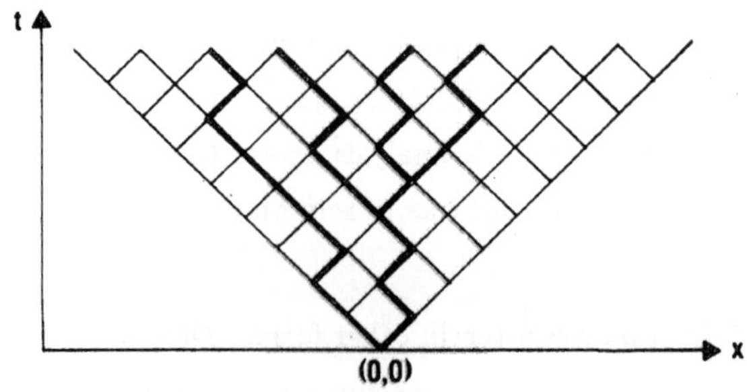

Figure 3. In this square lattice each bond is given a random value; at the level t there are t points and each of them can be connected to the apex of the triangle in a unique optimal way. A few local optimal paths are shown; one path is the overall best path.

expect the scaling behavior $x_c \sim t^{\nu}$, where the exponent ν is related to the above exponent z, $\nu = 1/z$.

If disorder is very strong we expect that only one path among all possible ones connecting $(\vec{0}, 0)$ to $(\vec{x}, t)$, dominates in the sum (6), so that it alone determines the scaling behavior. This is the so-called zero temperature phase. More sophisticated study[4] shows that in $(1+1)$-dimensions there is only one phase, i.e. the zero temperature phase persists for all disorder strength. Thus our problem is reduced to finding the "best" path, which maximizes the exponential in (6), subject to the constraint of fixed starting and ending points and continuity of the path. This is an optimization problem which can be solved numerically using a transfer matrix technique, and by various indirect analytical methods. If we move one end of the string $(\vec{x}, t)$ (the other end at $(\vec{0}, 0)$ is fixed), i.e. let $\vec{x}$ vary and keep t constant, there will be other local optimal paths. An illustration is drawn in the figure below.

The ensemble of the optimal paths is naturally organized into a hierarchical tree structure, which is not hard to understand: since there should be no two exactly equivalent optimal paths, loops should not appear. In Fig.4 we can see the tendency that two neighboring optimal paths try to join together as soon as possible. This is because it is very "costly" to have two optimal paths running parallel for too long a distance.

The hierarchical tree structure of our optimization problem is thus a result of "ecomonical" considerations. Such phenomena are not uncommon in natural circumstances: river basins, blood-vessels, tree or plant roots and even man-made highway networks, etc., all exhibit this hierarchical tree structure to some extent.

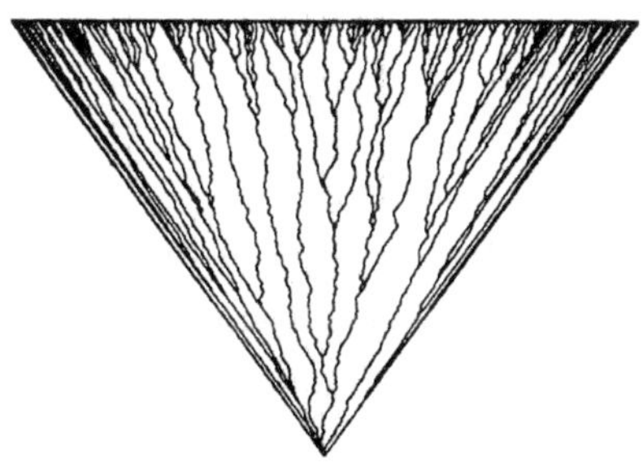

Figure 4. A collection of polymers of lowest energy directed along the diagonals of a square lattice with random bonds. Each polymer (crossing 500 bonds) has one end fixed to the apex of the triangle, the other to various points on its base, and finds the optimal path in between.

Among all the optimal paths with constant t, there is an absolute optimal path. It is this best of the best paths that is responsible for the transverse fluctuation of W, $x_c \sim t^{\nu}$, which can be regarded as its most probable location. Typically there is a weight advantage $\exp t^{\omega}$ for W at the absolute optimal path, with respect to $W(\vec{0},t)$ at the geometrical center. Both (ω,ν) can be measured numerically. ω is related to the above "surface" exponents by $\omega = \chi/z$. There is a heuristic argument to relate the two exponents ω and ν directly in the polymer language: The free energy $(-\log W(\vec{x},t))$ can be approximately written as

$$\frac{1}{2}\frac{x^2}{t} - t^{\omega}$$

where the first term is the entropy contribution which favors the geometrical center $\vec{x} = \vec{0}$, the second term is the energy gain due to randomness. Minimizing the free energy (with $x = t^{\nu}$) we obtain $x \sim t^{(\omega+1)/2}$, or the exponent relation $\nu = (\omega + 1)/2$. Note that this is equivalent to the above relation derived from Galilean invariance $\chi + z = 2$ $(\nu = 1/z, \omega = \chi/z)$.

We may ask more questions in our optimization problem.[7] For instance, how stable is the best path solution, if the random environment changes slightly? These changes may be caused by very slow time dependence of the system. In more general optimization problems, there are small allowed margins when the constraints are specified, we may want to know within these margins how much optimal solutions vary. We let each lattice bond vary independently by an infinitesimal amount, so that we have two almost identical random lattices. In our numerical simulations we have observed that the optimal path jumps a large distance due to the environment change $t^{\nu'}, \nu' = 0.83 \pm 0.01$. The motivation (i.e. energy gain) for this jump is numerically found to be $t^{\omega'}, \omega' = 0.67 \pm 0.01$.[8]

$1/f$ Noise

In this section we shall apply the above results to explain $1/f$ noise. The $1/f$ noise problem refers to the low frequency divergence (in the form $1/f^{\alpha}$) in the power spectrum of noise of many natural processes. What is remarkable of this divergence is that it is very close to perfect $1/f$ behavior (i.e. $\alpha \sim 1$), whether it is from an electric current in a carbon-resistor, from sand-flow in an hour-glass, or from levels of the Nile in the last 2000 years. This problem has proved a source of inspiration as well as frustration for theorists in the past few decades.[9]

Many specific mechanisms and models were proposed to explain particular phenomena. However, the general feeling is that there *ought* to be some *universal* explanation under general, mild conditions, to the level of the Central Limit Theorem which states that the sum of a large number of independent random variables follows (approximately) a gaussian distribution.

Recently it was suggested by Montroll and Shlesinger[10] that, if a process is multiplicative, $1/f$ noise follows naturally. For example, the probablity of a grand event P is a *product* of the probabilities of many sub-events p_i, $P = \prod_{i=1}^{n} p_i$ where p_i (n of them) are independent from each other, then it is easy to show that P follows a log-normal distribution,

$$D(P) \sim \frac{1}{P} \exp -|\log P|^2/n.$$

For large n, over a wide range of P the exponent is negligible, $D(P) \sim 1/P$, then the waiting time ($\tau \sim 1/P$) for an grand event to occur is distributed by $D(\tau) \sim 1/\tau$ and standard arguments[10] lead to the $1/f$ divergence in the power spectrum. This scenario is very appealing: from our daily experience many events can be thought of consisting multiplicative sub-events. On the other hand, however, in nature there are also processes which are *additive*: sub-events contribute to the grand event independently, i.e. they are alternatives to each other. This can be expressed by $P = \sum_i p_i$. It is clear that P will follow a gaussian distribution and there is only white noise.

We can symbolically depict a multiplicative process by a chain of many bonds, as shown in Fig.5. Each bond represents a sub-event. In order for a grand event to happen, all the bonds in the chain have to be crossed successfully. In the logical language this can be represented by $AND \cdot AND \cdot \cdots \cdot AND$. On the other hand, if all the sub-events are *additive*, i.e., they go in parallel, this can be represented by $OR \cdot OR \cdot \cdots \cdot OR$.

While it is natural to split any grand event (e.g. a macroscopic observation) into sub-events in a multiplicative way, it is also conceivable that many alternative, or parallel sub-events must also exist. For example, it is true that the flooding of the Nile depends first (for the sake of argument we start from here) on atmospheric conditions, then a rain drop has to be formed, then the wind, temperature, soil and forest conditions contribute in a sequential succession. In any case, there must be multiplicative contribution to the final level of the Nile near Cairo. However, one must admit that alternative, or parallel processes are inevitable at intermediate stages—if this drop of rain does not fall, some other

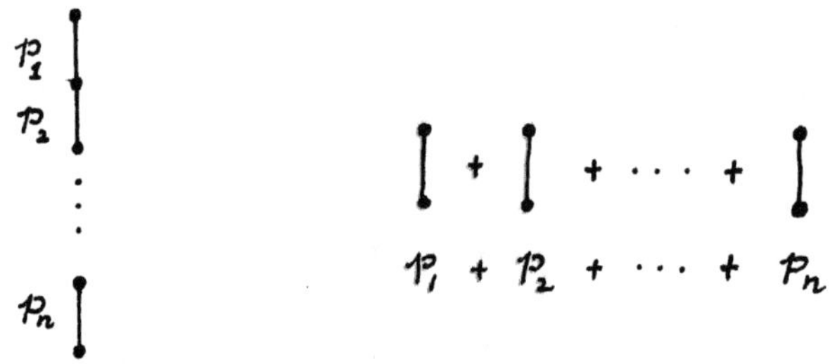

Figure 5.

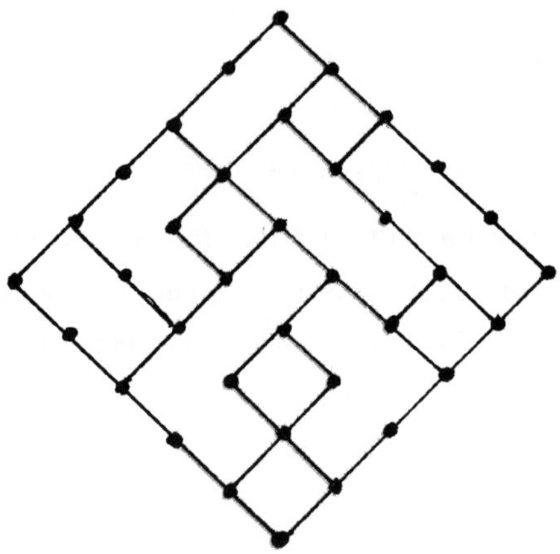

Figure 6.

will; if this tree blocks a drop, another tree may let it go through; the reader can continue this reasoning *ad infinitum*.

The above example helps us to arrive to the following conclusion: a grand event should be a mixture of multiplicative as well as alternative sub-events, with chain and branching structures occuring at all (space and time) scales, in a random way. In Fig.6 an artificial rendering is shown, to illustrate our point.

A single multiplicative chain gives rise to the log-normal distribution—hence $1/f$ noise, while for additive processes, a gaussian distribution—hence white noise. From the above discussion, we believe many natural processes are somewhere in between. For a random hybrid of both, such as shown in the above figure, what is the probability distribution of the grand event?

Here the result from studying directed polymers comes into play. On a regular lattice, rather than on a random structure, the expression discussed above

$$P = \sum_{path} \prod_{i \in path}^{n} p_i, \tag{8}$$

can be shown to have the distribution function[11]

$$D(P)dP \sim \frac{1}{P} \exp\{-a|\log P|^{\eta}/n^{\eta\omega}\}, \tag{9}$$

where a is a constant, n is the length of the products (t in the DP context), $\eta = 3/2$ for $d = 2$ (exact result). For $d > 2$ cases, η as well as ω can be inferred from numerical simulations.[11] According to the most recent work[12] on surface growth, we deduce that $\eta = (d+1)/d, \omega = 1/(d+1)$. However, the precise values of these exponents do not affect our conclusion. This implies that the $1/f$ noise will persist when branching, alternative sub-events are included, which changes only the power of the exponent η. It is in this sense the results for regular lattices should also apply to random structures, such as shown in Fig.6.

As for the log-normal case, when n is large for a large range of P, $|\log P|^{\eta}/n^{\eta\omega}$ is negligible, we have $D(P) \sim 1/P$, hence $1/f$ noise.

When can additive noise have the upper hand? For instance in *nature* there are processes with more alternatives (branchings) than multiplications, i.e., there is a large number of branchings (alternatives) *per* lattice node, wouldn't that behave more like a pure additive process? This is equivalent to increasing the dimensionality of the lattice. From the above formula (9) we see that, only when $d \to \infty$ (where $\eta \to 1$), is there a possibility that the exponential of a log comes down to spoil the $1/P$ law. For the precise transition from approximate $1/P$ to a gaussian distribution, one should make more careful analysis of the large d limit.

We conclude that when the probability P of a grand event is multiplicative, it has the universal behavior $D(P) \sim 1/P$. The behavior of a pure multiplicative chain (log-normal distribution) is qualitatively unaffected when branchings, or alternative sub-events are taken into account. Although we have only analyzed the "branching trees" on regular lattices, from above discussion it is clear that our conclusion is very general since it does not depends on the details (which only affect the exponents). In this sense we say that the $D(P) \sim 1/P$ law is very robust, which, in turn will lead to "robust" $1/f$ noise.[10] It is conceivable that many processes in *nature* are composed of sub-processes, multiplicative as well as additive (alternative), in a random way such as shown in Fig.6. It is under this "mild" assumption we can say that $1/f$ noise is inevitable.

Acknowledgement: I thank M. Kardar for sharing insight with me in our collaborations over the last few years.

REFERENCES

1. M. Eden in Proc. of 4th Berkeley Symposium on Mathmatical statistics and Probability Ed. F. Neyman (UC Berkeley 1961) Vol.IV.
2. M. Kardar, G. Parisi, and Y.-C. Zhang, *Phys. Rev. Lett.* **56** (1986), , 889.
3. S. F. Edwards and D. R. Wilkinson, *Proc. Roy. Soc. London Ser.* **A381** (1982), 17.
4. E. Medina, T. Hwa, M. Kardar, and Y.-C. Zhang, *Phys. Rev.* **A39** (1989), 3053; and references therein.
5. D. Forster, D. R. Nelson, and M. J. Stephen, *Phys. Rev.* **A16** (1977), 732.
6. M. Kardar and Y.-C. Zhang, *Phys. Rev. Lett.* **58** (1987), 2087.
7. Y.-C. Zhang, *Phys. Rev. Lett.* **59** (1987), 2125.
8. M. V. Feigel'man and V. M. Vinokur, *Phys. Rev. Lett* **61** (1988), 1134.
9. For a review see: W. H. Press, *Comments Mod Phys. Part* **C7** (1978), 103; or, P. Dutta and P. M. Horn, *Rev. Mod. Phys.* **53** (1981), 497.
10. E. W. Montroll and M. F. Shlesinger, *Proc. Natl. Acad. Sci (USA)* **79** (1982), 3380.
11. Y.-C. Zhang, *EuroPhys. Lett.* **June** (1989), .
12. J. M. Kim and J. M. Kosterlitz, *Phys. Rev. Lett.* **62** (1989), 2289.

Part 8

Large Scale Distribution of Matter in the Universe

THE FRACTAL NATURE OF THE GALAXY DISTRIBUTION

Paul H. Coleman

Kapteyn Astronomical Institute, University of Groningen
Postbus 800, 9700 AV Groningen, The Netherlands

ABSTRACT

The extent of the small scale fractal structure of the universe is examined. Previous analyses using the two point correlation function $\xi(r)$ as a description of galaxy clustering, indicate that the universe becomes homogeneous for length scales which are a few hundred times the size of a typical galaxy. Those analyses require an *a priori* assumption of homogeneity on length scales smaller than that of the sample analyzed. A statistical indicator which does not depend on this assumption is tested and used to reanalyze the galaxy distribution. Results of this reanalysis of the CfA galaxy catalog, the best published catalog for this purpose, show that the distribution of galaxies remains a fractal up to the largest length scales probed by this catalog. These maximum length scales are much larger than the value at which the universe was previously believed to become homogeneous. This invalidates the principle conclusions based on the use of $\xi(r)$: There is *no* evidence in the CfA catalog for the existence of a turnover to a homogeneous distribution on large scales. The universe remains a fractal out to the limits in size attainable with current catalogs. This fact is shown to clear up some of the puzzling features of the observed large scale structure of the universe.

INTRODUCTION

The distribution of galaxies in the universe is thought to be homogeneous for scales greater than the famous 'correlation length' r_0. This correlation length is defined as the length scale at which the 2–point correlation function $\xi(r)$ for galaxies equals one. Analyses of different catalogs of galaxies with $\xi(r)$ gave approximately the same result, $r_0 \sim 5\,h^{-1}$Mpc (Peebles 1980). This is roughly 15–30 million times the distance light travels in a year and a few hundred times the size of a typical galaxy. Although this is a rather large distance, it is still small compared to the largest distances measurable in our universe.

For length scales smaller than r_0, the distribution of galaxies is known to exhibit simple fractal behavior. By simple fractal behavior I mean that the average number density of galaxies falls off like a power law with a single exponent i.e., $n \propto r^{-\gamma}$. This power law, with measured exponent $\gamma \simeq 1.8$, is seen to hold for a range of 'small' length scales, from just greater than the size of a galaxy, to an upper limit ($\sim r_0$). This distribution, and therefore presumably all matter, is thought to move away from this small scale fractal nature and become homogeneous for length scales $\gtrsim r_0$. Galaxies separated by distances less than r_0 are highly correlated, while galaxies at greater separation should be essentially uncorrelated (homogeneously distributed).

Fractals' Physical Origin and Properties
Edited by L. Pietronero
Plenum Press, New York

Thus one expects to find large fluctuations in the density of galaxies for length scales smaller than the correlation length and small – if not negligible – fluctuations for length scales which are larger than the correlation length.

This expectation is not realized. Voids and structures which are much larger than $5\,h^{-1}$Mpc are observed in three dimensional galaxy surveys (cf. Zeldovic *et al.* 1982, Oort 1983, de Lapparent *et al.* 1986). Clumps of galaxies are found to be as large as the largest length scales which can be probed with the given sample of galaxies (e.g., the many contributions in Audouze *et al.* 1988). Furthermore, large anomalous streaming velocities which indicate very large, massive structures have also been reported (Burstein *et al.* 1986, Audouze *et al.* 1988). All of these observations are inconsistent with the claimed correlation length which is much smaller than the sizes of the structures reported. This growing body of evidence points out that some reconsideration of the traditional statistical analysis of galaxy clustering is required.

In this paper, I will examine the extent of the fractal structure of galaxies by stepping through a recently performed reanalysis of the galaxy distribution (Coleman *et al.* 1988) which reachs the somewhat startling conclusion – that in fact *no* turnover to homogeneity is observed. It will be seen that the previous analyses are flawed because the statistical test used depends on the untested assumption of homogeneity. An analysis which is free of all unnecessary assumptions has been performed on the best currently published galaxy catalog and the results indicate that the universe remains a simple fractal out to the limits in size obtainable with that catalog. I will also show how this fact helps to resolve some of the remaining contradictory features of the large scale distribution of galaxies.

THE TWO POINT CORRELATION FUNCTION

The usual correlation analysis of galaxy distributions in space is based on the 2–point correlation function

$$\xi(r) = \frac{\langle n(\mathbf{r}_0)\cdot n(\mathbf{r}_0+\mathbf{r})\rangle}{\langle n\rangle^2} - 1 \tag{1}$$

where $n(\mathbf{r}) = \sum_{i=1}^{N}\delta(\mathbf{r}-\mathbf{r}_i)$ is the number density of objects and N is the total number of objects in a volume V. The averages in equation (1) are just standard volume averages i.e., $\langle\cdots\rangle = \frac{1}{V}\int_V(\cdots)\,d\mathbf{r}_0$, and $\langle n\rangle$ is simply N/V.

The use of $\xi(r)$ and its interpretation are based on the *implicit* assumption that the galaxy distribution becomes homogeneous for length scales smaller than the size of the sample. If this assumption is true then $\langle n\rangle$ is a well defined quantity which is independent of the physical extent of the sample. If the assumption is false, then the use of $\xi(r)$ is inappropriate for that sample – unless it has already been shown that the distribution of galaxies homogenizes on scales probed by the sample and hence the average density of galaxies is known *a priori*. In other words, since $\xi(r)$ depends on the assumption of homogeneity, it cannot be used to prove that a sample is homogeneous. A simpler test is called for.

Pietronero (1987) introduces a description of the spatial distribution of galaxies which is independent of the assumption of homogeneity, the *conditional* density

$$\begin{aligned}\Gamma(r) &= \frac{\langle n(\mathbf{r}_0)\cdot n(\mathbf{r}_0+\mathbf{r})\rangle}{\langle n\rangle} \\ &= \frac{1}{N}\sum_{i=1}^{N}\frac{1}{4\pi r^2 dr} \times \int_r^{r+dr} n(\mathbf{r}_i+\mathbf{r})\,d\mathbf{r}\end{aligned} \tag{2}$$

and the *average* density as a function of length-scale

$$\Gamma^*(r) = \frac{3}{4\pi r^3}\int_0^r 4\pi r'^2\,\Gamma(r')\,dr' . \tag{3}$$

These two densities are not independent but analysis of a sample with both is sometimes instructive. The *average* density $\Gamma^*(r)$ is recommended as a check of general tendencies, since it is not as strongly affected by fluctuations as $\Gamma(r)$, which is more sensitive to features in the distribution.

From equations (1) and (2) we see that

$$\xi(r) = \frac{\Gamma(r)}{\langle n \rangle} - 1 . \tag{4}$$

Since $\Gamma(r)$ is the average number density as a function of radial distance from the galaxies in the sample, $\xi(r)$ is just that conditional density normalized by $\langle n \rangle$. Note however, that in view of the implicit assumption about the existence of $\langle n \rangle$, one cannot simply obtain $\Gamma(r)$ from a standard calculation of $\xi(r)$. If the sample becomes homogeneous for scales greater than some length scale, then $\langle n \rangle$ is simply the average value of $\Gamma(r)$ for those length scales. However, if this asymptotic value is not known or *does not exist*, then the normalization is *arbitrary* and hence the amplitude of $\xi(r)$ and the correlation length r_0, are also arbitrary.

Pietronero goes on to point out that this arbitrariness exists when $\xi(r)$ is applied to a simple fractal. Since a simple fractal is never homogeneous on any scale, it should never exhibit a true correlation length – yet analysis with $\xi(r)$, can determine a false correlation length. I present his analysis below.

The number density of a fractal in a sphere of radius r is

$$n(r) = \frac{3}{4\pi} B r^{-\gamma} , \tag{5}$$

where B is just a constant which depends on the small scale cutoffs of the fractal and $\gamma = 3 - D$, D being the fractal dimension. If the fractal is contained in a spherical volume of radius R_s then

$$\langle n \rangle = \frac{N(R_s)}{V(R_s)} = \frac{3}{4\pi} B R_s^{-\gamma} \tag{6}$$

i.e., the average density constructed for this volume will depend on the *size* of the volume. The conditional density of a simple fractal is a power law independent of any intrinsic length scales,

$$\Gamma(r) = \frac{D}{4\pi} B r^{-\gamma} , \tag{7}$$

while the 2–point correlation function

$$\xi(r) = \left(\frac{3-\gamma}{3}\right)\left(\frac{r}{R_s}\right)^{-\gamma} - 1 \tag{8}$$

is dependent on the maximum length scale in the volume. Furthermore, the correlation length

$$r_0 = \left(\frac{3-\gamma}{6}\right)^{1/\gamma} R_s , \tag{9}$$

also depends on the largest length scale which can be probed with the sample. The point at which $\xi(r)$ becomes zero ($\xi(r_0') = 0$), also depends on sample scale and will have the same form as equation (9) with the 6 replaced by a 3.

Therefore analysis of a fractal with $\xi(r)$ gives a well defined power law (slope $-\gamma$) at small r and has a 'correlation' length r_0 which depends on the largest length scale sampled. Furthermore, it will deviate from the power law for larger r and become zero at r_0', a value which is also dependent on the maximum length scale of the sample. In contrast $\Gamma(r)$ and $\Gamma^*(r)$ remain power laws with the same exponent ($-\gamma$) for all scales *independent* of the spatial extent of the sample.

For a system which is fractal up to a length-scale λ_0 and above it becomes homogeneous, $\Gamma(r)$ and $\Gamma^*(r)$ show a power law with exponent $-\gamma$ up to $r \simeq \lambda_0$. Beyond this length they become constant. The observation of this well developed constant behavior is the most clear and unbiased check that a distribution becomes homogeneous.

TEST DISTRIBUTIONS

Simulated distributions of galaxies can be created to test the predictive power of $\Gamma(r)$, $\Gamma(r^*)$, and $\xi(r)$ for finite samples of objects. Once a 'universe' of known distribution properties has been generated, a portion of it is extracted. This portion is chosen to mimic both the total number of galaxies in, and the boundaries of, the "CfA galaxy catalog" described below. This is done in order to assess the effectiveness of each of the statistical indicators and determine any possible effects which occur in the analysis due to the boundaries and the finite number of galaxies present in the sample. The numbers of galaxies are always about 200-450 and therefore some care should be taken to ensure that the statistics being used do not reflect the somewhat small numbers of objects.

The quantities $\Gamma(r)$ or $\Gamma^*(r)$ are calculated by counting the number of galaxies in a spherical shell or sphere (respectively) of small radius centered on each galaxy in the sample. These numbers are then divided by the appropriate volumes to obtain a density and averaged. If the shell around a galaxy crosses a boundary of the sample, the densities $\Gamma(r)$ and $\Gamma^*(r)$ derived for that galaxy are not included in the averaging. The radius of the sphere is then increased and the procedure is repeated. At each step the number of galaxies whose surrounding densities are used in the averaging decreases (due to the finite spatial extent of the total sample volume). $\Gamma(r)$ and $\Gamma^*(r)$ are averages taken about the surviving galaxies and hence the largest r values are determined by the galaxies in the center of the sample volumes. The largest r points in the figures which follow in this paper are the averages taken over the last ten galaxies which survive this process. An 'effective' sample radius R_s is defined to be the radius of the largest sphere centered on a galaxy which can be embedded in the survey volume.

This method of excluding galaxies which are too close to the boundaries decreases the statistical significance of the large r density determinations and limits the length scales which can be probed with the statistical tests. It has the advantage, however, of being completely assumption free. Other methods, such as weighting schemes (Davis and Peebles, 1983), are used to account for the boundaries of the catalog and to increase the range of length scales over which the 2-point correlation function can be used. These methods should not be used in an assumption free analysis however, since they depend on implicit assumptions of isotropy and/or homogeneity of galaxies not contained in the sample volume! By computing the densities in the way outlined above, the analysis contains no assumptions about the spatial distribution of galaxies inside or outside the catalog volume. The only legitimate way to increase the length scales analyzed is by observing fainter galaxies and constructing deeper complete catalogs.

Three types of distributions are of particular interest for the problem of interpreting the large scale structure of the universe, they are: a completely homogeneous sample; a sample which is a simple fractal; and a sample which is a fractal up to a certain length scale and homogeneous for larger scales. In the following sections, $\Gamma(r)$, $\Gamma(r^*)$, and $\xi(r)$ will be calculated for an example of each of these cases to investigate effects due to the boundaries and finite sample size on the statistical tests. I have already shown how $\xi(r)$ fails as a good statistical indicator for fractal distributions and this fact will be evident in the analysis which follows.

A Homogeneous Sample

A homogeneous distribution of galaxies was generated with a random number generator and distributed in a large spatial volume. A volume which matches the CfA volume was extracted and a random subsample of 442 galaxies were collected. This sample is plotted in Fig. 1 using an Aitoff equal area projection centered on the north galactic pole. As the name implies, this projection has the property that the same ruler can be applied with any orientation to any portion of these plots. This projection also has the added property that it does not deform the distribution, which means that it is especially good for depicting projected density enhancements. The human brain is often blamed for constructing structure where there is none. In 1905 for instance, Percival Lowell made now famous claims as to the existence and intricacy of martian canals, which have since been shown to be false. Lowell did not have the good fortune of having CCD detectors and fast computers to analyze the structures he 'saw'. We do however and, with this historical warning in mind, notice the uniformity of surface density of the galaxies in Fig. 1. We can now compare our perception with mathematically determined indicators of clustering by calculating $\Gamma(r)$ and $\Gamma^*(r)$ for this distribution.

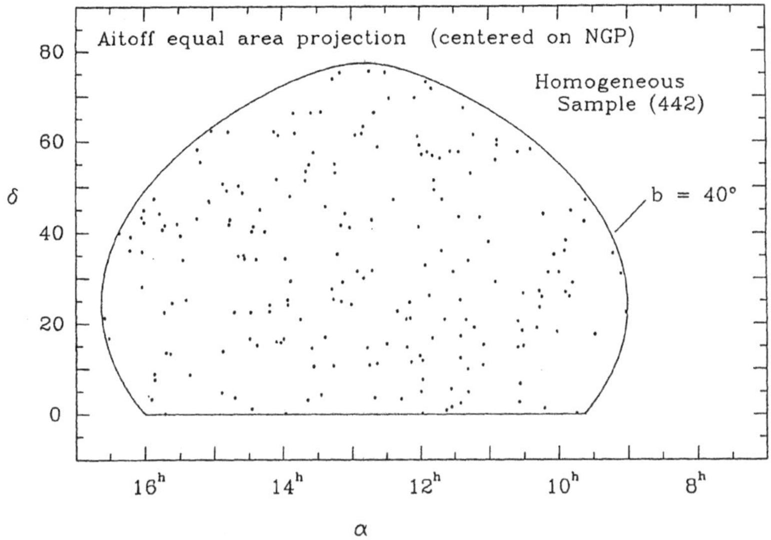

Fig. 1. A simulated homogeneous universe is shown in an Aitoff projection centered on the north galactic pole. The boundaries of the sample and the number of objects (442) are the same as those for one of the CfA galaxy subsamples which is analyzed later.

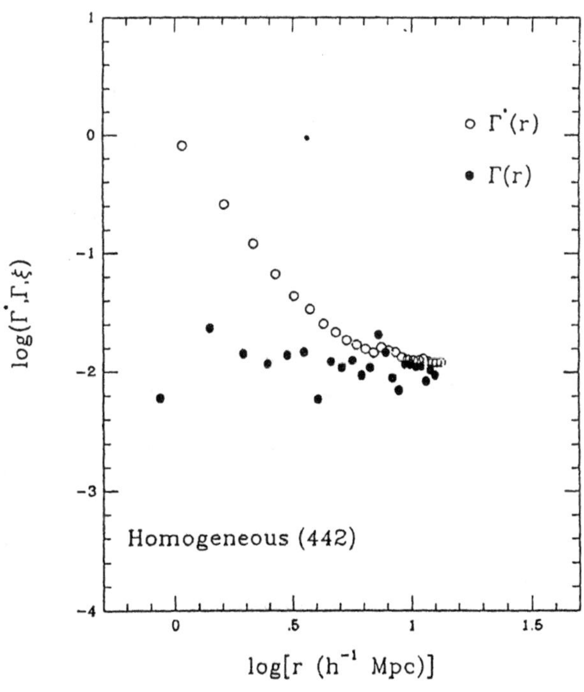

Fig. 2. The conditional density $\Gamma(r)$ and its 'integral' $\Gamma^*(r)$ plotted as functions of length scale for a simulated universe which is purely homogeneous.

Fig. 2 is a log–log plot of the result of applying $\Gamma(r)$ and $\Gamma^*(r)$ to this sample of objects. The filled circles ($\Gamma(r)$) show considerable fluctuations but are essentially flat throughout the range of length scales which can be tested i.e., they show a roughly constant density. The open circles ($\Gamma^*(r)$) drop steadily down to eventually level off to that same constant density for scales greater than $\sim 8\,h^{-1}$Mpc. The statistic $\Gamma^*(r)$ shows that for radii smaller than the typical Poisson separation of the galaxies in the sample ($\sim 2.5\,h^{-1}$Mpc), spheres about most of the galaxies do not include any neighboring galaxies. Thus the rapid decrease in $\Gamma^*(r)$ is nothing more than the r^{-3} in the definition of density. This effect (a rapid decrease in the 2–point correlation function for very small scales) has been misinterpreted in the analysis of galaxy catalogs and called "bi-fractality" i.e., that there are two fractal regimes with differing slopes. This effect is seen in pure single power law fractal samples and is just due to the finite numbers of galaxies present and the lower cutoff to the fractal regime.

At larger length scales more and more galaxies contribute a sensible density to the average and finally, for length scales greater than $8\,h^{-1}$Mpc, the statistic gives a reasonable signal. The homogeneous nature of the distribution is clear. Since this is constructed to be a purely random distribution of galaxies, there is no fractional power law (fractal) regime in the density. This is also fairly evident in Fig. 2.

A Fractal Sample

A pure fractal sample of 306 galaxies generated by the "Levi flight" algorithm (Mandelbrot 1983) is presented in Fig. 3. This algorithm is a fractional random walk with a stepsize l drawn from probability distribution:

$$\begin{aligned} p(l) &= 0 \qquad & l < l_0 \\ &= \mathrm{D}\, l_0^{\mathrm{D}}\, l^{-(\mathrm{D}+1)} \qquad & l \geq l_0 \end{aligned} \tag{10}$$

Where D is the fractal dimension and l_0 is just a minimum step size which can be scaled to any value. This algorithm, by its very nature, is not a very good volume filling algorithm. Often, even an exact number of galaxies can not be generated in certain volume with a single application of the generation process. It creates galaxies at each step of a 'drunkards walk' though a volume, often leaving portions of that volume with negligible probability of ever being reached by the algorithm. In principle, to obtain a well filled volume of space, an infinite number of galaxies must be created to ensure that all parts of the volume have been sampled by the algorithm. In practice, creating very large numbers of galaxies and picking randomly with equal probability from the final distribution, generates a more volume filling distribution of galaxies. The sample in Fig. 3 was constructed in that way with the same fractal dimension as the galaxy distribution, $\mathrm{D} = 1.2$ ($\gamma = 1.8$). This figure shows much more clumpy structure and larger void regions than that of Fig. 1.

The analysis of this sample proceeds as described previously except that $\xi(r)$ is also calculated by using equation (4) and the results of that analysis are presented in Fig. 4. Both $\Gamma(r)$ and $\Gamma^*(r)$ are simple power laws and the dashed line in Fig. 4 indicates the input power law $\gamma = 1.8$. The 2–point correlation function, indicated by the solid line, shows a rough power law, deviates, and then goes to zero. This function exhibits a 'correlation length' ($\xi(r_0) = 1$) of $r_0 \sim 4\,h^{-1}$Mpc for this sample which has no correlation length. These galaxies never become homogeneous on any scale by definition and therefore any correlation length derived is *spurious*. Thus we see once again that applying $\xi(r)$ to any arbitrary distribution can give misleading results. It will always give a 'correlation length', even if one does not exist.

A Fractal Sample with a Turnover to Homogeneity

A sample which is fractal on small scales and homogeneous on large scales is constructed as follows: A number of random locations are chosen in a large volume. Since the locations are Poissonly distributed, they will have an average separation λ_0 where $\lambda_0 \simeq 0.55n^{-\frac{1}{3}}$. Each of these locations is the starting point for constructing a fractal which samples length scales up to the limiting value λ_0. The standard catalog volume is extracted and, as a final step, a fixed number of objects (442) are randomly picked for the 'catalog'. This prescription ensures (by brute force) that the sample is a fractal on scales smaller than about λ_0 and homogeneous for

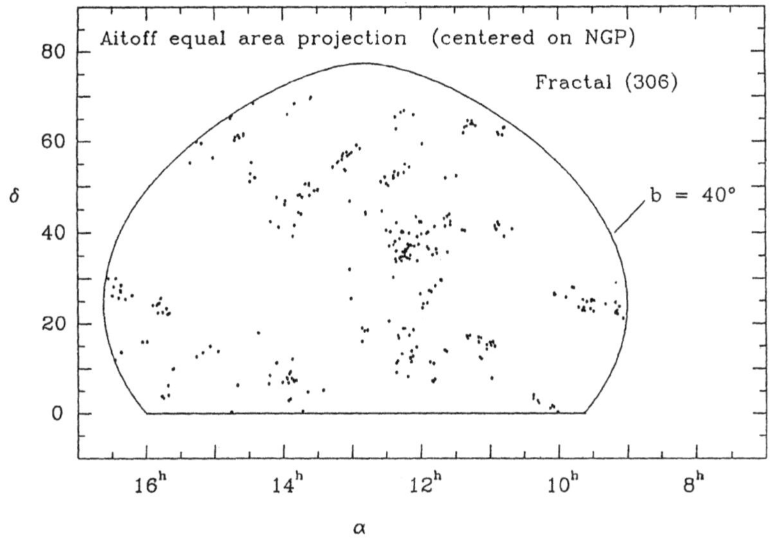

Fig. 3. A simulated fractal universe (dimension = 1.2) is shown in the same projection as the sample in Fig. 1. The number of objects (306) is a bit less than Fig. 1 due to the algorithm used to create the sample.

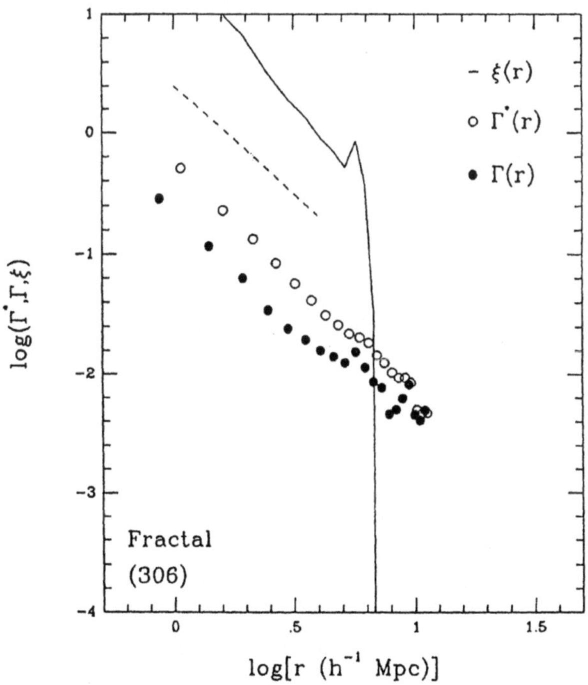

Fig. 4. $\Gamma(r)$, $\Gamma^*(r)$, and $\xi(r)$ plotted as functions of length scale for the simple fractal universe shown in Fig. 3. The dashed line indicates the input slope of -1.8.

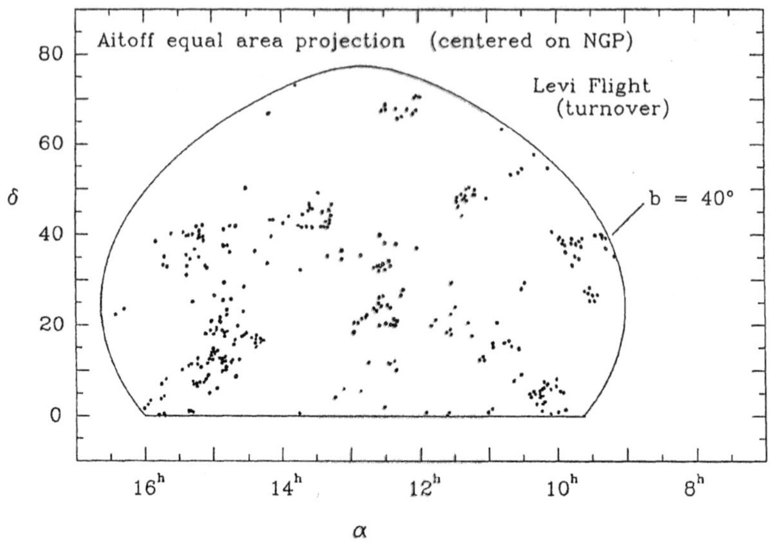

Fig. 5. A simulated universe which is fractal on small scales and becomes homogeneous for scales larger than the correlation length. It is presented with the same projective geometry as Figs. 1 and 3.

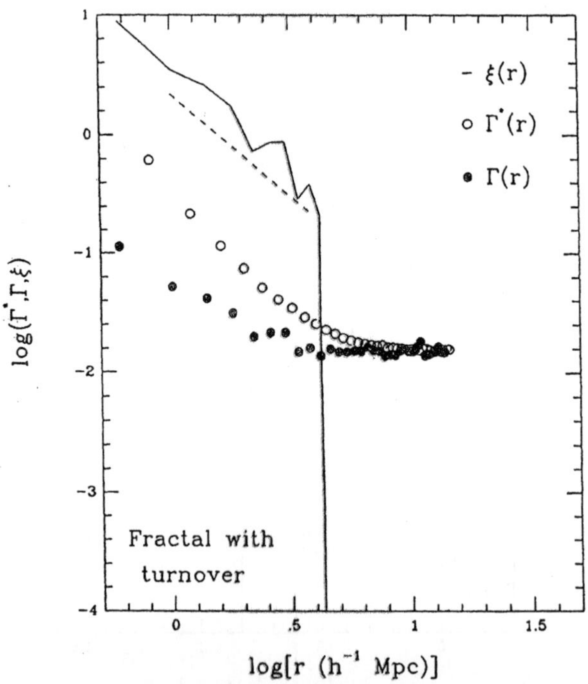

Fig. 6. $\Gamma(r)$, $\Gamma^*(r)$, and $\xi(r)$ plotted for the simple fractal universe on small scales which becomes homogeneous for scales of about 4–5 h^{-1}Mpc). The dashed line indicates the input slope of -1.8.

length scales greater than λ_0. An example of such a distribution is shown in Fig. 5. The value of λ_0 was arranged to be about $5\,h^{-1}$Mpc.

Both $\Gamma(r)$ and $\Gamma^*(r)$ flatten out at about that value in the analysis presented in Fig. 6. The 2–point correlation function indicates an r_0 of about $3\,h^{-1}$Mpc, if you average over fluctuations. If you do not, then the point at which $\xi(r)$ crosses one will just be at the point where $\Gamma(r)$ fluctuates below twice its assymptotic value for the first time. Notice that the value of of the correlation length tells one nothing about the point at which the distribution becomes homogeneous.

For the preceding three examples, $\Gamma(r)$ and $\Gamma^*(r)$ have indicated the true nature of the distribution tested. On the other hand, for the pure fractal distribution, $\xi(r)$ has given results which are misleading and blatently false. Therefore it is possible that previous analysis of galaxy catalogs with $\xi(r)$ has also given misleading results. In the following section, I describe one such galaxy catalog.

THE CFA CATALOG

The CfA (Center for Astrophysics) survey of galaxies, and in particular the subsample known as the "North Zwicky 40", is the most appropriate published catalog for investigating the spatial distribution of galaxies. It goes out to fairly large radial distances from our galaxy and also covers a respectable solid angle of the sky. It is a subset of a larger survey of all galaxies in the northern hemisphere compiled by Zwicky *et al.* (1961) and is presented in Fig. 7.

The noticeably high density area at the bottom of the plot is the nearby Virgo cluster. The galaxies shown are brighter than a certain *observed* level (i.e., each has an apparent magnitude which is less than 14.5), have a galactic latitude greater than forty degrees, and are in the northern hemisphere. Most of the other published galaxy catalogs are lists of the angular coordinates of galaxies without any information about the radial distances to each individual galaxy. The analysis of such catalogs with correlation function or other techniques always requires a few extra assumptions in order to go from the observed angular separations to true spatial separations. The radial distances to each of the galaxies in the CfA sample, on the other hand, is known thanks to a monumental effort by a large collaboration of researchers.

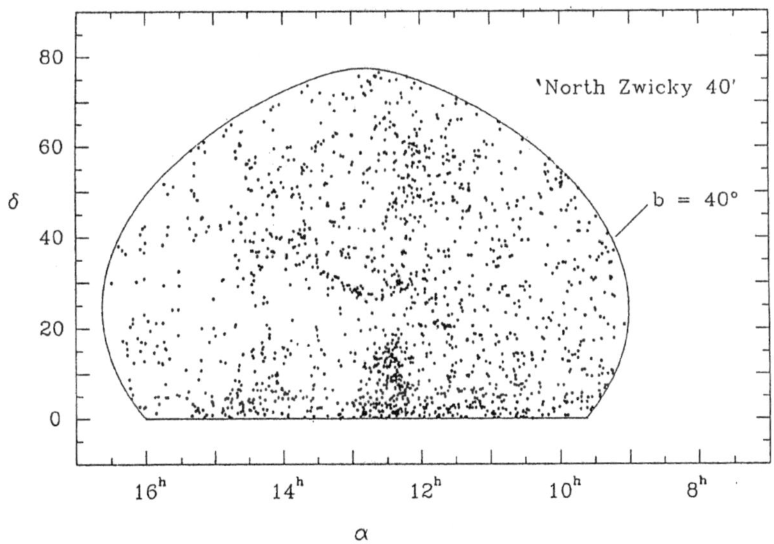

Fig. 7. A subset of the CfA galaxy catalog shown in an Aitoff projection centered on the north galactic pole. The sample is the $\sim$ 1800 northern hemisphere galaxies with apparent visual magnitude brighter than 14.5.

The distances to the approximately 1800 galaxies has been measured by various methods, but primarily by the observation of spectral lines which have been doppler shifted to longer wavelengths (redshifted) from the rest frame wavelength of that spectral line.

In the standard Hot Big Bang model of the universe, galaxies are rushing away from us and each other as a result of a catastrophic initial explosion. This expansion of the universe is observed in the redshifting of spectral lines of galaxies. The distance from us to each galaxy is simply the velocity inferred from this doppler shift divided by the so called Hubble 'constant', H_0. The Hubble constant has the units km/s · Mpc and is thought to be anywhere from 50 to 100 km/s · Mpc. Distances in this paper are reported in units of h^{-1}Mpc where h is simply the Hubble constant in units of 100 km/s · Mpc. I will also refer to distances in terms of the recession velocities (km/s) of the galaxies and in order to convert a velocity into a distance (h^{-1}Mpc), simply divide the velocity by 100.

The radial distance to a galaxy, along with its angular position (right ascension α and declination δ – the celestial analogs of longitude and latitude), fixes its position in three dimensions. Surveys which have redshifts and are very deep but cover a very small solid angle of the sky essentially provide 1–dimensional probes of the galaxy distribution (cf. Kirshner *et al.* 1979, Shanks *et al.* 1983). Typically the largest scale transverse to the line-of-sight is comparable to the claimed correlation length. The CfA survey, on the other hand, covers a large fraction of the sky, and in this sense is more representative; it is the most 3–dimensional of the existing surveys in that it is much larger in all three dimensions than the claimed correlation length. Moreover the large volume of the CfA survey and completeness down to apparent magnitude 14.5, assures a reasonable number of galaxies for statistical evaluation.

Previous analysis of the CfA Catalog (Davis and Peebles, 1983) made use of the 2–point correlation function which showed a power law with exponent −1.8 for values of r up to 10–15 h^{-1}Mpc. For larger r, there is a breakdown from the power law behavior and $\xi(r)$ becomes zero and eventually negative. Since $\xi(r)$ is an improper function to use, as demonstrated above, a reanalysis of the CfA catalog in terms of $\Gamma(r)$ and $\Gamma^*(r)$ is required. This was done by L. Pietronero, R. Sanders, and myself (Coleman *et al.* 1988) and I will present and expand upon the result.

THE ANALYSIS OF THE CFA

Fig. 8 presents the absolute magnitudes (luminosities) of the galaxies included in Fig. 7 plotted against their recession velocities (radial distances). Minimal corrections for Virgo cluster infall have been made to some of the velocities in the catalog (Davis and Huchra 1982) and each velocity is determined in the preferred frame of the Cosmic Microwave Background Radiation. Galaxies with higher velocities are further away and galaxies with smaller absolute magnitudes are brighter. Thus in Fig. 8, distance increases to the right and source luminosity increases going up. An important selection effect exists, in that at every velocity in this apparent magnitude limited survey, there is a definite lower limit which is the absolute magnitude of the faintest galaxy which can be seen at that distance. Hence at large distances, intrinsically faint objects are not observed whereas at smaller distances they are observed. For example, a less luminous galaxy of absolute magnitude $M = -14 + 5\log h$ can only be seen out to a velocity of about 500 km/s corresponding to a distance of 5 h^{-1}Mpc. Whereas an intrinsically bright galaxy, $M = -21 + 5\log h$, could be seen at velocities of $\sim$ 12,500 km/s (125 h^{-1}Mpc).

In order to analyze the distribution of galaxies, a catalog which does not suffer from this selection effect must be used. So called 'volume limited' subsamples must be extracted and two such subcatalogs are depicted in Fig. 8. The first subsample has a velocity limit 8000 km/s (80 h^{-1}Mpc) and an absolute magnitude limit $M \leq -20.0 + 5\log h$. Every galaxy which is more luminous than that limit is in the sample – there is no incompleteness. The sample consists of 226 galaxies and occupies the region of the plot in the upper left corner – separated by the solid lines. The second sample occupies the smaller volume defined by $v \leq 4000$ km/s($\lesssim 40\, h^{-1}$Mpc) with $M \leq -18.5 + 5\log h$ and contains 442 galaxies. That subsample, whose boundary is shown by the dashed line in Fig. 8, is plotted in projection in Fig. 9. I have arranged to have the numbers of objects in the simulated samples be comparable to the number in this subsample, so that the reader may compare directly Figs. 1, 3, 5, and 9.

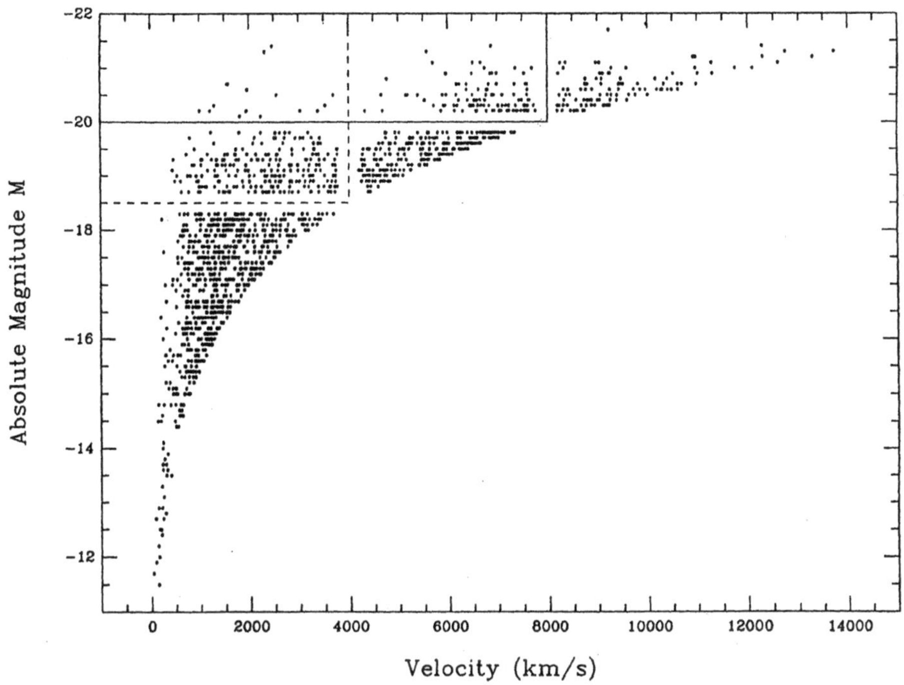

Fig. 8. The absolute visual magnitude of each of the galaxies shown in Fig. 7 is plotted as a function of its recession velocity. The solid- and dashed-line borders in the upper left corner, enclose the two complete subsamples which are tested. Luminosity increases going up and radial distance, in h^{-1}Mpc, to each galaxy is simply the velocity divided by 100.

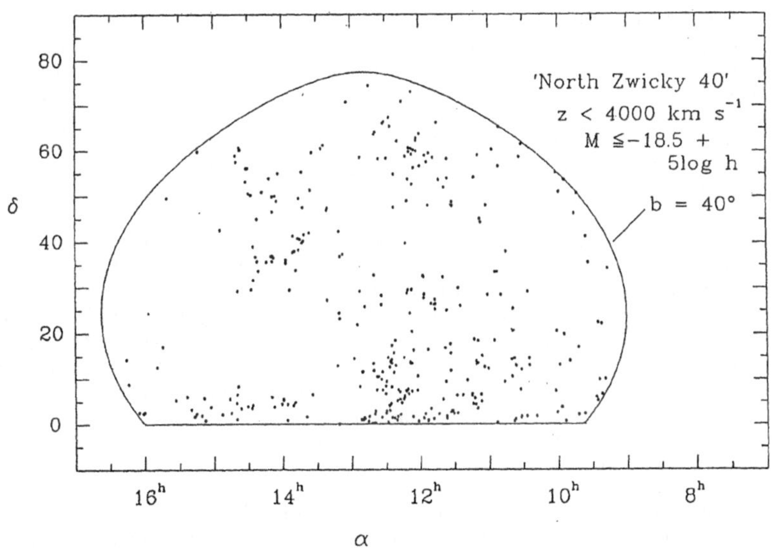

Fig. 9. A complete subsample of the CfA galaxy catalog shown in an Aitoff projection centered on the north galactic pole. The sample is all northern hemisphere galaxies with expansion velocities $v \leq 4000\,km/s(r \lesssim 40\,h^{-1}Mpc)$, galactic latitude $b \gtrsim 40°$, and $M \leq -18.5 + 5\log h$. 442 galaxies are selected by these criteria.

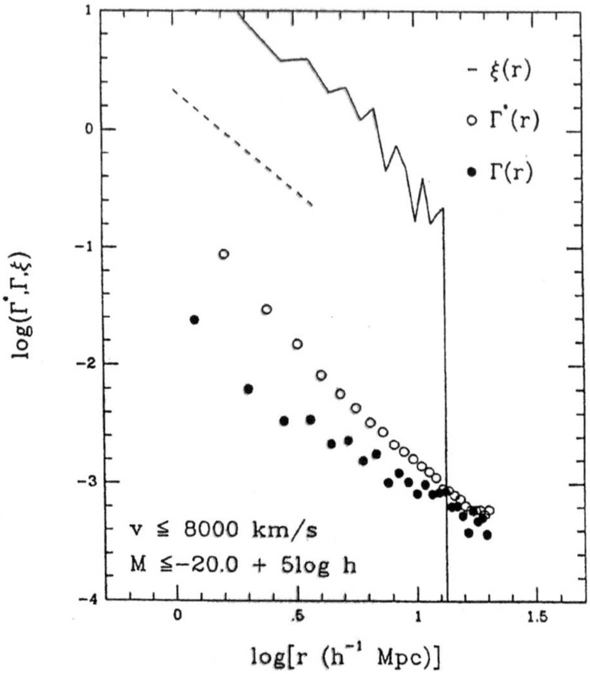

Fig. 10. $\Gamma(r)$, $\Gamma^*(r)$, and $\xi(r)$ plotted as functions of length scale for the CfA catalog limited to $v \leq 8000\,km/s$; $M \leq -20.0 + 5\log h$. The dashed line indicates a reference slope of -1.7.

The analysis with $\Gamma(r)$, $\Gamma^*(r)$, and the corresponding $\xi(r)$ of the CfA sample up to 8000 km/s is shown in Fig. 10. As expected the function $\Gamma^*(r)$ is less affected by fluctuations than $\Gamma(r)$ or $\xi(r)$ and shows a well developed power law up to about $20\,h^{-1}$Mpc or $0.7R_s$, where $R_s \simeq 28\,h^{-1}$Mpc. The so-called 'correlation length' of this sample obtained from $\xi(r)$ is $r_0 \simeq 7\,h^{-1}$Mpc. Note that no deviation from the power law is observed for $\Gamma(r)$ around this point, where the usual interpretation of r_0 would have implied an abrupt flattening of $\Gamma(r)$ from just greater than r_0 up to the sample limits. In addition the value of $r_0' \simeq 14\,h^{-1}$Mpc ($\xi(r_0') = 0$) is about half of the effective sample radius R_s, as predicted for a fractal structure with this exponent (Pietronero 1987).

Fig. 11 shows the same analysis for the second subsample ($v \leq 4000\,km/s$). Most of the discussion of Fig. 10 can be repeated for Fig. 11 Note however that in Fig. 11 the characteristic lengths derived from $\xi(r)$ are $r_0 \simeq 4\,h^{-1}$Mpc and $r_0' \simeq 7\,h^{-1}$Mpc, that is they are smaller by a factor of two for a sample whose effective radius has been reduced by a factor of two. The slight tendency for $\Gamma(r)$ and $\Gamma^*(r)$ to flatten on scales larger than $10\,h^{-1}$Mpc is not the signature of an approach to homogeneity on these scales as is seen by the absence of such a feature at that length scale in the 8000 km/s sample. The correction for peculiar velocities of infall into the Virgo cluster makes very little difference to these results; if the correction is not made, the form of $\Gamma(r)$ and $\Gamma^*(r)$ remains a power law out to the largest significant distance but the value of the exponent (γ) is reduced somewhat.

Figs. 10 and 11 show quite emphatically that the conditional density calculated for the CfA is completely consistent with a fractal structure extending to the maximum scale which can be reasonably probed with the catalog ($\sim 20\,h^{-1}$Mpc). It has been argued that the CfA volume is not a 'fair sample' of the universe due to the proximity of the local supercluster; that we sit in a region near a particularly large positive density fluctuation (Davis and Huchra 1982). While it is true that the CfA catalog is not homogeneous and therefore the use of the two point correlation function on the CfA catalog is conceptually wrong, it is not necessarily

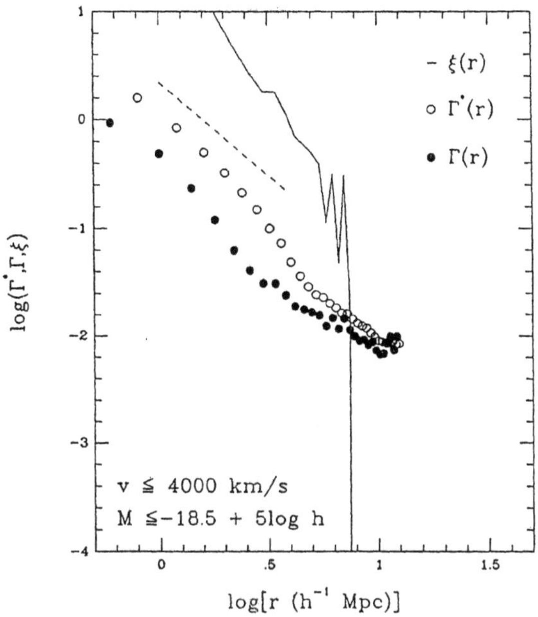

Fig. 11. $\Gamma(r)$, $\Gamma^*(r)$, and $\xi(r)$ plotted as functions of length scale for the CfA catalog limited to $v \leq 4000\,km/s$; $M \leq -18.5 + 5\log h$. A reference slope of -1.7 is indicated by the dashed line.

true that the distribution of galaxies in the CfA catalog is in any way anomalous. If we adopt the point of view that we do not sit in a special spot in the universe, then the CfA is a fair sample in terms of estimating the universal run of density as a function of distance from any galaxy – the conditional density. No 'characteristic length' can be defined in this system and no trend towards homogeneity is present. The characteristic length $r_0 \simeq 5\,h^{-1}$Mpc previously derived from the two point correlation function is thus a *spurious* result due to the erroneous *a priori* (and often implicit) assumption that the universe is homogeneous on a scale which can be probed with the CfA catalog.

In the next section, I discuss how this new insight resolves some of the other puzzling features of the standard picture of the large scale structure of the universe.

PUZZLES

Einasto *et al.* (1986) were the first to find that r_0 for the CfA catalog depends on sample depth. This conclusion was quite contrary to the usual picture where r_0 is thought to be a constant. Those investigators did not realize that this is the natural result for a fractal system which does not attain homogeneity on any length scale of the sample. This was pointed out by Pietronero (1987) and can be seen in equation (9) above. Both r_0 and r_0' will depend on effective sample radius (or more loosely – sample depth) simply because there is no average density for the sample.

As a simple consistency check and illustration, Coleman *et al.* (1988) analyzed other complete subsamples ($M < -18.5 + 5\log h$) limited to velocities of 2000, 2500, and 3000 km/s (20, 25, and $30\,h^{-1}$Mpc). The effective sample radii for these three subsamples were $R_s = 7, 8.75$, and $10.5\,h^{-1}$Mpc, respectively. Fig. 12 presents that analysis and clearly shows a linear dependence of r_0 and r_0' on R_s in full agreement with the properties of a fractal structure and implies that the current interpretation of r_0 as an intrinsic 'characteristic length' of the galaxy distribution is incorrect. The constant ratio $r_0'/r_0 \simeq 1.5$ is also that expected for a fractal with $\gamma = 1.8$.

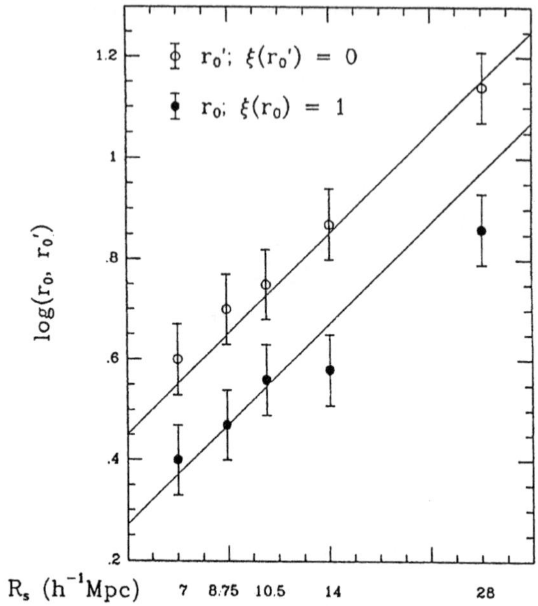

Fig. 12. 'Characteristic length scales' r_0 ($\xi(r_0) = 1$) and r_0' ($\xi(r_0') = 0$) plotted as functions of effective sample radius R_s.

Another problem with the usual analysis of galaxy distributions is the fact that clusters of galaxies seem to have different clustering properties than galaxies themselves. This is a puzzle since the only force involved with either distributions is gravity, which is thought to have no scale dependence i.e., it is a $1/r^2$ force. Furthermore the distribution of clusters should only trace the high density peaks of the distribution of galaxies - the so called 'skeleton' of the galaxy distribution. The 2–point correlation analysis of clusters of galaxies gives approximately the same value of γ (the slope) but considerably larger value of amplitude for $\xi(r)$ (see Bahcall 1988 and the references therein). The amplitude of $\xi(r)$ for clusters A_c is factor of 18 times the amplitude of $\xi(r)$ for galaxies A_g i.e., $A_c = 18A_g$.

Pietronero (1987) points out that if the cluster distribution is drawn from the same self similar (fractal) structure as the distribution of galaxies, then the simple relation

$$\frac{A_c}{A_g} = \left(\frac{R_c}{R_g}\right)^{\gamma} \tag{11}$$

holds, where R_g and R_c are the 'depths' of the catalogs for galaxies and clusters respectively. The depth of the cluster catalogs is known to be $\sim 5R_g$ which when inserted in equation (11) along with $\gamma = 1.8$, gives the factor of ~ 18 in a quite natural way. Thus there is no mystery to the amplitude difference and in fact this simple test indicates that perhaps the universe is a simple fractal for even larger length scales than the modest $20\,h^{-1}$Mpc limit obtainable with the CfA galaxy catalog.

The final feature I wish to comment on is the very large scale structures seen in the universe and their average mass densities. The average mass density of our galaxy is a few times 10^{-21} kg/m^3. The average mass density of the region of space which encloses the local group of galaxies is of order 10^{-25} kg/m^3. A typical supercluster volume has mass density $\sim 10^{-26}$ kg/m^3. So for each increase in scale there is a corresponding decrease in mass density. If galaxies have a typical mass, then this decrease in mass density is really just a decrease in number density. In this simple fractal picture, such structures and decrease in number density are natural and require no further explanation. An observer in such a universe will generally see a 'local supercluster'. The largest structure or void will always be comparable to the largest scale probed by the survey and estimates of mass density will always decrease as a function of length scale.

CONCLUSION

The analysis presented has shown that the structure of the universe (as probed by the best published 3–dimensional catalog, is fractal out to the limits in length scale imposed by the limitations of the catalog. There is no evidence for a turnover to homogeneity for length scales greater than $5\,h^{-1}$Mpc and quite a bit of evidence that *if the turnover exists*, it occurs on length scales larger than ten times this claimed 'correlation length'. Although there are some strong arguments and religious beliefs for why the universe should become homogeneous on large scales, the distribution of galaxies offers no evidence of this. The length scales probed by the currently published catalogs are not large enough to see any approach to homogeneity. The next set of deeper catalogs (when they become available) will extend the length scales which can be examined by considerable factors and perhaps they will show evidence of homogeneity on scales of $\gtrsim 100\,h^{-1}$Mpc. However, that remains an open question for future investigation.

This analysis has shown that the work being done on fractals across the world in physics departments, in solid state laboratories and on sophisticated computer graphics systems, has some very far reaching, large scale applications indeed! I eagerly await a theory of fractal growth which can be applied to galaxies in the universe.

REFERENCES

Audouze, J., Pelletan, M., Szalay, A.: editors of *Large Scale Structures of the Universe IAU Symp. #130*

Bahcall, N. A.: 1988, *Ann. Rev. Astron. Astrophys.*, **26**, 631

Burstein, D., Davies, R. L., Dresler, A., Faber, S. M., Lynden-Bell, D., Terlevich, R., Wegner, G.: 1986, in *Galaxy Distances and Deviations from Universal Expansion,* eds. B. F. Madore, R. B. Tully, Reidel, Dordrecht, p. 123

Coleman, P. H., Pietronero, L., Sanders, R. H.: 1988 *Astron. Astrophys.*, **200**, L32

Davis, M., Huchra, J.: 1982, *Astrophys. J.*, **254**, 437

Davis, M., Peebles, P. J. E.: 1983, *Astrophys. J.*, **267**, 465

Einasto, J., Klypin, A. A., Saar, E.: 1986, *Monthly Notices Roy. Astron. Soc.*, **219**, 457

Giovanelli, R., Haynes, M. P., Chincarini, G. L.: 1986, *Astrophys. J.*, **300**, 77

Huchra, J., Davis, M., Latham, K., Tonry, J.: 1983, *Astrophys. J. Suppl.*, **52**, 89

Kirshner, R. P., Oemler, A., Schechter, P. L.: 1979, *Astron. J.*, **84**, 951

de Lapparent, V., Geller, M. J., Huchra, J. P.: 1986, *Astrophys. J. Lett.*, **302**, L1

Mandelbrot, B. B.: 1983, in *The Fractal Geometry of Nature,* Freeman, New York

Oort, J. H.: 1983, *Ann. Rev. Astron. Astrophys.*, **21**, 373

Peebles, P.J.E.: 1980, *The Large Scale Structure of the Universe* Princeton, Princeton University Press

Pietronero, L.: 1987, *Physica*, **144A**, 257

Shanks, T., Bean, A. J., Efstathiou, G., Ellis, R. S., Fong, R., Peterson, B. A.: 1983, *Astrophys. J.*, **274**, 529

Zeldovic, Ya. B., Einasto, J., Shandarin, S. F.: 1982, *Nature*, **300**, 407

Zwicky, F., Herzog, E., Wild, P., Karkowicz, M., Kowol, C.: 1961, *Catalog of Galaxies and of Clusters of Galaxies* Vols **1-6**, Pasadena, California Institute of Technology

INDEX

MIX
Papier aus verantwortungsvollen Quellen
Paper from responsible sources
FSC® C105338

If you have any concerns about our products,
you can contact us on
ProductSafety@springernature.com

In case Publisher is established outside the EU,
the EU authorized representative is:
Springer Nature Customer Service Center GmbH
Europaplatz 3, 69115 Heidelberg, Germany

Printed by Libri Plureos GmbH
in Hamburg, Germany